APRAXIA OF SPEECH IN ADULTS

D0931963

Apraxia of Speech in Adults
The Disorder and its Management

Robert T. Wertz, Ph.D.

Chief, Audiology and Speech Pathology, Veterans Administration Medical Center, Martinez, California; Adjunct Associate Professor, Department of Neurology, University of California School of Medicine, Davis, California

Leonard L. LaPointe, Ph.D.

Professor and Chairman, Department of Speech and Hearing Science, Arizona State University, Tempe, Arizona

John C. Rosenbek, Ph.D.

Chief, Audiology and Speech Pathology, William S. Middleton Memorial Veterans Administration Center, Madison, Wisconsin. Adjunct Professor, Department of Neurology, Medical School and Department of Communicative Disorders, University of Wisconsin, Madison, Wisconsin.

S SINGULAR PUBLISHING GROUP, INC.
SAN DIEGO, CALIFORNIA

Singular Publishing Group, Inc.
4284 41st Street
San Diego, California 92105

© 1984 by Allyn and Bacon
© 1991 by Singular Publishing Group, Inc.

All rights, including that of translation, reserved. No part of this publication
may be reproduced, stored in a retrieval system, or transmitted in any form
or by any means, electronic, mechanical, recording, or otherwise, without the
prior written permission of the publisher.

Library of Congress Catalog Number 83-49100

International Standard Book Number 1-879105-54-3

Printed in the United States of America

To Donna and Beth

To Corinne, Adrienne, and Chris

To Susan and Wendy

Contents

Preface

The term "apraxia of speech" may have been coined by the Blackfoot Indians, because its name has changed every season or two. Or perhaps a worshipper of the Babylonian god Marduk, who had 50 names denoting his various attributes, assisted in formulating the term. We use "apraxia of speech" to describe a pattern of behavior that others have observed but may call by a different name. Our experience with the disorder has taught us that it is like nursery stock: it can be bought bare-root or container-bound. The bare-root stock—Broca's aphemia, Darley, Aronson, and Brown's motor speech disorder—is more fragile and may not survive academic storms. The container-bound stock—a pattern of motor behavior that coexists with or without a language disorder and requires a specific method of management—we believe to be more hardy and to respond to clinical cultivation.

We write about adults and not about children. The efforts of Yoss and Darley and others have revolutionized the way we look at abnormal articulation in these little folks. They echo the distant drum of Morley and those who saw what she did. We acknowledge the disorder, developmental apraxia of speech, but we manage adults; our focus, therefore, is on the adult who was a talker but is no longer, and not on the child who attempts to become one.

This book is an attempt to take stock of our knowledge of apraxia of speech in adults, to determine exactly where we stand in regard to it, to inquire about the conclusions that the accumulated facts seem to justify, and to ascertain in what direction we may look for fruitful inquiry in the future. Most of all, however, we have attempted to take apraxia of speech out of the classroom and laboratory and into life, to see if our science has influenced our service, to see whether our data are reflected in our deeds. We built our book like a triangle. Treatment constitutes its base.

There is no ordering of authors except that required by print. Each of us has contributed an ingredient here, another there; some thought; some organization; some experience; a question. When names must be put in order, one goes first, another second, another third. Most important are the names that do not appear on the cover—those who taught us, disagreed with us, permitted us to practice with them, and those who permitted us to practice on them. Their contributions, filtered correctly and incorrectly through the biases of our abilities, constitute our book's contents.

Of course, every effort like this contains its cast of those who perform the Fifth Business, those who make the things happen. Zelda Ballantine, Bette Laccoarce, Boyd Johnson, Shirley Lamm, Iris Tanney Kraemer, Kathy Lindgren, Ardith Pierick, and Linda Mader turned our scrawl into print. Beverly Bowling assisted in library research, and Deb Shiman proofed our prose.

We are not so beknighted as to believe unflinchingly in any of the things that we have written. The years may erase the term apraxia of speech from the taxonomy of neurogenic communication disorders. Or new approaches to language and language disorders may impose an entirely new system on these communication disorders so that oldtimers will recognize apraxia of speech as one does an old friend seen disappearing around a corner and into a crowd.

One can only hope for such a fate, for with new systems will come new diagnostic tools and therapies. Perhaps, too, they will be better. For now, this is the way it seems to us.

We hope it helps.

Reason and Rationale

I have had a strange warning. I have felt the wind from the wing of imbecility pass over me! (From the journal of French poet Baudelaire, shortly before he suffered a stroke. Reise, W., 1977, p. 29.)

His mind has worked too hard, he is worn out before his time. Though his tongue is not paralyzed, he has lost the memory of sound . . . he listens to and understand all that is said to him. I tell him things about his childhood; he understands me and listens to me attentively. And then when he wants to answer me, the futile efforts that he makes to express himself throw him into a rage. . . what makes him lose his reason is not being able to speak. Some Paris friends wish to share expenses in order to take him there and care for him. . . . For his part he does not want to leave or go out. He wants to talk. (From a letter describing the condition of Baudelaire, written by his mother. Reise, W., 1977, pp. 34–35.)

There are cases in which all of the muscles—including those which subserve phonation and articulation—are under voluntary control, the auditory apparatus is intact, and the general faculty of language remains unaffected, but in which, nevertheless, a cerebral lesion abolishes articulate speech. It seems to me that this loss of speech in patients who are neither paralyzed nor demented is singular enough to warrant a special designation; therefore, I shall name this symptom aphemia *because these patients lack only the ability to articulate words.* (Pierre Paul Broca, in Rottenberg & Hochberg, 1977.)

The poet Baudelaire's strange warning and eventual "loss of memory for sound" and Broca's description of the disorder he called aphemia are interwoven by several common threads. The commonalities and intricacies of this tapestry capsulize some of the concerns and ideas we shall deal with in this book.

We shall examine the ideas of Broca and the extended issues surrounding those functions subserved by the cortical area which bears his name. We shall concern ourselves with other areas of the brain as well, particularly those that relate to the complex behaviors of speech and language; those uniquely human characteristics that allow all other achievements, from science and technology to the maintenance of human intimacy. We shall look upon communication in disruption, and attempt to make sense of the tangled symptomatology that results when brain cells die or are compromised.

Just as Broca and countless others have struggled with the essence or nature of disrupted "articulate speech," we shall present our view of it. In a broader sense, we shall examine, deflate, and perhaps stimulate hypotheses about the nature of articulate speech and its correlates in the nervous system. These are the broader concerns that intrigued Broca, enraged Baudelaire, frustrate our patients, and continue to provide a never-ending stream of questions and delights that allow the expression of the strategies of science and the eventual prospect of understanding what one portion of the world is really like and how we can improve both it and us. But there is a more mundane, though no less important focus of this book. That is encompassed in the concern that we, as speech–language pathologists, have for discovering ways of restoring communicative effectiveness to people with damaged brains. We have no difficulty accepting the premise that communication is a primary ingredient to a favorable quality of life. Therefore, we believe that efforts to restore it are important and should assume a high priority. Without communication between and among humans, quality of life sinks to levels of mere existence; and existence without communication is vacuous.

Our biases will not be subtle. They will permeate the chapters of this book and the least subtle of these will be our clinical concern and commitment. Therefore, much of this book will reflect our attempts to synthesize and transduce concepts which allow us to understand, to assess, and to treat more efficiently those people afflicted with neurogenic disorders of speech. Our biases and our suggestions will come partly from our appreciation of the past and our attempts to understand the writings that reflect the struggles and revisions of others; but as much, they will spring from our own struggles, failures, and successes in the clinic with people who have come to us with disrupted speech. We hope we can avoid the pretense of authority and instead convey the impression of clinicians. We are acquainted with the literature and have fenced and wrestled the issues and debated perspectives both in print and private. Ultimately, though, our views are bathed in the biases of those who are charged with the responsibility of doing something about the disorder as well as discussing it.

This book is directed to all who have an interest in the speech and language disturbances that accompany brain damage. This does not limit it to any single profession. If ever there were an area where interdisciplinary study is appropriate it is that of brain organization and communication. The term "neurolinguistics" is gaining popularity to describe investigation of language—brain relationships, and the search for meaningful answers and sound theory in this area has been pursued by researchers and clinicians in such disciplines as speech—language pathology, linguistics, psychology, and neurology. No single discipline can strike a claim on the brain or on human language, and without doubt *trans*disciplinary cooperation will prove to be the most effective and economical means to prevent us from getting bogged down in incomplete technologies or parochial and checkered understanding. All of the disciplines mentioned above may find something useful in this book, but those who confront and attempt to modify disrupted speech perhaps will be most interested.

Speech—language pathologists in hospitals, rehabilitation clinics, private practice, and academic setting are most frequently charged with the chore of doing something about aberrant speech. A rich variety of clinical suggestion, some successful and some not so successful, is encompassed in this work. Not all of it is atheoretic or floundering without benefit of principle, but much of it is pragmatic and sorely in need of being put to the clinical test. Much of it also may smack of deja vu. Most clinical strategies have been written about before and tried by others. We make no claims of originality and have based many of our ideas on concepts and procedures of others. Wherever we can discern it, we have attempted to document this debt.

This book is also directed to students in the above disciplines. Though we make no claims to be free of the bias and influence of our training and experience, we have attempted to insert balance, reasonableness, and perspective into the development of controversial themes and issues. Students, particularly those who have completed the basic curriculum and are ready to assume the mantle of clinical responsibility, should find not only specific direction on how to procede with a clinical assignment, but ample material for molding opinions.

More than anything, we would hope that this work serves as a catalytic force to inspire others to seek the answers we have missed, or to straighten out the issues we have bungled. We doubt that a cataclysmic breakthrough will solve the riddles in this area. More likely, the gradual accumulation of knowledge, particle by particle, will allow a cohesive understanding to evolve.

Since one thesis of this book is that a significant portion, if not all of the problems in the selection and sequencing of speech sounds, may be due to a fundamental impairment in programming neuromuscular movements, we will discuss some of the issues related to nonspeech disturbances of movement. These generally are treated in the literature under the rubric of "apraxia," a disturbance of purposeful movement that cannot be accounted for by lack of comprehension, paralysis, or muscular weakness.

The descriptive term used to label the disorder discussed in this book is "apraxia of speech." We choose this label for several reasons. First, we feel that it focuses on what appears to be the underlying dynamics of the disorder. Our conceptualization of this may change with additional study and interpretation but for now at least "apraxia of speech" appears to direct one's attention explicitly to the neuromotor aspects of positioning the speech musculature for the production of speech sounds. It also indicates a discrepancy between execution of the speech act and relative intactness of semantic and syntactic linguistic features. Disrupted morphosyntax and execution of the movements necessary for speech sound production can coexist, and frequently do, but they can exist as well in relative isolation. Furthermore, we feel the term apraxia of speech is gaining favor in the literature, and increased usage occasionally serves the pragmatic function of improving clarity of communication. If labels have unambiguous referents, trans- and intradisciplinary communication will no doubt be enhanced. We define apraxia of speech as a neurogenic phonologic disorder resulting from sensorimotor impairment of the capacity to select, program, and/or execute in coordinated and normally timed sequences, the positioning of the speech musculature for the volitional production of speech sounds. The loss or impairment of phonologic rules of the native language is not adequate to explain the observed pattern of deviant speech, nor is the disturbance attributable to weakened or misdirected actions of specific muscle groups. Prosodic alteration, that is, changes in speech stress, intonation, and/or rhythm, may be associated with the articulatory disruption either as a primary part of the condition or in compensation for it.

Over a dozen speech and nonspeech behaviors have been categorized as characteristic of apraxic speech, and these will be elaborated upon in subsequent chapters.

We have presented the purposes this book is intended to achieve, the terminological confusion surrounding the disorder we choose to call apraxia of speech, and our definition of the disorder. We feel the state of the art is such that future research and interpretation will clarify the issues and answer some of the questions. In the meantime we can synthesize what is known, adopt a reasonable theoretic and clinical stance, an open mind, and an unfettered scientific attitude toward evidence that does not support our views, and get on with the task of attempting to help those people afflicted with the condition in the best way contemporary technology and knowledge will allow.

1

A Historical Perspective

EARLY TIMES: GODS, SPIRITS, AND HUMORS

The concept of apraxia is relatively new. The concept of an apraxia affecting the movements necessary for speech is even newer. But the idea that perhaps the secret organ encased in the skull might somehow be related to movements of the mouth and communication has been around for a long time. We can assume, without too much anthropologic fantasy, that since the dawn of man and the remarkable advent of oral communication the emerging faculty of speech has been susceptible to disruption or compromise. The age of mysticism and superstition contributed many a persistent notion about the relationship between brain and behavior; but even in this time of attributing diseases to gods or spirits one can see the embryonic concepts of clusters of symptoms associated with the head, if not the brain.

The Golden Mean, the Silver Median

The Age of Pericles, or the Golden Age of Greece, was responsible for many changes in rational thought, and the area of disease and affliction was no exception. Hippocrates' revolutionary writings provided a firm mooring for many aspects of contemporary medicine. The Hippocratic treatise, *On the Sacred Diseases*, written about 400 B.C., was remarkable in that it disavowed the superstitions associated with epilepsy and other brain diseases and for the first time in history assigned the brain an exclusive role in mental functions.

It was during this time as well that the unique and specific relationship between speech and the brain was emerging. In his aphorisms on apoplexy (the old name for stroke) Hippocrates observed that "... persons in good

5

health are suddenly seized with pains in the head, and straightway are laid down speechless . . ." (McHenry, 1969, p. 11).

In *Epidemics* he described hemiplegia and loss of speech in what McHenry (1969) calls probably the first written description of neurogenic communication impairment; the speech description ['the tongue unable to articulate . . . her speech was delirious . . . speech was indistinct. . ." (McHenry, 1969, p. 11)] could be aphasia, one of the dysarthrias, the language of hallucinations, or perhaps even apraxia of speech.

Galen (131–201 A.D.) furthered the science of neuroanatomy, in particular our knowledge of the cerebral ventricles and some of the cranial nerves, but even with the passing of six centuries, the physiology of the nervous system was thought to be based on the action of animal spirits within the ventricles (Meyer, 1971).

THE 1800s: TURNING POINT

In the 1800s a great deal changed. The inactivity of several dormant centuries ended. The impact on our understanding of the brain and behavior is unprecedented. Pierre Paul Broca, the French anthropologist and surgeon, is the name most closely linked with the surge of interest in the brain and speech, and 1861 has become the year of turning; the milestone by which we divide the age of relative enlightenment from the dimness of the early centuries. But Broca's contributions, while not insignificant, were not entirely pioneering, and several of his predecessors and contemporaries deserve equal recognition. As early as 1820, Lordat described "alalia," a disorder of the synergy of the muscles used for speech (Riese, 1947).

Head Bumps and Misdirection

Franz Joseph Gall (1757–1828) was as much a harbinger of a new era as anyone; but Gall is saddled with a bad reputation. His very real contributions to understanding the brain and behavior were hobbled by his subsequent fanaticism about phrenology, that pseudoscience that correlated behavioral and personality traits with bumps on the skull.

As Critchley (1970) has stated, Gall and the 1800s saw the pendulum of opinion swing well across from the holistic early views of brain function. But with phrenology, many thought the pendulum had swung too far and stuck too long. The concept of phrenology may have been overdrawn, but important ideas sprung from it. So the doctrine of speech as a localized function became the center of controversy, first in France, and then else-where. The heat and fury of this controversy provided the catalytic environment for breakthroughs in brain and behavior that were to have impact well into the twentieth century.

Bouillaud, Auburtin, and Broca

Bouillaud

The medical and scientific community of Paris aligned itself either for or against the ideas of speech as a localized function, and one of Gall's strongest advocates was an influential dean of medicine, Professor Bouil-laud. In 1825 Bouillaud first published his views on the issue. He adopted Gall's views of the plurality of cerebral organs and called the anterior lobes the "legislative organ of speech" (Riese, 1947). Bouillaud distinguished for the first time (and this distinction is germane to current issues surrounding apraxia of speech) the faculty to create words as signs of ideas and to retain them in memory, from the faculty to articulate them. Loss of speech, according to the teachings of Bouillaud, might be due to a loss of either of these facilities. Controversy raged for more than a decade with opponents of Bouillaud attempting to discredit him by associating him with Gall and phrenology, despite Bouillaud's presentation of several carefully observed cases in support of his views.

Though Bouillaud was a true pioneer in promulgating his views for a score of years through a series of publications, he apparently had not settled entirely on the precise localization of speech. The anterior lobes, bilaterally, were suggested as vital, and he was so convinced that he offered to forfeit 500 francs to anyone who could produce a brain of one who had lost speech during life but showed no frontal lesion. (Critchley, 1970, p. 61). According to Critchley, a gentleman named Velpeau appears to be the only one to have claimed the prize, when in 1843 he showed a specimen with bifrontal tumors, and the patient was reported to be not only nonaphasic before his death but extremely talkative. Bouillaud's mistake, of course, was in not realizing that lesions to some areas of the frontal lobes would not cause speech disruptions.

After the flurry of controversy from 1825 to the 1840s, the issue of the locus of speech was somewhat quiescent, despite the advocacy of Bouil-laud, until 1861 when the problem of speech and cerebral localization was again introduced to repeated sessions of the Anthropological Society of Paris by Ernest Auburtin. The roles of both Bouillaud and Auburtin have not been accorded the recognition they so rightly deserve, according to some historians (Stookey, 1963).

Auburtin

Ernest Auburtin was born in 1825 (the year Bouillaud first published his doctrine on the frontal lobes and speech), the son of mirror makers. Critchely (1970) characterized Auburtin as a "deep thinker with a reflective turn of mind" who was a member of the newly formed Anthropological Society. Auburtin was an advocate of Gall's views on the locus of speech in the brain, and eventually supported the views of Bouillaud as the controversy churned among the great thinkers of Paris. No doubt Auburtin had occasion to discuss the issue at some length at the home of Bouillaud.

Some have characterized April 4, 1861 as the most important date in the history of the study of the brain and language (Critchley, 1970, p. 61). At the age of 36, Auburtin dared to challenge the views of his colleagues, most of whom were his senior with established reputations and professionals with considerable power. He argued, rebutted, and interpreted published pathological reports; but perhaps his most dramatic evidence was the unprecedented experiment on a living patient at the Hospital St. Louis. This patient apparently had attempted suicide with a pistol and had completely shot away the frontal bone so that the anterior lobes of the brain were laid bare but not damaged. Intelligence and speech were intact and the patient survived several hours during which the following experiment was undertaken. In the words of Auburtin:

> While the patient was being interrogated the flat surface of a large spatula was lightly applied; on gentle pressure speech was suddenly suspended; a word begun was cut in two. Speech returned as soon as pressure was removed. The pressure thus exerted produced neither paralysis nor loss of consciousness and was exercised in such manner as to compress only the frontal lobes. (Stookey, 1963, p. 1026.)

Auburtin recognized that one cerebral lobe could be unmolested and speech be retained, but the precise area crucial to speech remained to be determined, despite his rather innovative pancake turner approach to neurolinguistic research.

Broca and Tan Tan LeBorgne

Upon hearing Auburtin's views, the young secretary of the Anthropological Society of Paris, Pierre Paul Broca, apparently became intrigued. He approached Auburtin after his lecture and invited him to see a patient of his at the Bicetre Hospital.

In the translated words of Broca:

> On April 11, 1861, a fifty-one-year-old man named LeBorgne suffering from a diffuse gangrenous inflammation of the entire buttocks, was admitted as a surgical patient to the general infirmary of the Bicetre. When I questioned him

the next day about the onset of his illness his only response was the mono-syllable "tan", repeated twice in succession and accompanied by a move-ment of the left hand. (Rottenberg & Hochberg, 1977, p. 138.)

The patient LeBorgne had little time left, and Broca reported that "the patient died at 11 P.M. on April 17." The autopsy was performed 24 hours later and the brain was shown to the Anthropological Society "a few hours after it was taken."

In presenting this classic case to the Society, Broca labeled it "aphemia of twenty-years duration produced by a chronic, progressive softening of the second and third convolutions of the superior part of the left frontal lobe."

Within a few months a second patient was admitted to Broca's surgical service at Bicetre due to a hip fracture. He had suddenly lost his speech five months earlier, being able to say only *oui, non, trois, toujours,* and *Lelo,* an attempt at his name, LeLong. Twelve days after admission, Lelong died, and Broca presented the autopsy findings before the Anthropological Society in November, 1861. The brain showed a more circumscribed lesion in the left third frontal convolution with only slight involvement of the second convolution, thus corresponding to the early period of Tan LeBorgne's illness (Stookey, 1963).

Whether or not these early patients and Broca's description of aphemia are early descriptions of what is now referred to as "apraxia of speech" remains moot. Certainly, the paucity of verbal output and the few reduplicated, stereotypic phrases or words attributed to both patients is not in keeping with the contemporary notion of the phonologic impairments of apraxia of speech, though some would argue that LeBorgne and LeLong were simply severe cases of apraxia of speech whose phonologic selection and sequencing disruption was masked by the severity of their condition. At any rate, these cases are of historical import in tracing the evolution of thought about brain damage and subsequent disruptions of speech, and Bouillaud and Auburtin deserve as much recognition for their courageous views as does Paul Broca.

Dax and Son

The question of priority of Broca's pronouncements has arisen peri-odically since 1861. Not the least of these controversies surrounds the claims of the French father and son named Dax. Marc Dax, the father, apparently had stated the conclusions of Broca publicly as early as 1836 at a medical meeting. So claimed his son, who even produced his father's manuscript that had been distributed to several of the senior Dax's col-leagues and then filed away in a bureau drawer to remain unpublished.

The younger Dax carried on a vigorous campaign to have his father's contributions recognized as being earlier than those of Broca and lamented the fact that later writers continued to pay no heed to his father. As Broca was alleged to have said, "I don't like questions about priority. . .," and the alleged original paper was not available to him, despite the younger Dax's later protests (Critchley, 1970, p. 63).

Controversy on the nature of the disorder followed Broca for years. Etymological purists chastized his choice of "aphemia" as a label, and Trousseau and Broca exchanged heated letters over proper Greek derivatives for "aphasia" versus "aphemia." The heart of the argument was whether the disruption was semantic or language based, or one of articulatory realization. Some issues change very little through the years.

DISORDERED MOVEMENT AND HUGO LIEPMANN

Apraxia of speech has a fundamental component—disturbed volitional movement that results in disrupted speech. The work of Hugo Liepmann at the turn of the century provided the basis for a more thorough understanding of the conditions of disturbed volitional movement that would eventually be called "apraxia." The term apraxia had been used earlier perhaps by Steinthal (1870, cited in Hecaen, 1972b) but Liepmann was first to describe the attempt to clarify the nature of the disorder. At the very onset of his now classic case report (Liepmann, 1900) he stated,

> So far as I know, it has not been observed—or at least not yet reported—that a human being might act with his right extremities as if he were a total imbecile, as if he understood neither questions or commands, as if he could neither understand the value of objects nor the sense of printed or written words, yet prove by an intelligent use of his left extremities that all of these seemingly absent abilities were in reality present (p. 15)."

Liepmann described the impairment of his case, Mr. T., from the standpoint of his limb impairment and elaborated in considerable detail about the differences in performance between Mr. T's right and left hands. Liepmann says, for example,

> On April 8, on being handed a toothbrush at a time when he was not accustomed to brush his teeth, he nevertheless employed it correctly with his left hand; with his right hand he used it as if it were a pen. On another occasion he put the handle into his mouth. On a third attempt he laughed in embarrassment, used the brush as if it were a spoon, shoveled with it, and put it into his mouth. Nor was he successful in using a trumpet or a harmonica (Rottenberg & Hochberg 1977, p. 171).

Liepmann described in considerable detail his case's speech function, movements to spoken command, imitation of movements, writing and drawing ability, performance on single and complex one- and two-handed tasks, sensory abilities, and motility. All of this description is Liepmann's attempt as he stated it, "...to prove that a syndrome exists as a pure entity, that my patient is apractic in the strictest sense of the word, and, more specifically that he is unilaterally apractic" (160). He summarizes by stating, "Apraxia is, in short, the inability to act, i.e., to move the moveable parts of the body in a purposeful manner, though motility is preserved" (p. 160).

Though Liepmann did not attempt to explain the speech and language impairment of Mr. T., and it may or may not have been what we now call apraxia of speech, at the very least he stimulated a good deal of further attention to the disorder that triggered comment by later writers such as Lord Brain, Derek Denny-Brown (1958), S.A.K. Wilson (1908), and more recently Norman Geschwind (1975). But it was Hugo Liepmann's pioneering work in the early 1900s that is most linked to the condition of apraxia. Liepmann's careful observations provided a foundation and methodological guide not only to subsequent researchers in the early 1900s but to contemporary writers as well.

Further observations on disrupted volitional movement have been made by Hughlings Jackson (Taylor, 1932), Marcuse (1904), Pick (1905), and later work again by Liepmann (1920). A resurgence of interest in apraxia was evident in the 1960s and the work of Geschwind (1965) and Hielman, Schwartz, and Geschwind (1975) has spawned a variety of definitions, interpretations, and analyses of the nature, extent, and neuroanatomic correlates of the disorder.

"Who knows only his own generation remains always a child" is an aphorism engraved above the entrance of the Norlin Library at the University of Colorado. We are prodded by that wise advice to study and appreciate the contributions of those who preceded us and to respect the history of an issue. Perhaps this time-lapse tracing of the evolution of concepts related to apraxia will stimulate additional interpretations or rekindle inquiry of issues that piqued the curiosity of our forebearers.

2

Phonology: The Study of
Sound Patterns in Speech

Observation of the motions of some of our speech organs to determine how sounds are made is fairly easy, but it is not as easy to observe and characterize the operations of the mind. Linguists are fond of saying that a speaker who has mastered his or her native tongue knows a lot more about the rules of language than any linguist. Serious fissures exist in our knowledge of language, and they extend well into the area of speech sound production. Behavioral science will not be daunted, though, and clinics and laboratories are adding daily to the accumulation of information in the area of phonology.

Two basic approaches exist to the study of speech sounds, structural phonology, and generative phonology. Structural phonology concerns itself with description and analysis of the make-up of the sounds of language, from articulatory, acoustic, and semantic viewpoints. Generative phonology is concerned with theoretical aspects of this structure and how it relates to other aspects of language.

The lobby of the United Nations building in New York is as good a place as any to be struck by the richness of the variations heard across languages. The clicks of Xosi, the nasals of French, and the tonal swoops and sweeps of Southeastern Asian all illustrate dramatic and easily extractable differences in producing speech. Linguists and clinicians are interested not only in these differences, but in the regularities and universals that can be sifted from these streams of mouth emissions. Phonology is the study of the ways in which speech sounds form systems and patterns in human language.

Ned W. Bowler, whom we worked with at the University of Colorado, is an example of a phonetician. His phonatory interest revolves around events at the physical, articulatory, and acoustic levels. He observed, and taught us to observe, the physical aspects of people speaking and how they produced these sounds. He recorded the sounds with a symbol system that could be interpreted by himself and others; and his trained ear, sometimes aided by instruments, indicated to him those sounds that were perceivably different. The careful phonetician, and Ned Bowler is no exception, cautions against confusing utility and reality in the study of differences in speech sounds. No two people speak exactly alike, and even the sound waves from a word spoken by the same person on repeated occasions will not be identical. Thus the phonetician must arrive at compromises of judgment and perception to serve his or her purposes. Sometimes one is interested in gross differences among utterances and may simply use a standard chain of phonetic signs to represent what is heard. Sometimes one wishes to paint with a finer brush and draw more detailed distinctions. If for example, there is interest in capturing the aspects of stress, intonation, or duration of speech sounds, a phonetic sign system can be embellished with a series of diacritical marks.

The phonetician's interest revolves around the physical aspects of the smallest speech segments that play a part in communication. As Colin Cherry (1968) has pointed out, though the semantic and syntactical aspects that help form a language grammar do not come directly under his microscope, the phonetician sees them out of the corner of his eye.

The skills and interests of the phonetician are vital to those who would study and remediate disorders of speech and language. The observable differences that occur in the speech of the person afflicted with apraxia of speech are apparent in the physical aspects of his or her utterances. The astute clinician must be able to observe, capture, preserve, and analyze these utterances, and this is where the study and appreciation of phonology becomes more than academic. It can be a useful daily tool in the evaluation and diagnosis of speech production disturbances and can provide a basis for analyzing and understanding some of the obvious and not so obvious reasons for the disruption. This chapter is included to present some basic concepts in phonology and also to speculate on aspects of phonology that may serve to clear up some of the controversy that has plagued the study of apraxia of speech. No doubt much of the scholarly discord can be attributed to unclear referents; poor descriptions and definitions of behavior; and, sometimes, a cursory and unsophisticated appreciation of the terms and methods of phonology.

SEGMENTS, PHONETICS, PHONEMICS

"There is a curious paradox . . .," as Gilbert and Sullivan were fond of pointing out. In phonology, one such curious paradox is the fact that a speech signal is physically continuous, but we seem to hear it as a sequence of discrete units. An underlying assumption of the phonetician is that we can represent our mutterings as a sequence of discrete units. This assumption allows us to discuss segments and sequences of segments and to use a sign system (usually the International Phonetic Alphabet) to represent these segments. Some argue, though, that the discrete units of speech are an artifact of analysis, something invented by phoneticians to allow them to play around with language and avoid work in the yard. Instrumental analysis and careful listening have demonstrated that speech sounds tend to merge and blend into one another. Analysis of a spoken sentence such as "Cowboys sometimes listen to symphonies," reveals that during the articulation of the initial consonant the tongue is already anticipating the following diphthong and even the lips are beginning to move slightly to get ready for the /b/ sound. Why is it, then, that as listerners we tend to hear speech in distinct though rapidly produced segments or units? Shane (1973), among others, has attempted to explain this phenomenon. If a speaker for some reason decides to say, "Cowboys sometimes listen to symphonies," the vocal mechanism is put together in such a fashion that in saying this sentence it does not produce one sound; stop; produce the next one; stop; and so on, but instead functions in a steady stream of motion, moving from one sound to the next, and even preparing for a sound in advance. This is more efficient. As listeners we are not required to wait around for hours for a person to finish a long sentence though it sometimes seems so. However, this stream of motion produces transitions—as Shane (1973) says, a series of slurrings and blurrings—and these transitions must be dealt with by a listener. How does the listener deal with utterances that are slip-sliding away in a continuous stream of sound? Somehow, the listener perceives it as discontinuous. Some heavy thinkers have guessed that this is the only way the human mind is capable of organizing language. There is good evidence that humans perceive this apparently continuous phenomenon as discontinuous. In writing, for example, even if a word such as "buns" is written cursively and all the letters are connected, we still perceive it as containing four separate letters, as if it were printed. It's what you "think" that counts, says Shane (1973). Despite the fact that X-rays and spectrograms show speech as being physically continuous, in this aspect of language the perceptual, the subjective, and the discrete override the physical, the objective, and the continuous.

Another fundamental concept in phonology, and one that has no little importance to the issues surrounding the disorder of apraxia of speech, is the necessary distinction between *phonetic* and *phonemic* descriptions of speech. Phonetics and phonetic description refer to variations in the basic components of speech sounds without reference to meaning. Some speech sounds are produced in slightly varying fashions depending upon context. For example, the first segment in the word "tar" is the same as the second in "star" and the last in "rat." But subtle variations exist in the production of each /t/ in the words. The initial /t/ in tar is phonetically aspirated. "Aspirated" does not mean swallowed and choked on but rather produced with a puff of air. Less aspiration is apparent to the careful listener on *star* and the final /t/ in *rat* may be aspirated or unaspirated (no air puffs). These differences in production are *phonetic variants* or *allophones*.

In addition to the phonetic aspects of allophonic variations in production, speech sounds can be looked upon as being comprised of sets of properties or components. These properties have been called distinctive features, and their use in the analysis of the production of brain-injured individuals may be a fruitful area for discovering subtle differences in the coordination and timing of the speech musculature. Distinctive features are considered in more detail below.

Phonemics and phonemic description are related to phonetic differences, but with an important addition. When the difference in the production of two sounds results in changes in meaning, that change is phonemic. The changes in production of the initial segment in the productions *fickle, mick'll, tickle, pickle* have a direct influence on meaning. These are phonemic changes. Knowledge of a language includes knowing which variants in production are phonemic and which are nonphonemic, and every speaker uses this knowledge and demonstrates it in speech. Schools of thought and diversity of opinion exist in linguistics and phonology as well as in speech pathology, and the concept of phonemics has not escapted rich and heated controversy. One theory holds that phonemes are not exactly classes of speech sounds that share common phonetic features, but that they exist only in the abstract sense in terms of the opposition of distinctive features. According to Lesser (1978), a group of linguists from Prague in the 1920s and 1930s proposed the concept of phonemes not being themselves real (the phonemes, not the linguists), but mere abstractions. In speech–language pathology we have grown accustomed to the practice of referring to phonologic segments which change the meaning of utterances as "phonemes." We can better appreciate Buckingham's (1978) criticism of the liberal and, to his way of thinking, untidy use of the term "phonéme" in the apraxia of speech literature if we understand the historical controversy that has surrounded the development of the concept of the phoneme in generative phonology. Even though the real nature of the phoneme is elusive, usage has dictated widespread use of the word to refer to changes in sound production that signal differences in meaning.

Distinctive Features

The series of binary contrasts which have come to be called distinctive features are an important aspect of generative phonology and may have more application in solving some of the riddles of neurogenic phonologic disruption than meets the ear. A variety of systems have been proposed to capture the distinctive features of speech sounds. Originally, about 12 sets of binary contrasts were proposed, but more sets have been added over the years.

Chomsky and Halle (1968) pioneered this distinctive feature approach to phonologic analysis. Far from universal agreement exists on the precise features that should be used and how many are necessary. The utility of distinctive feature analysis to pathologies of speech has been questioned by some, but the approach has been used with neurologically impaired persons by La Pointe and Johns (1974), Blumstein (1973), and Martin and Rigrodsky (1974b). Some of the features are based primarily on acoustic characteristics, while others derive from articulatory factors.

In keeping with the binary nature of characterizing each feature, phonemes, or more accurately, phones, are assigned either a plus or a minus for any given feature. Table 1 presents a fairly standard distinctive feature matrix for the sounds of American English. It is adapted from MacKay (1978).

Distinctive features are defined, usually in acoustic and/or articulatory terms, as follows (MacKay, 1978):

Consonantal (cons):	Low degree of acoustic energy; obstruction at some point along the vocal tract.
Vocalic (voc):	Unobstructed vocal tract except for vocal fold vibration; presence of acoustic format structure.
Continuant (cont):	Produced without total blockage of oral cavity at any point (*non*continuant sounds totally block oral cavity).
Nasal (nas):	Velum is lowered, introducing nasal cavity as a resonance chamber; lowered intensity of formants.
Anterior (ant):	Produced in front part of oral cavity (alveolar – palatal region is dividing line).
Coronal (coron):	Produced with tongue blade arched above its neutral position.
High (hi):	Dorsum (not tip) of tongue is raised.
Low (lo):	Tongue is lowered below neutral position.
Back (ba):	Produced with retraction of body of tongue.
Voice (vc):	Produced with vocal fold vibration.
Tense (tns):	Produced with tongue root advancement; great energy spread acoustically (applies only to vowels).
Strident (stri):	Acoustically, a greater proportion of sound is noise (aperiodic).
Sonorant (son):	Produced with relatively free passage of sound or air through vocal tract.

Table 1
Matrix of Distinctive Features for English Phones

	p	b	t	d	k	g	tʃ	dʒ	f	v	θ	ð	s	z	ʃ	ʒ	m	n	ŋ	r	l	h	w	j	i	I	e	ɛ	æ	u	U	o	ɔ	ʌ	a
Consonantal	+	+	+	+	+	+	+	+	+	+	+	+	+	+	+	+	+	+	+	+	+	−	−	−	−	−	−	−	−	−	−	−	−	−	−
Vocalic	−	−	−	−	−	−	−	−	−	−	−	−	−	−	−	−	−	−	−	+	+	−	−	−	+	+	+	+	+	+	+	+	+	+	+
Continuant	−	−	−	−	−	−	−	−	+	+	+	+	+	+	+	+	−	−	−	+	+	+	+	+	+	+	+	+	+	+	+	+	+	+	+
Nasal	−	−	−	−	−	−	−	−	−	−	−	−	−	−	−	−	+	+	+	−	−	−	−	−	−	−	−	−	−	−	−	−	−	−	−
Anterior	+	+	+	+	−	−	−	−	+	+	+	+	+	+	−	−	+	+	−	+	+	−	−	−	−	−	−	−	−	−	−	−	−	−	−
Coronal	−	−	+	+	−	−	+	+	−	−	+	+	+	+	+	+	−	+	−	+	+	−	−	−	−	−	−	−	−	−	−	−	−	−	−
High	−	−	−	−	+	+	+	+	−	−	−	−	−	−	+	+	−	−	+	−	−	−	+	+	+	+	−	−	−	+	+	−	−	−	−
Low	−	−	−	−	−	−	−	−	−	−	−	−	−	−	−	−	−	−	−	−	−	+	−	−	−	−	−	−	+	−	−	−	+	−	+
Back	−	−	−	−	+	+	−	−	−	−	−	−	−	−	−	−	−	−	+	−	−	−	+	−	−	−	−	−	−	+	+	+	+	+	+
Voice	−	+	−	+	−	+	−	+	−	+	−	+	−	+	−	+	+	+	+	+	+	−	+	+	+	+	+	+	+	+	+	+	+	+	+
Strident	−	−	−	−	−	−	+	+	+	+	−	−	+	+	+	+	−	−	−	−	−	−	−	−	−	−	−	−	−	−	−	−	−	−	−
Sonorant	−	−	−	−	−	−	−	−	−	−	−	−	−	−	−	−	+	+	+	+	+	+	+	+	+	+	+	+	+	+	+	+	+	+	+
Tense	−	−	−	−	−	−	−	−	−	−	−	−	−	−	−	−	−	−	−	−	−	−	−	−	+	−	+	−	−	+	−	+	+	−	+

Adapted from MacKay, 1978, with permission.

17

The phonetic symbol /t/, as an example, is a shortcut used to represent the bundle of features unique to that sound. To capture the features unique to /t/, it could as well be written as

+ cons
− voc
− cont
− nas
+ ant
+ coron
− hi
− lo
− ba
− vc
− son

Questions have arisen as to the utility of distinctive features. The case can be made that they are truly a *distinctive* way of isolating the similarities and differences among phones. Some of these similarities and differences might well have been obscured by the old terminology and phonetic taxonomy. For a long time, phoneticians and clinicians were content to classify speech sounds along the traditional lines in articulatory phonetics of manner, place, and voicing. Manner of articulation is described using one of five categories (plosives, fricatives, affricates, nasals, or glides); place of articulation utilizes the names of various locations in the vocal tract where points of articulation are produced (bilabial, dental, alveolar, palatal, velar, lingual, glottal); and voicing refers to whether or not the vocal folds are vibrating during the production of a consonant.

The utility of the distinctive feature system has the potential to make some very practical contributions to understanding phonologic impairment that accompanies brain damage. As we comb the surf we can expect the loss of fewer sea creatures if we select a seine with a fine mesh, though we may entrap a crab or a squid along the way. Similarly, by using more sensitive tools of observation and analysis perhaps we can prevent information loss that affects not only our understanding of clinical syndromes, but the very theories on which these syndromes are based. MacKay (1978) presents an example in mathematics that may be analogous to our problem in articulatory phonetics. In mathematics, most people are familiar with Roman numerals and can write a few of them. We are equally aware that these numerals are quite useless for performing mathematical calculations. To divide LVII by XXIX without converting to Arabic is cumbersome if not impossible. The Arabic numerals do not represent simply another means of recording the same information as Roman numerals (just as with distinctive feature analysis), but within the Arabic numeral system are certain sophisticated conventions that allow the user to gain insights into the properties and workings of numbers. Advanced mathematics is made possible through the recording system selected. Likewise, MacKay (1978) suggests, the distinctive feature notation system will allow us to understand phonologic processes that might otherwise escape our attention if traditional classification systems (nets with wider mesh) were used. Thus, the early adaption of a narrower phonetic transcription system may have prevented some of the problems that plague us today in the study of apraxia of speech.

Markedness

A concept of linguistics that has gained some attention in recent years is that of *markedness*. Application of descriptive linguistics to the disrupted output of the brain-damaged population has fostered both applied and theoretic interest in this concept. First of all, it serves to reinforce the compulsive nature in some of us that drives us to attempt to impart some degree of order or system on the seeming chaos of the speech of the brain damaged. Garbled speech is easier to deal with if it seems to be patterned, organized into a system, or categorized. Even if the system we adopt to impose organization is rather arbitrary, we are comforted by increased order and can grasp and discuss complexities with somewhat greater ease. So utility and order are strong motivations to study disrupted speech by such descriptive linguistic strategies as markedness. But, in addition, and on a more theoretical level, markedness has been proposed as an explanatory principle underlying the normal organization of language, and researchers such as Ulatowska and Baker (1975) have suggested that it also may have explanatory force regarding what persists and what is susceptible to loss in the language of the brain damaged. These writers, as have others before them, argue that beneath the surface diversity of languages, there exist structural similarities which are determined by biologically and neurologically based constraints on what form a language can take.

The notion of markedness essentially holds that features of language, from phonology to morphosyntax, can be analyzed in dichotomous fashion in order to determine whether a component or aspect is present or absent. In phonology, for example, speech segments or phones can be characterized by the presence or absence of certain distinctive features. Thus, the /z/ segment may be designated as either marked or unmarked for the feature of voicing. /z/ is voiced of course, since the vocal cords are activated audibly, so it is designated as marked for voicing. /s/, on the other hand, is unmarked for voicing. This binary categorization scheme has been explained during the discussion of distinctive features. The point to be made here is that a system of markedness can be used to explain relative complexity of speech segments. The unmarked member of this system of phonologic opposition is characterized as being (a) more "natural" in the sense that the vocal and articulatory apparatus is positioned relatively closer to the phonetically neutral position; (b) usually more frequently occurring; and (c) usually earlier in arriving during the process of language acquisition.

Ulatowska and Baker (1975) explain and urge the use of markedness analysis in the attempt to grasp an understanding of disrupted phonology and hint that there is a strong tendency in the dissolution of phonology for marked structures to be impaired, in contrast to the relative preservation of unmarked structures.

An interesting application of markedness analysis was performed on a single case by Wolk (1978). She devised a markedness table based on values suggested by Cairns (1969) and Chomsky and Halle (1968), and concluded that error analysis revealed that ". . . many of the utterances consisted of phonemes and phoneme sequences in which the value of the features in the target system were retained." Wolk even enters the arena of terminologic controversy and suggests that phonologic errors are systematic, more likely to be less complex, and therefore ". . . inseparable from the general aphasia disorder . . ." (p. 97).

A further application of markedness analysis to the phonemic substitution errors in ten speakers with apraxia of speech was conducted by Marquardt, Reinhart, and Peterson (1979). They concluded that more errors were produced on sounds high in markedness; some changes in markedness were from marked to unmarked; and errors and directional changes in markedness were positively correlated with "ease of articulation."

The concept of markedness analysis is no doubt a valid and useful strategy for aiding our understanding of phonologic disruption. But it cannot be a singular filter through which we let pass the speech behaviors that we are interested in viewing. Some limited linguistic approaches have failed to analyze some of the nonlinguistic behaviors, such as articulatory groping, initiation difficulty, restarts, retrials, self-corrections, and on-line changes in production. These features are as much a part of the condition as are the segmental selection and seriation difficulty, and they must be considered when attempting to explain or describe the disorder. They will not go away merely by ignoring them or leaving them unanalyzed.

Phonologic Rules

Most of us who have a basic knowledge of linguistics are aware that there are certain rules or statements about some aspects of how language works. We are familiar with certain conventions and their violations related to semantics and to syntax and that these conventions serve as the grammar of our language. We learn these conventions of language for the most part inductively, that is, we infer and use the rules by being exposed to them repeatedly during the acquistion of language. Few rules are specified or verbalized for us (presented deductively) with the exceptions of some syntactic universals drilled home to us by Mrs. Chard and our other English teachers.

Phonology is bound by conventions and rules as well. Certain aspects of pronunciation and the use of speech sounds can be stated in a formal way to prevent ambiguity and to foster study and understanding of this aspect of language. Very little analysis of the deviant speech patterns of the neurologically impaired has approached the disorder from the standpoint of phonologic rule violation. When segments and, for that matter, suprasegments undergo change, we are interested in at least three issues: (1) which segments or suprasegments change; (2) how they change; and (3) under what conditions they change.

Shane (1973) stated that phonolgic rules can be summarized under four categories: feature changing rules; rules for deletion and insertion; rules for permutation and coalescence; and rules with variables. We will not attempt to list or explain all of the phonologic rules that have been suggested by scholars of American English; some are complex, sequential, and interdependent; and some are nondistinctive and do not result in change in meaning. A few examples might be useful, however. The rules of phonology have been summarized by many linguists, including Fromkin and Rodman (1974).

Feature Adding Rules

Aspiration Rule—Voiceless stops are aspirated at the beginning of a word.

This rule applies to certain conventions of pronunciation in English. The small puff of air that the careful listener hears after the /k/ in the word "kid" can be distinguished from no aspiration in words such as "skid." In skid, no aspiration is apparent because the rule states that it follows a voiceless stop *only* at the beginning of words. The aspiration rule is nondistinctive, that is, violation of it normally will not change meaning, but it is a good example of the influence of phonetic environment on the specification of added features in English.

Assimilation Rule—A vowel is nasalized when it occurs before a nasal consonant.

This is a phonologic rule that is so common it is believed to be universal in the languages of the world. A rule such as this dictates the influence relative to feature change that one segment has on another segment. Adjacent phonemes become more similar when this rule is involved and, no doubt, this similarity is caused by articulatory and physiologic limitations or "the path of least amount of effort."

Plural-Formulation Rule—(a) Insert (ə) before the plural ending when a regular noun ends in /s/, /z/, /ʃ/, /tʃ/, /dʒ/, or /ʒ/; (b) change voiced /z/ to voiceless /s/ if regular noun ends in a voiceless sound.

To form regular plural forms in English (irregular plurals such as children and oxen are exempt from the rule), the speaker adds either a /z/, /s/, or /əz/.

The final phoneme of the word determines which sound one selects; and rules or regularities determine which of these endings we use. These plural –formulation rules guide us in adding /s/ to rat, /z/ to hog, and /əz/ to kiss.

Feature Changing Rules

Homorganic Nasal Rule—Within a word, a nasal consonant assumes the same place of articulation as a following consonant.

This is also an assimilation rule in that the phonetic environment influences application of the change in feature. Homorganic means that two sounds have the same place of articulation. The phonetic form of the prefix meaning "not" is a good example of the phonetic variance that this rule dictates. These variations in production are realized as (in) before a vowel or alveolar consonant (inappropriate, indefinite); (im) before a labial consonant (impossible); and /ŋ/ before a velar (inconsequential).

Feature Deletion Rules

Deletion Rule—Delete a /g/ when it occurs before a final consonant.

With this rule, we can properly pronounce, with the appropriate /g/ deletion, such words as sign, resign, or malign. Knowledge of the limits of this rule (only before a *final* consonant) allows us to produce the /g/ when a suffix is added to the root or stem word and properly contrast sign/signature, resign/resignation, and malign/malignant.

/b/—Deletion Rule—Delete a word-final /b/ when it occurs after an /m/. Knowledge of this rule allows us to omit correctly the production of the word-final /b/, and to contrast such pairs as bomb/bombay and crumb/crumble.

This selection of phonologic rules of American English is representative but certainly not exhaustive. As Fromkin and Rodman (1974) point out, some of the rules may be complex but they are never too complex to be learned. They indicate to us what speakers of a language know, from the basic units of our spoken language (the phonemic segments) to the circumstances under which these constructs are realized. No one makes us memorize these rules. We learn them by listening to our mothers, uncles, teachers, fathers, butchers, and everyone else in our environment who uses our native tongue. In writing and formulating these rules, linguists are not just attempting to dazzle us by demonstrating a firm and obfuscating grasp of the obvious. They are attempting to provide devices by which we can study language under controlled conditions, in the laboratory, in the field, or under a "microscope." These strategies hold some hope for furthering our understanding and fostering explanations of the mechanisms involved when the phonology of language is in disarray. The degree to which knowledge of phonology contributes to the efficiency of our management of apraxia of speech patients remains to be seen. At best, it will help us solve some of the riddles that have plagued us; at the very least, it will share the rationale our grandmothers used for milk-toast therapy: "It can't hurt." We should realize full well, though, that many of the aberrant behaviors in apraxia of speech cannot be captured by phonologic rule violation. Many are nonlinguistic compensations and disruptions of speech movement and cannot be neglected by sole reliance on a linguistic notation system.

SUPRASEGMENTALS

"It's not *what* you said; it's *how* you said it." This is a frequent comment of an offended party in an argument. "How we say it" can be manipulated in several ways. The same sentence can be invested with many meanings. In addition to individual phonemes or segments, speech is composed of identifiable characteristics that cross the boundaries of segments and are referred to as *suprasegmentals.* Authors do not universally agree on what to call the components of the suprasegmentals, but stress, rate (timing), and intonation are common features. The collective effect of stress, rate, and intonation is often called "prosody" or the "prosodic features" of speech. In some of the early writings in phonology and speech − language pathology, one gets the impression that the attitude toward prosody is that it was regarded as sort of the frosting on the speech cake or the after-six formal wear of speech; nice to have for a party but not essential for utilitarian communication tasks. This attitude may not reflect the very real contributions of prosody to meaning. Some feel (Rosenbek & LaPointe, 1978; Weintraub, Mesulam, & Kramer, 1981) that the role of prosody is not so much the *formal* wear but closer to the foundation garments or *underwear* of speech. It may be going too far to suggest that the increased loudness necessary for contrastive stress should be called "Fruit-of-the-Boom," however. Prosody and the suprasegmentals allow us to say the same string of words in different ways. Although psycholinguists argue about the notion of "linguistic intonation," there is little doubt, as Egan (1980) has pointed out, that different judgments based on prosodic change reflect more than just the enrichment and embellishment of declarations. Meaning is manipulated in a rich variety of ways by changes in prosody, and such semantic dimensions as credence, option, salience, arousal, connotations, emotional associations, and social meanings have been studied by psycholinguists (Egan, 1980).

Since certain strategies of therapy in apraxia of speech (and in the dysarthrias as well) are based on carefully controlled manipulations of prosody (contrastive stress, for example), some fundamental concepts related to suprasegmentals and prosody are presented.

Stress

Stress is the feature of speech we used to call "emphasis" or "accent." These terms, emphasis and accent, are too ambiguous and ill-defined for most phoneticians, and "stress" has replaced them. Acoustically, relative stress is accounted for by measurable changes in intensity, duration, and fundamental frequency.

Stress comes in many forms. Stress collapses bridges, gastrointestinal walls, and sentence ambiguity. The phonetician is apt to be more interested professionally in semantic stress than in the bridge or the gut, though, and considerable research on the contribution of word, phrase, and sentence stress has accumulated (Langacker, 1968). In English, *word stress* operates phonetically on the syllable (MacKay, 1978) to aid us in distinguishing among word meanings. *Cón*vict and conv*íct* are differentiated by changing syllabic stress. Subtle and synchronous changes in duration, loudness, and pitch allow us to perceive and attribute the proper meanings to these words.

Phrase stress. In phrases, the semantic or syntactic relationship among words determine that some of them take a distinctive stress pattern. In phrases and sentences, the terms primary, secondary, and tertiary are assigned to portions of the utterance in descending relative prominence. For sentences or discourse, phoneticians use the marks /, \, and ∧ to indicate primary, secondary, and tertiary stress, while weakly stressed syllables or words are left unmarked. The careful phonetician, then, has a way of distinguishing four levels of stress. In phrases of adjective–noun combinations, the adjective usually assumes a secondary stress role, while the information-bearing noun receives primary stress. For example: "He's in the grèen hoúse." The primary and secondary stress roles are reversed, though, in compound words made up of two nouns or an adjective plus a noun. Notice the difference in "He's in the greénhoùse."

Differences in phrase stress allow us to attach very different meanings to such contrasts as *hot dog* (a weiner or a show-off on skis) and *hot dog* (a Schnauzer that has just run a mile); *black bird* (any bird that is black; a crow for example) and *blackbird* (the red-winged variety we used to see sitting on cattails in the swamp behind the Channing roundhouse); *French teacher* (teacher of the French language) and *French teacher* (the nice teacher from Nice).

Sentence stress. Rules govern stress placement in words and phrases, and sentence stress is distributed lawfully as well. Information-bearing or content words (most often nouns, verbs, adjectives, and adverbs) receive greater stress than the functors (articles, conjunctions, prepositions) in a sentence. MacKay (1978) presents a useful explanation of this and uses the sentence example, "The couple came to the party." Here, the content words receive noticeably greater stress than function words, but MacKay is quick to point out that, occasionally, words change their grammatical role as in "The unconscious man came to." In this example, the word *to* is stressed more than in the earlier example, since *to* is now part of the verb and carries more information. A simple test of this relative semantic value in each sentence is to produce each one and omit *to* while noting the change in meaning.

Contrastive (emphatic stress). Contrastive stress occurs in spoken English in relation to certain well-specified conditions of discourse. In subsequent chapters it will be shown how it can be used as a facilitator of phonologic integrity. One use of contrastive stress in conversation is to eliminate confusion between two people with the same name. For example we might stress the family name in: "Elmo DWERK will bring the champagne," to prevent confusion with Elmo SCOTT who is scheduled to bring the ribs.

Sometimes, certain individual words in a sentence must be stressed in order to change emphasis. Fairbanks (1954) has a series of good examples in his *Voice and Articulation Drillbook* involving herds of horses. MacKay (1978) illustrates this function of contrastive stress as well. Notice the change in meaning in the following sentences.

Jay is not involved in the Red Zinger Bicycle race.
(factual statement)

Jay is not involved in the Red Zinger bicycle race.
(but somebody is)

Jay is *not* involved in the Red Zinger bicycle race.
(wouldn't be caught dead there)

Jay is not *involved* in the Red Zinger bicycle race.
(though he may know about it)

Jay is not involved in the *Red* Zinger bicycle race.
(the *Blue* Zinger, maybe?)

Jay is not involved in the Red *Zinger* bicycle race.
(he's in the Red *Cross* race)

Jay is not involved in the Red Zinger *bicycle* race.
(he's involved in the foot race)

Jay is not involved in the Red Zinger bicyle *race*.
(though he may be involved with a Red Zinger bicycle)

Contrastive stress may be used as well when we feel that the listener may have expected to hear something else. For example: The *whales* are responsible for water pollution. This stress would clear up confusion if the listener had expected the speaker to accuse chemical plants or swimmers.

Rate (timing).   Speech rate can be analyzed from at least three vantage points. Overall rate may be determined, or one may wish to measure pause time or articulation time. Certainly, social and contextual discourse influences speed of speech. The emotional or fatigue state of the speaker ("I've got great news! It's a father, I'm a boy!"); the urgency of the message ("I believe your pants are on fire!") and the formality of the situation ("Mr. President . . . Honored Guests . . . Mother Teresa . . . Prince Charles . . . Stevie Wonder . . . Welcome to our Awards Banquet") all have modulating influences on speech rate.

A certain amount of rate manipulation is possible through prolongation of articulation time, principally on vowels. However, careful use of silence is less distorting. As MacKay (1978) suggests, we tend to overestimate the number of pauses in speech, perhaps because we are conditioned by writing, where spaces neatly separate words. Spoken language is not so choppy, in fact is quite fluent, though we hear prolongations of speech sounds and occasional verbal filler ("uhhh . . .," "ahhh . . .," "er–ah," "hwahmmm . . ."), particularly by nervous speakers or those whose speech is filled with "verbal tics" ("like, ah . . .," "you know . . .").

Pauses *are* used in discourse, however, for both emphasis and meaning distinction. For example,

She didn't ride because the jockey was there.
(she rode, but not just because the jockey was there to watch her)

She didn't ride because the jockey was there.
(she didn't ride; the jockey did)

The pause, coupled with stress and prolongation, imparts a very contrasting meaning to these sentences. Pauses also are a natural consequence of normal speech during word retrieval or temporary memory lapse; this fact must be considered during the speech analysis of a brain-damaged individual who might well present coexisting word retrieval deficit or memory loss. Normal speakers also use pause for emphasis or dramatic effect.

An aspect of rate and rhythm of speech indicated by MacKay (1978) that may sometimes be relevant in our judgments of prosodic abnormality in people with neuropathology is that of *stress-timed rhythm* and *syllable-timed rhythm*. The rhythm of English is dramatized by a staccato pattern of uneven and varying numbers of syllables between successive beats (strongly stressed syllables). Other languages, and French is an example, have a distinctive rhythm based on the total nymber of syllables in a sentence. This pattern is called a *syllable-timed rhythm*, and if it is imposed on spoken English, the result will sound abnormal and stilted. Some have suggested (MacKay, 1978) that the hearing-impaired have a tendency to use such a rhythm and give equal weight and time to all syllables. Sometimes, imposing a syllable-timed rhythm, such as the pacing imposed by speaking with a metronome or other pacing device, can be used as a facilitator to improve intelligibility. Much more will be presented on this potential for remediation in subsequent chapters.

The neural mechanisms of prosody are not completely understood, but we do know that certain cerebellar−cortical connections, along with right-cerebral-hemisphere areas, may share a good portion of the responsibility for prosodic integrity. Kent and Rosenbek (1982) have reviewed some of the neurophysiologic bases of prosody.

Intonation

Intonation is one of the more endearing aspects of the suprasegmentals. Perhaps the inherent asthetic quality of intonation is related to its closeness to its first cousin, music. As Bolinger (1975) has said, "Intonation is the broad undulation of the pitch curve that carries the ripples of accent on its back" (p. 48).

To Bolinger, accent is what we refer to as stress. Intonation and stress together are often called speech melody, and this may be more than a metaphor. Speech melody and the melody of music may share a common origin and some linguists have written essays on the close ties between the music and language of cultures (Bolinger, 1975).

Tomes have been written on tone, and an example is the comprehensive work edited by Fromkin (1978). In her book *Tone: A Linguistic Survey,* she has called upon a number of clever linguists to address such questions as What are the physiological and perceptual correlates of tone? How do tonal and nontonal features interact? What are the necessary and sufficient tonal features? Should tone be represented segmentally or suprasegmentally in a lexicon? What is the nature of tone rules and are they similar to or different from other phonologic rules?

The production mechanism of tone has fascinated speech scientists for years, as is pointed out by Ohala (1978), and laboratory experiments have ranged from the early Halloween-like measurements of the results of externally generated air streams though the larynges of cadavers to today's sophisticated use of computers and microcircuitry to plot frequency contours.

The mechanism of tone is explained in many texts on basic phonetics. MacKay (1978), for example, explains the relationship of vocal fundamental frequency to intonation. Fundamental frequency is the speed of vibration of the vocal folds. Normal fundamental frequency is dependent upon the age and sex of the individual but, fortunately, is under the control of the speaker and may vary at will within a certain range. This is done by our subtle little adjustments that allow changes in the tension of certain muscles in the laryngeal region. The normal fundamental frequency of the adult male is approximately 125 hertz (Hz) but ranges from about 80 to 200 Hz. Adult females have a fundamental frequency nearly an octave higher at about 225 Hz and a range of from 150 to 300 Hz.

Fundamental frequency is relatively independent of the resonant or formant frequencies of vowel sounds. As MacKay (1978) points out, this means that the fundamental frequency of the voice can be changed without changing the speech sounds themselves. Vocalists are grateful for this phenomenon, since that is exactly what happens during the process of singing. When Pavarotti, Leontyne Price, or Corinne sing the vowel /a/ in a Puccini opera, the phone /a/ stays the same even though the fundamental frequency changes with low, middle, or high notes. The listener hears the same vowel at different musical pitches. These changes in pitch are perceived in spoken words as well as words that are sung, and when sentences or words are spoken in certain patterns of pitch change, linguistic significance is imposed. For example:

"You're finished."

"You're finished?"

These statements have the same speech sounds and words but very different patterns of pitch. These tonal patterns or contours of pitch change are called intonation and are a vital part of speech prosody.

Varieties and, sometimes, subtle shades of meaning are carried by intonation changes. Sometimes, the intonation is as subtle as the hint of tarragon in a salad; sometimes it is as fundamental as lettuce or spinach and alters the nature of the salad entirely. The number of different contours is great, but a few basic types recur.

In declarative sentences, simple statements, the intonation contour is fairly level with a slight rise near the end and a fall at the termination of the utterance:

"Adrienne and Chris are not at home."

Interrogatives, or questions, take the contour of a slight fall near the end followed by a rise at the very end:

"Where is your banana?"

Exclamatory utterances have a pattern similar to declaratives, except that they are usually louder and there is a more severe pitch descent at the end:

"You can't have it!"

In extremely short sentences of only one or two words, the entire intonation pattern seen in longer sentences is retained, but it is usually temporally compressed. For example:

"Jeat chet?" "Uh uh." "Uh huh?" "Uh uh!"
(Did you eat yet?)

If the sentence is relatively long, the phrases, clauses, and other syntactic features may dictate variations in intonation.

"If he doesn't bring the monkey, the organ grinder will have to dance alone."

Lists or enumerated sequences of items have a distinctive intonation pattern. Intonation aids us in separating the individual items of the list and also in concluding that the last item has been named.

"For the party he has to bring champagne, Mexican pastry, sushi, cheese, strawberries, and chocolates."

MacKay comments on how automatic the use of intonation is. He gives the example of how easy it is to discern unnatural intonation in acting or dramatic reading when one is trying to imitate the intonation pattern of a person who is being interrupted. When a person knows that he or she is going to be interrupted, as in acting, it is very easy not to betray that you know by letting the pitch fall just before the interruption. Good actors have mastered the technique of not tipping off the anticipated interruption by a fall in pitch. Sarcasm, irony, and various types of humor are also dependent upon intonation changes.

It is important to emphasize that all of the components of prosody interact. The suprasegmentals of stress, rate, and intonation are constantly used together in speech and combined in appropriate ways to produce the desired linguistic effect. That does not mean, though, that they cannot be understood or dealt with in at least relatively isolated fashion. This is very important for management of the patient with apraxia of speech for, as you will see, we feel that an understanding of fundamental concepts of phonology and manipulation of the suprasegmentals is a powerful tool for the restructuring of disrupted speech.

PHONOLOGIC PROCESS ANALYSIS

Traditionally, speech production errors were analyzed using a rather uncomplicated system. "Articulation" could deviate from usual production in a number of ways, and the strategy of differentiating speech errors was to identify and isolate individually deficient speech sounds, or phones, and describe the manner of their errant ways with the use of such terms as distortion, substitution, omission, addition, and the like.

This system of error analysis and description is still widely used, but some writers are advocating an approach that may have some advantages for both explanation and economy of description. Phonologic process analysis is a method of speech analysis that is influenced by advances in generative linguistics and apparently is preferred by clinical researchers with a strong orientation to linguistics. Some advantages and disadvantages of the system are readily apparent. The disadvantages appear to be that it is strongly rooted in the belief that phonologic speech errors are the result of phonologic rule violation, an assumption that is yet to be demonstrated unequivocally. Another disadvantage, particularly in the analysis of apraxia of speech, is that not all of the error behavior can be accounted for by purely linguistic behavior. Initiation difficulty, restarts, retrials, silent groping of the articulators, and the directional and timing errors that result from inadequate positioning and shaping of the valves and cavities of speech cannot be attributed to phonologic rule violation, and, therefore, much of the aberrant behavior in certain pathologies of speech can be lost to both description and explanation. However, the fact that most speech production in daily living occurs in the context of discourse or connected conversation argues strongly for a system of analysis that incorporates the combinatory phenomenon of speech. Co-articulation and assimilation are two of the many factors that occur in discourse. When speech segments or phones are combined to produce words, phrases, sentences, and eloquent bits of persuasive debate, other combinatory phenomenon are in operation as well. MacKay (1978) explains some of these, and there is no doubt that many of them have been neglected in past analyses of apraxic speech. Some of these follow.

Dissimilation. This is the process of simplifying speech by inserting phonetic contrasts in sequences that contain very similar nonadjacent sounds. Some of us used to conceive of phonetic complexity as being maximal when segmental sequences had markedly different phonetic contrasts. Just the opposite may be true. Difficulty appears to be the result of too many similar sounds too close together. This would explain the difficulty we find in spitting out tongue twisters at a rapid rate, such as "Mrs. Smith's fish sauce shop seldom sells shellfish," or "I slit a sheet; a sheet I slit; upon a slitted sheet I sit."

Inaccurate production of these articulatory obstacle courses can take a variety of forms with both phonetic and social consequences, but one way of characterizing the result is by dissimilation.

Elision. This is the process of leaving out one or several speech sounds during pronunciation. Thus, the edge on the top of a ship or boat is called a "gunnel" although it is spelled "gunwhale." If the novice seaman were to scream "Watch the gun whale!," the captain might think he was attempting to call attention to a huge migratory mammal with a revolver.

Elision can occur in deviant speech as well, and may not be specifically attributed to one given class of segments, but to context.

Epenthesis. This is the addition of a vowel sound, usually to separate a group of consonants, such as saying /filəm/ for "film." The epenthetic vowel has been noted in apraxic speakers and called the "intrusive schwa" (/pəliz/ for "please") by writers such as Johns and Darley (1970) and LaPointe and Johns (1975).

Haplology. This process is similar to elision except that in haplology an entire syllable is left out. "Probably" may become "probly."

Metathesis. This is the process of segmental inversion within a word. Two speech sounds swap places. This phenomenon has been described by LaPointe and Johns (1975) in apraxic speech. When the inversion involves the speech sounds across word boundaries, the term "spoonerism" is usually used.

This lawfulness or system of rule violation that appears to underly at least some of the errors seen in apraxic patients has been commented upon by a number of researchers. Kearns (1980) suggests that phonologic process analysis has been used as a basis for gaining a better theoretical appreciation of the seemingly random errors that result from brain damage. He cites the work of Blumstein (1973), Lecours and Lhermitte (1969), Martin and Rigrodsky (1974a, 1974b), Schnitzer (1971), and others as contributing to our theoretical understanding of phonologic disruption, but he laments the relative lack of clinical application of the strategy. Kearns (1980) presents an example of the application of phonologic process analysis to the speech of a 57-year-old patient who had suffered a single, left-hemisphere cerebrovascular accident.

Kearns cautions that the clinical usefulness of this technique has yet to be established firmly and must await the collection of additional empirical data, but he points out that traditional methods of analysis of his patient would not have revealed across-phoneme error patterns or a number of deletion errors. The treatment implications of application of this system are intriguing.

Phonologic process analysis also has been advocated for the analysis of apraxic speech by Crary and Fokes (1979). They undertook a reanalysis of data previously published and suggested that apraxic speakers systematically simplify their articulatory performance. Considering the disadvantages inherent in formulating conclusions from data gathered by other researchers, the advocacy of Crary and Fokes grows somewhat exuberant (e.g., ". . . the evidence overwhelmingly supports the feasibility and practicality of employing this approach," p. 11).

As Kearns suggests, proponents of phonologic process analysis of children's speech errors use the system because it suggests that treatment would focus on the elimination of processes that are creating error patterns. This would eliminate the need to target single sounds in treatment and instead would focus on processes that affect entire classes of sounds. Hypothetically, if these processes could be altered, training would become more generative and more efficient. In our view, hypotheses of this nature are worth testing.

3

Praxis and Apraxia

"Praxis makes perfect." That paraphrase of the old axiom has more than a grain of meaning in it. First of all, the Greek word "praxis" means action, and a common definition found in medical dictionaries is 1. practice, or 2. the performance of action. (Stedman's, 1966). Praxis, or the performance of action or movement patterns, can go awry in the face of central nervous system damage, and this disruption of movement control can affect a single limb, the whole body, constructional abilities, ocular movements, probably the legs and genitals (although these conceivable disorders are neglected in the clinical literature), or the components of the motor speech system. When a movement cannot be performed accurately on a volitional basis and is not due to muscular weakness, fatigue, or the reduction of range or direction of movement (that is, paralysis or paresis) it is called "apraxia"; when it affects the speech system, systematic practice has been shown to improve it. Hence "praxis makes perfect" is more double-meaning truism than pun.

This chapter will review some aspects of normal volitional movement or praxis; general concepts of motor control and motor skill learning; speech production models and speech motor control; and some of the more common types of apraxia described in the clinical literature.

MOTOR CONTROL

The mechanism and principles involved in how the central nervous system produces coordinated or patterned motor output has been a topic of increasing concern to a variety of researchers interested in motor performance and motor skills. Physicians in sports medicine, neuropsychologists, behavioral neurologists, speech and language researchers, and exercise physiologists who attempt to teach us to use Nautilus equipment without rupture have pooled their talents and energies in a cross-disciplinary assault on the secrets of motor performance. As Stelmach (1976) has suggested, motor control is a relatively new area of study for the behaviorist seeking to understand skilled movement. In other times this area was considered nearly the exclusive domain of the neurophysiologist, but recent efforts succumbed to the inevitability that skill execution cannot be divorced from cognitive factors, memory trace, the internal representation of sensory information, perceptual trace, and other behavioral phenomenon. This realization has demanded that a cross-disciplinary approach be taken. As Kelso and Stelmach (1976) have noted, the orientation in motor behavior has shifted only recently, from a global view of task analysis and product performance to an attempt to understand the processes underlying movement.

As in so many areas, the state of the art is rapidly evolving and permits only a few conclusions about underlying mechanisms, even for the simplest of movements. Typical of this interdisciplinary approach is the collection of works entitled *Motor Control: Issues and Trends* (Stelmach, 1976). This source summarizes work on the central and peripheral mechanisms of motor control, the schema approach to motor learning, spatial location cues and movement production, the structure of motor programs, attention and movement, memory and movement production, and dimensions of motor task complexity. All of these issues, though they are more general and relate to a variety of movement patterns, have relevance to the discrete patterns necessary for speech.

A particularly informative treatment of speech production models as they relate to apraxia of speech is presented by Mlcoch and Noll (1980). They review and present a critique of closed-loop associative-chain models and open-loop preprogramming models of speech production. The closed-loop associative-chain model utilizes information provided by ongoing sensory feedback, whereas the open-loop preprogramming models assume that all information needed to explain production of a speech utterance is planned and specified within the central nervous system prior to actual speech production. As Mlcoch and Noll (1980) point out, each set of models provides convincing arguments, but neither offers adequate proof that any single model can account entirely for the control or facilitation of speech in all possible situations. As with so many areas of understanding, a combination of the principles from both approaches may offer a better explanation. Perhaps in some situations sensory information associated with fine motor control is necessary, while in other instances during which extremely fast speech patterns predominate, preprogramming is essential. This amalgamation of the major speech production models may be more useful in allowing us to analyze and classify the errors produced by individuals who have apraxia of speech.

In another attempt to explain the nature of afferent influences on speech motor coordination and programming, Abbs and Cole (1982) also arrived at the conclusion that both explanatory views may be relevant. They conclude that

1. autogenic or closed-loop feedback processes may not play a significant role in speech motor programming, except during learning or in adaptation to unusual disruptions, and
2. afferent influences are nevertheless very important in speech control and may be acting through open-loop, feed-forward pathways to reduce the coordinative complexity associated with the rigid timing requirements for multiple speech movements and to allow for predictive error correlation in the process of speech production.

Earlier work on speech motor control relied on explanations based on stored motor commands, but as the early work by MacNeilage (1970) pointed out, perfectly intelligible speech can occur with spontaneous reorganization of the movement pattern of the tongue and lips, for example, in the case of a teeth-clenching pipesmoker. MacNeilage suggested that pehaps stored spatial location information was all that was needed to free models of motor speech from being solely dependent upon storage of discrete movement patterns. This approach to the regulation of movement has been supported in more recent work by Russell (1976).

In recent work directly related to an explanation of the apparent difficulties that apraxic speakers have with both positioning of the articulators and response sequencing, Kent and Rosenbek (1983) extend some of the early work on spatial location storage, as well as concepts proposed by Schmidt (1976) on motor schema theory. Kent and Rosenbek (1983) attempt to relate the disruption of speech in apraxia to disintegrations of temporal schemata that aid in the control of movement sequences, and of spatial targets defined by a space coordinate system of the vocal tract. They suggest that the inaccuracies of place of production described in apraxia of speech might be taken to mean either that the speaker's access to the space coordinate system for target speech sounds is impaired, or that the generalized spatio-temporal schema cannot reliably use spatial information in generating response specifications. Initiation errors in the apraxic speaker, they suggest, could reflect a general failure of the schema to specify motor commands given the intended motor responses, the current state of the articulators, or motor experience in meeting similar demands. Kent and Rosenbek also review some of the concepts on apraxia proposed by Roy (1978), including an explanation that would account for several types of apraxic disturbance.

The evidence appears to be mounting that many of the speech errors and nonspeech gropings of the apraxic subject can be explained by models of motor control and programming. The relative influences of syntactic, semantic, and other behavioral variables no doubt will be clarified by continued study.

MOTOR SKILL LEARNING

A wide variety of factors may influence motor skill learning. Not all of the principles generated by research on motor learning and human perform-ance are directly applicable to treatment of the speech apraxic individual, but many of them are easily translatable to our purposes. Singer (1980) has outlined a number of prepractice, practice, and postpractice conclusions which he has drawn from the empirical research on motor skill learning. While some of them may appear as a firm grasp of the obvious and are routinely utilized by practicing clinicians who deal with neurogenic pathologies of communication, others bear review and may be useful guides as we formulate our intervention plans with patients who present disrupted control of speech movements. As Singer indicates (p. 412) moti-vational influences permeate the learning of new skills or the reorganiza-tion or facilitation of these skills. Motivation influences selection of a preference for an activity, persistence, effort, and adequacy of perform-ance relative to a set of standards. Singer identifies four dimensions of motor activities that relate to motivation: complexity, physical demands, appeal, and meaningfulness.

Programs or activities a clinician can manipulate to ensure maximal motivation include systems of rewards and reinforcers, the use of knowl-edge of results of performance, patient involvement in goal setting, and high levels of clinician enthusiasm.

Other principals based on motor skill research that relate directly to task practice or the nature of therapy sessions include the following.

1. Practice sessions should be briefer and distributed over a longer time rather than larger and concentrated in a short time span
2. Massed practice and distributed practice often lead to similar reten-tion performances, but distributed is superior to massed practice in immediate effects
3. Whole practice is favored when tasks are relatively simple or well organized, but part practice is more efficient for complex tasks
4. Mental practice, without any overt motor activity, is more effective in learning a motor skill than no practice at all
5. Emphasis on speed reduces accuracy and emphasis on accuracy reduces speed, and practice performance conditions should simulate

actual performance conditions as much as possible (that is, if speed and accuracy are equally important, both should be emphasized in practice)

6. When a sequence of events comprise an activity, the last and first learned are usually retained best
7. The instructional methods of either drill or problem solving can be equally effective, depending upon training objectives
8. Programmed self-learning encourages independent and individual rates of work
9. Highly prompted learning is expedient when learning a new task, but discovery learning may create better retention and generalization
10. Overlearning a task—that is, beyond criterion—will lead to better retention

Many of these principles of motor learning, which have been elaborated upon and supported by a list of documented studies by Singer (1980), are drawn from the literature related to individuals with a normal nervous system. The learning characteristics of individuals with cortical lesions may vary considerably. Nevertheless, these ideas may guide our intervention and task design and can be put to the test and either confirmed or denied. They deserve to be considered as we formulate the clinical decisions necessary for proper management of the individual with motor speech impairment.

TYPES OF NONVERBAL APRAXIA

The nonverbal apraxias would hold little inherent relevance to communication specialists, other than that they represent a peculiar and puzzling range of disorders, if it were not for the possibility that they represent a neurobehavioral phenomenon that may aid us in understanding the nature of a movement disorder that may well have an analog in speech. Also, some of the nonverbal apraxias are a part of the behavioral sequelae package that accompanies cortical damage and may affect gesture, signing, pointing, or other aspects of motoric behavior.

Nonverbal apraxia is considered to be an impairment of the ability to perform preplanned, volitional purposeful movements in the absence of paralysis or weakness, sensory loss, comprehension deficit, or ataxia. The impairment may be evident as an inability to perform pretended actions, to use common objects, to respond to spoken commands, or to engage in spontaneously generated movement patterns.

The behavior pattern of the person with apraxia is varied, but the nature or quality of the response is important in determining whether or not the impaired movement is apractic. The response varies as follows:

1. the desired response may be absent;
2. the person may produce haphazard, unrelated movements that result in an altered version of the desired response;
3. the appropriate movements of two or more gestures may be combined into a single gesture;
4. the desired response may be accurately completed after several groping false starts.

Goodglass and Kaplan (1963) have labeled and discussed other behavioral characteristics that may be observed in apraxic patients:

Gestural enhancement is embellishment of the desired gesture with additional facial or body movements.

Pantomimed context is the performance of actions that are part of the situation in which the desired gesture is embedded. For example, a patient who is asked to demonstrate "lighting a match" may pantomime opening a package of cigarettes, withdrawing one from the pack, and placing it in his or her mouth.

Body part as object is the use of a part of the body as an object in pretended action such as stirring coffee with an index finger; using a fist as a hammer; or using the leg as a screwdriver.

Liepmann (1905) distinguished three varieties of apraxia: (1) ideational apraxia; (2) ideomotor apraxia; and (3) limb apraxia.

Ideational apraxia, according to Liepmann, is characterized by correctness of individual elements of a complex act without accomplishing the desired objective. The patient fails to apply the elements to a purpose or ideational plan (e.g., patient puts a match into his or her mouth or strokes it on the sole of a bare foot in trying to light a cigarette; or tries to drink from a cup by leaning over or under it). The normal sequence of the overall act may be altered, resulting in inaccurate and sometimes bizarre performance. As the desired action becomes more complex, the disorder appears more severe. An apraxic person may substitute one action for another or omit one or several steps. Imitated actions may be performed in an altered manner or reordered. Perseveration of one action into another is common.

In ideomotor apraxia isolated gestures are impaired, but the overall purpose may be preserved. A patient may have difficulty performing volitional acts with the nonparalyzed hand, although performance of automatic movements with the same hand is not impaired (e.g., a patient cannot wave goodbye with the nonparalyzed hand on command, but does so in response to the examiner's departure). The disorder rarely presents itself during spontaneous activity, and is often detected by tests of verbal command or of imitation. Performance to imitation may be preserved more intactly than that to command.

Associated clinical symptomatology for both ideomotor and ideational apraxia includes aphasia, constructional apraxia, intellectual impairment, sensory disorders, and finger agnosia. Dominant hemispheric posterior parietal and temporoparietal lesions play an important role in the production of ideomotor and ideational apraxia. De Ajuriaguerra, Hecaen, and Angelergues (1960) found ideomotor apraxia to be associated with parietal and temporal lesions, and ideational apraxia with large posterior (parietal, temporoparietal) lesions.

Ideomotor apraxia does not usually accompany ideational apraxia; however, there is considerable disagreement over whether ideational apraxia can occur independent of ideomotor apraxia. Hecaen and Gimeno (1960) reported 8 cases of ideational apraxia in a series of 47 cases of ideomotor apraxia.

Liepmann (1905) and Kleist (1934) proposed that ideational and ideomotor apraxia represent different degrees of severity of the same basic problem. Some authors consider ideational apraxia to be a defect in the handling of objects; others define it as a defect in the performance of serial movement. A defect in the handling of objects also has been considered a severe form of ideomotor apraxia.

Heilman (1973) asserted that ideational apraxia represented a separate disorder. He described three patients who were completely unable to respond to command, unlike patients with ideomotor apraxia who respond to commands with appropriate motions, although with difficulty. These patients performed flawlessly on imitation, unlike patients with ideomotor apraxia who improve slightly with imitation. In making these types of inferences about the existence and relationship of esoteric types of apraxic disturbances, the examiner must carefully control and account for deficits in auditory comprehension and other factors that might confound results. Untidy examination and ignoring or discounting behaviors that fly in the face of pet theories can generate misleading conclusions.

Constructional Apraxia

Kleist (1934) identified a separate variety of apraxia that he named "constructional apraxia." This refers to an impaired ability to perform visuospatial tasks such as drawing, assembling stick designs, and constructing three-dimensional block arrangements, and is uncovered by giving the patient drawing or constructional tasks (using blocks or sticks), by verbal command, or by imitation. Defects of drawings or construction may include simplification of the model; the closing-in phenomenon, in which the drawing or the construction is placed very close to the model; misalignment on the page; and spatial disorientation.

In a study of subjects with verified lesion localizations (Hecaen & Assal, 1970) a significant correlation for constructional apraxia was found with parietal lobe lesions. Split-brain studies have indicated that the right hemisphere plays a dominant role in visuoconstructive activities (Gazzaniga, Bogen & Sperry, 1967; Bogen, 1969; Dimond, 1972).

Warrington, James, and Kinsbourne (1966) studied drawing disabilities in relation to lateralization of the cerebral lesions. They concluded that constructional apraxias following right-hemisphere damage were due to a defect in visuospatial perception. Performance did not improve with learning during the test procedure. The constructional apraxias following left-hemisphere damage were due to a defect in motor executory control, a defect in programming the action. Visual cues and learning improved performance. Visual cues appear to compensate for the deficit by providing a program for the action. These types of findings on facilitory or compensatory routes of accomplishing an action may be relevant to treatment approaches for apraxia of speech.

Constructional apraxias following left-hemisphere lesions are sometimes accompanied by the fluent aphasias, elements of the Gerstmann syndrome, or the entire syndrome (acalculia, agraphia, right −left disorientation, and finger agnosia).

Dressing Apraxia

With dressing apraxia, the semiautomatic motor ability for dressing oneself is lost. The patient handles clothing haphazardly and is unable to organize the gestures necessary to establish the appropriate relationship between his clothes and his body. He may attempt to put a leg through the arm of a T-shirt, put socks on the hands or interchange shirt and pants. A person who appears in public misdressed in this fashion unfortunately will be perceived by some as being at the very least, socially eccentric. In mild cases clothes may eventually be put on properly, although the patient is unable to tie a necktie or shoelaces.

Like constructional apraxia, dressing apraxia is related to the visuospatial difficulties of the nondominant hemisphere. Dressing apraxia frequently occurs as a result of lesions in the parietal and occipital lobes (Hecaen & Assal, 1970). It occurs less frequently than constructional apraxia in a ratio of 1:4.

Oral Apraxia

As with so many of the disturbances associated with volitional movement disorder, oral apraxia is also a condition in search of a consistent label. It has been observed for decades in patients with cerebral damage and has been called oral nonverbal apraxia, buccofacial apraxia, lingual apraxia, and dozens of other names.

The first to comment on it was the British neurologist Hughlings

Jackson in 1878. Jackson did not saddle the condition with a label but, in keeping with his usual cautious nature, carefully described it and attempted to relate it to the obvious speech and language impairment in which it was cloaked. Jackson has been characterized by some writers as not an experimentalist but a clinician. His more than 300 papers include extremely careful and detailed observations of the clinical, pathological, and physiologic aspects of neurologic disease. His essay entitled "Remarks on nonprotrusion of the tongue in some cases of aphasia" was typical (Taylor, 1932). In it, he described a patient of his who was unable to protrude his tongue on command, but was able to move it about spontaneously and freely and was able to lick his lips accurately after eating or drinking. Not only did this report document a puzzling paradox, but it offered some tentative explanations and stimulated a good deal of further research interest.

It remained for Liepmann (1900) to associate defective volitional movement with apraxia, and to define the disturbance as the incapacity to act or move various parts of the body volitionally. To fit the description of apraxia, this incapacity could not be the result of paresis, paralysis, or auditory incomprehension.

The proximity of the characteristics of oral apraxia to the apparent movement disturbance seen in apraxia of speech has proved to be an enticing subject for study. The temptation to draw correlates and formulate causal inferences on the relationship between the two conditions has been strong. Many have been seduced by observing the frequent coexistence of oral apraxia and speech apraxia into a Jacksonian hierarchical inference of dependence. "If the motoric programming of the nonspeech movements of the mouth goes, so does the speech" is a simple way to view it. In reality the relationship probably is not that simple.

Nonverbal apraxia of the oral mechanism has been defined in a number of ways. Eisenson (1954) views apraxia as a defective volitional use of tools, and when those tools are the tongue, lips, and velum, oral apraxia is the result.

De Arjuriaguerra and Tissot (1969) called the condition buccofacial apraxia and defined it as

> A disturbance in carrying out of voluntary swallowing movements; of movements of the tongue toward the chin, the nose, the corners of the mouth; of movements in making clicking sounds; movements in making the apico-dental tsk-tsk; of the voluntary mimicry of laughter, of anger, etc.; and of the action of whistling (p.48).

Geschwind (1965) characterized the condition in the following way:

> The patient usually does most poorly in carrying out facial movements to verbal command. He may simply fail to perform at all or may make an incorrect movement, e.g., he may open the mouth when asked to protrude the

tongue, or blow instead of suck. He may make movements with one of his limbs to carry out the demanded task; thus, he may pretend to stub a match in an ashtray or stamp on it with his feet when asked how he would blow out a match. He may remove imaginary crumbs from his lips with his fingers and not use his tongue even when asked repeatedly to use his tongue; he may even insist that he has always performed this action with his hand. Most interesting of all, the patient may echo the command or produce onomatopoetle responses. Thus, when asked to blow out a match he may say 'blow'; or even 'blow out a match'; or 'puff' (p.613).

Most of the descriptions of oral verbal apraxia list qualitative characteristics of the defective movement. Few simply describe it as a range of motion or strength disturbance, because to do so would lose the essence of the impairment. Instead, the hallmarks appear to be disrupted volitional, elaborative motoric oral motor behavior that spares automatic, over-learned, or reflexive motoric function. The impaired oral movements may be associated or unassociated with the desired target and are frequently random, bizarre, and irrelevant; often with vocal and/or verbal overflow. As Jackson noted, the patient frequently has "power in his muscles and in the centers for coordination of muscle groups" (Taylor, 1932). The condition may coexist with sensory disturbances, gestural disturbances, aphasia, or apraxia of speech, but inferences of interdependence are most likely related to neighborhood lesion affects.

Though oral nonverbal apraxia has been described by authors representing a wide variety of orientations and nationalities (Nathan, 1947; Bay, 1957; Denny-Brown, 1958; Alajoulanine & Lhermitte, 1964; Luria, 1970), only in recent years have systematic studies addressed the condition.

Several key questions have been investigated in these recent studies. Hypotheses have been formulated on the prevalence of oral apraxia in various samples of brain-damaged people; on the relationship of oral apraxia to site of lesion and to types of aphasia; on the underlying mechanisms that might result in the disorder and thereby explain it; and by the existence of qualitative differences or types of oral apraxia.

DeRenzi, Pieczuro, and Vignolo (1966) studied the relationship of oral apraxia to "phonetic-articulatory" impairment and to various aphasia types. They suggested a strong association between impaired nonverbal movements of the mouth and phonemic-articulatory disturbances, but just as importantly, found that these disorders can occur independently. They found that many patients also had a phonemic articulatory problem with no oral apraxia; but found as well four subjects who presented oral apraxia with no impairment in speech. This would lend evidence against a hypothesis that proposed phonemic-articulatory disruption, or apraxia of speech as being a reflection of a more basic apraxic disturbance of nonverbal oral movement.

LaPointe and Wertz (1974), in an article based on the doctoral dissertation of LaPointe (1969), found oral apraxia in 14 of 28 brain-injured subjects who presented articulatory impairment. This apraxic disorder was apparent on both isolated oral motor movements and on tasks of oral motor sequencing. They suggested that the groping, irrelevant responses described by DeRenzi, Pieczuro, and Vignolo (1966) as oral apraxia may be more prevalent than expected and that a need existed for systematic appraisal of its presence and severity in brain-injured patients.

In a study based on a doctoral dissertation by Moore (1975) at the University of Colorado, Moore, Rosenbek and LaPointe (1976) reported on the development of an oral, nonverbal gesture battery. A relatively wide range of error behavior was documented on eight subtests.

These eight subtests ranged from matching the oral gestures depicted in photographs to production of oral gestures in response to demonstration, auditory command, and written description. Subjects displayed a relatively wide range of error behavior, the most frequent of which were semantic substitution (operationally defined as the replacement of the target oral gesture by another discrete oral movement or noise; e.g., puffing the cheeks in response to "open your mouth"); body substitution (replacement of target oral gesture by other body part movement; e.g., one subject kicked his leg when asked to stick out his tongue); verbal substitution (replacement of the target oral gesture with a verbal response); noise substitution (e.g., one subject whistled in response to "pucker your lips"); augmentation (movement or noises produced in addition to the target oral gesture); oral augmentation (oral movements produced in addition to the target); body augmentation (body movements in addition to the target oral gesture); and noise augmentation, (e.g., a sipping noise accompanying a smile to "show me your teeth."

A third category of errors, defined in detail by Moore (1975), included those errors categorized by deficient performance. These included no response, fragmentary execution (omission of any part of the target oral gesture), and distorted execution (any movement judged to be marred by disturbances in range, force, or velocity of movement). The remaining categories included perseveration, groping, delay, self-correction, correct, and unintelligible oral responses (not clasifiable in any of the other categories).

Using this array of subtests, stimulus items, and scoring nuances, Moore (1975) studied the response of ten subjects with aphasia, ten with aphasia and coexisting apraxia of speech, and ten subjects free of neurologic disease. No appreciable differences were observed between the two brain-injured subgroups in this study, but it pointed the way to more systematic appraisal of the conditions and to the future search for how oral apraxia relates to the speech disruption that so often accompanies it.

Other researchers (Poeck & Kerschensteiner, 1975) have looked carefully at the quality of errors on an oral apraxia test and found no distinctive profiles that correspond to aphasia subgroups. Brown (1977) on the other hand, reported two different forms of facial apraxia and suggested that subjects with anterior lesions displayed errors which he called "dyspraxia" (clumsy errors) and subjects with posterior lesions displayed "parapraxia" or errors of movement substitution for a target gesture.

Tasks more akin to speech movements (for example, the multiple sequential oral movement of several articulators) were designed and used by LaPointe (1969) and reported by LaPointe and Wertz (1974). They were the first to report impairment on these oral motor sequencing tasks, and since then a number of researchers have pursued this line of inquiry. Mateer and Kimura (1977) studied simple and multiple, unfamiliar oral movement productions of 13 right- and 23 left-hemisphere-damaged subjects and found that only nonfluent aphasic patients produced lower scores in imitating simple discrete movements. Both fluent and nonfluent aphasic subjects were impaired on multiple, unfamiliar oral movements, though, when their performances were compared with nonaphasic right- and left-hemisphere-damaged subjects. These researchers suggested that this impairment was not related to impaired memory or perceptual deficit, nor by the presence of lingual sensory deficit. Mateer and Kimura suggested that these deficits in reproducing nonverbal oral movements were fundamental to most aphasic impairment, and that at least two systems were responsible for the motor control of speech: one for relatively discrete movements, and one for the transition from one movement to the next in a smooth and orderly fashion. These authors proposed anatomical areas corresponding to such a schema roughly analogous to the anterior and posterior speech zones.

Further evidence for heterogeneous oral apraxia was provided in an article conducted by Japanese researchers and reported in French (Ohigashi et al., 1980). This question has been studied further by Watamori, Itoh, Fukusako, and Sasanama (1981). They point out the difference between simple, isolated oral movements (postural acts) such as touching the upper lip with the tongue or pursing the lips, and the more complex acts of spitting, kissing, whistling, and clicking the tongue. Luria (1970) called these latter acts "symbolic" and suggested that they were more impaired in the brain damaged because of their relationship to the symbolic impairment of aphasia. Watamori et al. (1981), however, looked upon these complex acts not so much as being "symbolic" but as involving much more demanding temporal and spatial coordination. The act of whistling, for example, demands the careful and smoothly coordinated temporal and spatial movements of inhalation, accurate positioning of the tongue and lips, and release of the air stream while monitoring and adjusting the position and movement of the tongue and lips. Johns and LaPointe

(1976) stated that tasks such as "cough," "clear your throat," "blow," and "whistle" were the most likely items on their test to be failed because they demanded careful coordination of the breath stream and/or phonation with oral movement.

Watamori et al. (1981) studied this issue with considerable care, along with several related questions. These researchers attempted to determine the relative incidence of oral apraxia among several subgroups of aphasic subjects who had lesions identified by CT scan. They also studied the error patterns associated with subgroups of aphasia and attempted to correlate the effects of task difference (i.e., "postural" or elemental versus "symbolic" or coordinated tasks) with aphasia subgroup. The subjects included 35 aphasic patients and ten matched controls who were free of neurologic disease.

Watamori et al. confirmed that oral apraxia is commonly seen in subjects with left-hemisphere damage (DeRenzi et al., 1966; LaPointe & Wertz, 1974) and its presence across type of aphasia (Poeck & Kerschensteiner, 1975). Subjects with Broca's aphasia comprised the highest percentage of orally apraxic patients (55%). Error analysis revealed different profiles for anterior subjects ("Broca I" and "Broca II" aphasia; i.e., mild language impairment and coexisting mild-to-severe apraxia of speech, or moderate-to-severe language impairment complicated by apraxia of speech) and for posterior (conduction and Wernicke's aphasia) subjects. When the tasks were analyzed in terms of the nature of the movements (elemental versus coordinated), Watamori et al. reported strikingly different error patterns. The anterior aphasic subjects (both subgroups of Broca's) presented more difficulty with coordinated movements in the verbal as well as the imitative mode. This tendency for coordinated movements to be more impaired in anterior aphasic subjects can be explained by relating it to the findings of Itoh et al. (1979; 1980) that a primary disturbance in apraxia of speech is a disruption in temporal organization among the coordination of different articulators. This is also consistent with the clinical impression of Johns and LaPointe (1976) and the suggestion of Luria (1970) that "symbolic" acts are more susceptible to disruption. The Wernicke's aphasia subgroup showed a clear discrepancy between the two stimulus modes, verbal and imitative. Auditory comprehension deficit was positively correlated with the oral apraxia score in the verbal mode only, thus indicating the influence of auditory comprehension on the accurate execution of movement in the verbal mode. Familiarity seemed to have assisted the performance of the posterior aphasic subjects in executing the required movements of this study, but such familiarity did not appear to improve the anterior aphasic subjects' performance. This also lends credence to the view that the anterior aphasic subjects' difficulty appears to stem from lesions in the premotor area that disrupted the motor programming involved in careful coordination of the temporal sequencing of the movements of several articulators. This careful study has shed a good deal of light on the relationship of oral apraxia to coexisting speech and language impairment. Researchers who follow the lead of Watamori et al. and meticulously control and analyze the subject and task variables related to oral movement disruption can expect fruitful return.

Oral apraxia by itself has little clinical importance. The existence of a disorder that disrupts volitional oral movements such as blowing or licking the lips cannot be expected to engender roars of public outcry or sympathy. The importance of this condition, however, exists in its potential relationship to the much more devastating disorder of the movement sequences necesssary for speech. Suffice it to say that the systems that program and control nonverbal oral movements and that control the complex and delicate sequences necessary for speech may be distinct and separate systems. Unlike what some researchers have assumed (Heilman, 1979) those of us who believe that apraxia of speech exists as a separate entity do not believe so because we feel it is a reflection of a more basic underlying apraxia of the oral mechanism. That belief would be simplistic. Other reasons and rationales abound in the neurolinguistic literature.

Unilateral Limb Apraxias

Liepmann (1900) discussed two types of unilateral left-sided apraxias. The first type, *sympathetic apraxia,* was associated with a right hemiplegia and motor aphasia. Gestures performed by the left arm and leg were severely impaired and were present both to command and on imitation, although there was improvement on imitation. The second type resulted from an anterior callosal lesion that deprived the right motor cortex of verbal commands coming from the left hemisphere. Thus, verbal commands could be carried out by the right hand but not by the left hand. The left hand could imitate gestures of the examiner. The patient with limb apraxia may exhibit difficulty in demonstrating such action as waving goodbye, using a hammer, and flipping a coin.

Hecaen and Gimeno (1960) discussed three forms of unilateral left-sided ideomotor apraxia. The first form was characterized by the absence of spontaneous activity of the left extremities. The second form was characterized by abnormal movements and tonic perseveration. The third form was characterized by normal object manipulation and impairment of activities that required coordination of both hands.

Whole-Body Apraxia

Apraxia of gait is often accompanied by what has been referred to as "trunco-pedal" apraxia, that is, apraxia of whole-body movements, such as lying down, sitting, standing up, or rolling over. Geschwind (1965; 1975) prefers the term frontal gait disturbance to apraxia of gait, since he believes that the gait disorder that follows frontal lesions reflects impairment of motor mechanisms and therefore should not be defined as an apraxia.

Geschwind has stressed the preservation of whole-body movements in apraxic patients. A patient with severe oral apraxia and severe bilateral limb apraxia may carry out whole-body movements such as standing up and turning around with little or no sign of impairment. Geschwind suggested that the corpus callosum is not necessary for the integration of these types of movements and that whole-body movements may be controlled as integrated acts at the level of the brain stem.

Geschwind (1975) proposed that recovery from apraxia is more common than recovery from aphasia. Unlike the aphasias, the nonverbal apraxias are not immediately obvious to the examiner. The failure of many aphasic patients to respond appropriately to commands is sometimes interpreted as a comprehension deficit. The converse is true as well. Careful examination is necessary to avoid misinterpretation and assure accurate identification of the nonverbal apraxias.

Perhaps this review of praxis and apraxia will provide a foundation for better appreciation of the disorder when it affects the finely timed and coordinated movements necessary for speech production. If so, the clinician should be better prepared to understand the condition and understand the patient.

4

Characteristics of Apraxia of Speech

An articulatory disorder resulting from impairment, as a result of brain damage, of the capacity to program the positioning of speech musculature and the sequencing of muscle movements for the volitional production of phonemes. No significant weakness, slowness, or incoordination in reflex and automatic acts. Prosodic alterations may be associated with the articulatory problem, perhaps in compensation for it (Darley, 1969).

Like chickens and eggs, all things have beginnings. For apraxia of speech, contemporary clinical interest probably began with Darley's presentation to the 1969 annual meeting of the American Speech and Hearing Association. And, like the name of that organization, the definition of apraxia of speech has been modified by time. Nevertheless, Darley gave us our contemporary start. He included in his presentation a list of "traditional characteristics." These are listed in Table 1. And, like the definition, the characteristics have been modified as we learn more and more. Today, we know more about apraxia of speech than we did in 1969, and we know that some of what we knew was not correct. Also, because progress can pervert as well as purify, we are less comfortable with that we know. That is good.

Today, we are in our third generation of listing characteristics that typify apraxia of speech. The first was characterized by Darley's (1969) observations drawn from the literature, his clinical experience, the Johns (1968) dissertation, and a soon to be published pivotal paper (Johns & Darley, 1970). The second generation included a rash of activity during a ten-year period when many probed and prodded apraxic patients to verify and expand the early observations. The third (and current) phase has taken patients into the laboratory to look for acoustic and physiologic confirmation or rejection of the earlier results that relied, primarily, on the percep-

Table 1.
Rules We Have Lived By: Traditional Characteristics of
Apraxia of Speech

Phonemic errors are prominent: omissions, substitutions, distortions, additions, repetitions of phonemes.

Some errors appear to be perseverative, others anticipatory.

Errors are seemingly off-target approximations of the desired production made in an effortful groping for the correct position or sequence of positions.

Errors are highly inconsistent.

Errors vary with the complexity of the articulatory adjustment.

Errors increase as words increase in length.

There is a discrepancy between the articulatory accuracy displayed in automatic–reactive speech performance and the inaccuracy displayed in volitional–purposive performances.

Imitative responses are particularly poor.

The speaker is usually aware of his or her errors but is typically unable to anticipate or correct them.

Monitoring of speech in anticipation of errors leads to prosodic disturbances: slowed rate, even stress, even spacing.

Oral apraxia is often, but not always, observed in association with apraxia of speech.

After Darley, 1969.

tion of the observer. This chapter creeps through that chronology in an attempt to accept, reject, or modify what we have learned in the past 13 years.

SOME CAUTIONS

No matter how you look at the apraxic patient's behavior—via acoustic analysis, physiologic instrumentation, or the ear and eye of the clinician— all measures are perceptual. Someone reads the results—after having selected what will be read—and interprets what was seen or heard. No one method is better than another unless better is qualified by a purpose. Next, most of the perceptual studies were done with broad phonetic transcription which tends to collapse errors into the number of bins available. Thus, the most frequent error identified in perceptual studies was an error of substitution. Recent acoustic and physiologic investigations indicate that the prominent error is one of distortion. Apraxic patients seldom use one sound to replace another. Broad transcription did not know that. On broad transcription's perceptual continuum, no sign indicates leaving substitution and entering distortion. Perhaps narrow phonetic transcription would have revealed many of the features that are now being identified by instrumental analysis. Finally, there is always the danger of confusing description with explanation. Such confusion results in academic arguments about the nature of the disorder. For example, some (Bowman et al., 1980; Martin, 1974) have suggested that substitution errors can be described, explained, and predicted by natural process analysis, therefore apraxia of speech is a linguistic disorder. The conclusion is spurious, especially if one considers the recent instrumental evidence that indicates that what we have been calling substitutions are really distortions. Moreover, our purpose in listing the characteristics of apraxia of speech is management—identification and treatment—not argument. Thus, what looks like a distortion on a spectrogram or EMG record may sound like a substitution to the ear. Currently, the instrumental techniques supplement the ear of the clinician; they do not replace it. Careful research can guide and explain but not manage.

What follows may be, in part, fiction, but we believe it is, for the most part, useful fiction to assist appraisal, diagnosis, and focusing treatment. We use what we have until it abuses patients. When it does, we discard it.

RULES WE HAVE LIVED BY

Darley's 1969 model of apraxia of speech was described by the characteristics listed in Table 1. It was known by its prominent phonemic errors—omission, substitutions, distortions, additions, and repetitions. Some of the errors appeared to be perseverative, while some appeared to be anticipatory. When errors were made, they were "in the ballpark," slightly off-target approximations of the desired production. An apraxic patient said "frigerette" for "cigarette," not "didakus." The errors were highly inconsistent. Sometimes the patient was correct, and sometimes incorrect. But even when incorrect, the same error was not always made. This behavior, we believed, differentiated this patient from the more consistent dysarthric patient. Errors varied with the complexity of articulatory adjustment. The more complex adjustment required, the higher the probability of an error. Errors seemed to increase as words increased in length. We saw more errors on "jabber" than on "jab," and if we were feeling particularly malicious, we asked the patient to say "jabbering." We observed more errors in volitional–purposive speech than in automatic–reactive performance. The numerous misarticulations noted in picture description or giving history lessened or vanished when counting, saying the days of the week, or commenting on difficulty: "God damnit, I can't say that." Imitation appeared to create problems. Of course, we loaded our stimuli to be imitated with sounds requiring difficult articulatory adjustments and long words, and we had patients do a lot of imitating. Circular and biased? What is not? We noted that the apraxic patient seemed to be aware of his or her errors, but this awareness did not appear to help in anticipating or correcting the difficulty. Prosody sounded abnormal. The apraxic patient used a slow rate, even stress, and even spacing. We thought this resulted from attempts to monitor speech and compensate for anticipated problems. Finally, when we had patients make nonverbal, oral gestures, many of them had difficulty doing so. Therefore, we concluded that oral, nonverbal apraxia frequently, but not always, coexisted with apraxia of speech.

We knew these patients by their characteristics. And we began to find a lot of them, at least in certain parts of the country. Because we had some rules to live by, we began to do what all clinicians do, or should do: test them. This was done in public, in the literature, because many of our patients were breaking the rules daily in the privacy of our clinics. We began to obtain some conflicting results. Not all of the rules withstood the rigor of empirical tests in group studies; these were like nature. They were careless with individuals within the group. Some patients were sacrificed— their performance submerged in the group mean—to protect, preserve, and promote what we were learning about the disorder. A few conservationists began to report on single cases that questioned the group data. We welcomed both, because without both the future was blank. Thus, we entered the second generation of describing the patient with apraxia of speech.

SECOND GENERATION CHARACTERISTICS

By the middle 1970s sufficient data had been accrued to confirm some of the early observations and to modify or reject others. Darley, Aronson, and Brown (1975) listed eight "behavioral characteristics," nine "factors influencing apraxic speech behavior," and four "factors not influencing apraxic speech behavior." Rosenbek and Wertz (1976) categorized what we knew about the apraxic patient into "articulatory characteristics in apraxia of speech, phonological influences on articulation, nonphonological influences on articulation, prosodic characteristics, and nonarticulatory characteristics." We will discuss these latter groupings and examine how they have withstood the test of time.

Articulatory Characteristics

Table 2 lists ten articulatory characteristics adapted from Rosenbek and Wertz (1976). These are distilled from evidence in the literature and filtered through clinical experience. Some are being refuted by recent acoustic and physiologic studies. We believe that they are useful for patient management, however.

Substitution Errors

When apraxic patients make errors, the most frequent ones are errors of substitution. Most, not all, of the perceptual studies support this belief. Recent acoustic analysis challenges it, however. Instrumentation permits us to see what our ears do not hear. Nevertheless, most researchers

Table 2.
Articulatory Characteristics in Apraxia of Speech

Substitution errors are more frequent than other error types.

Error sounds are more likely to differ from the target by one phonetic dimension than by two, three, or four.

Errors are most likely errors of place, followed by errors of manner, voicing, and oral–nasal.

Voiceless-for-voiced substitutions are more frequent than voiced-for-voiceless substitutions.

Some errors are anticipatory, some perseverative, and some metathetic with anticipatory errors probably predominating.

Errors are more likely on consonant clusters than on singleton consonants.

Apicoalveolar and bilabial sounds are more often correct than sounds produced at other places.

Affricatives and fricatives tend, as classes, to be more often in error than plosives, laterals, nasals, and vowels, although order varies with the position in the utterance.

Consonant errors are more likely than vowel errors; however, some patients may make no more consonant errors than vowel errors.

Many substitutions appear to be of more "difficult" combinations for "easier" ones.

Adapted from Rosenbek and Wertz, 1976.

(Shankweiler & Harris, 1966; Johns & Darley, 1970; Sasanuma, 1971; Trost & Canter, 1974; LaPointe & Johns, 1975; Klich et al., 1979) identified more substitution errors in their patients than errors of distortion, addition, repetition, and omission. All used broad (IPA) phonetic transcription. Also, Shankweiler and Harris (1966) cautioned that "broad transcription admittedly ignores features of speech which may have real importance for a physiological understanding" (p. 283), but they suggested "it has the virtue of allowing the features to stand in bold relief."

Substitution errors abounded in these reports—91% in Sasanuma's (1971) patient, 61% in the Klich et al. (1979) sample, 67% in Trost and Canter's (1974) patients, and 32% in the Johns and Darley (1970) sample. Only Square et al. (1982) question the earlier results. Their sample of "pure apractic" patients—no significant coexisting aphasia—showed more distortion errors than substitution errors, and the major problem appeared to be in "initialization and transitionalization."

While most of the reports on substitution errors focused on consonants, Lebrun et al. (1973) gave special attention to vowels. They observed that vowels were never substituted for consonants or vice versa in their two patients, and back vowels were never replaced by front vowels or the converse.

Do apraxic patients make more substitution errors than other types of errors? Probably, if one listens and uses broad transcription to jot down what one hears. Probably not, if instrumental analysis or narrow transcription is used. The latter approach is good for the theory, and the former assists in management.

Phonetic Dimensions

Several investigations have analyzed errors according to how they differ in phonetic dimensions—place, manner, voicing, oral−nasal—from the target sound. Compared with the agreement obtained among reports on substitution errors, these data lose their syzygy. Reports range from Trost and Canter's (1974) conclusion that "Errors are close approximations to their target sounds" (p. 76) to Shankweiler and Harris' (1966) observation that there is "An apparent unrelatedness of many of the substituted sounds to their targets" (p. 289). One-third of the errors they observed, the largest category, were unrelated substitutions and omissions. Let us examine this discrepancy.

Probably the most exhaustive analysis of phonetic dimensions is found in Trost and Canter's (1974) report. They analyzed four dimensions: place, manner, voicing, and oral−nasal. Errors of place were indicated by substitution of a sound for another produced at a different place; for example, substitution of a /t/ for a /p/. An error of manner crossed classes; for example, substitution of a stop for a fricative. Six classes—stops, affricates, fricatives, laterals, glides, and vowels—were analyzed. Voicing errors compared substitution of a voiced sound for a voiceless sound (e.g., /d/ for /t/) or vice versa (e.g., /t/ for /d/). The oral –nasal analysis also looked in both directions; substitution of an oral sound for a nasal, for example, /d/ for /n/, or a nasal for an oral, /m/ for /b/. Thus, errors could differ from the target by from one to four phonetic dimensions. For example:

/t/ for /p/ = error of place, one dimension
/f/ for /k/ = error of place and manner, two dimensions
/v/ for /t/ = error of place, manner, and voicing, three dimensions
/h/ for /m/ = error of place, manner, voicing, and oral –nasal, four dimensions

In addition, Trost and Canter constructed scales to determine the degree of place and manner errors. These are shown in Figure 1. For place errors, they used a scale that ranged from bilabial through dental, alveolar, palatal, velar, and glottal. This indicated the "distance" an error was from its target. For example, if the target was the bilabial /p/, substitution of the alveolar /t/ would be off 2 degrees in place; substitution of the palatal /k/ would be off 3 degrees; and so on. Similarly, the manner scale utilized a range of oral, articulatory constriction. It ran from complete constriction in plosives through affricate, fricative, lateral, glide, and vowel. Substitution of a fricative /s/ for a plosive /p/ would be off 2 degrees in manner, and substitution of a vowel /u/ for /p/ would be off 5 degrees in manner.

Trost and Canter's results indicate that over half of the errors their patients made were one-dimension errors, and 88% were limited to one- or two-dimension errors. Errors of place were most common, 61%, followed by manner errors, 53%, voicing errors, 36%, and oral –nasal errors, 6%. The percentages add up to more than 100% because some errors included more than one feature, e.g., /f/ substituted for /p/ would be two errors, one of place and one of manner. Analysis of place errors on the scale shown in Figure 1 indicated that errors were close approximations to the targets. More than half were off by only 1 degree, and an additional third were off by only 2 degrees. The manner analysis indicated less systematic data. Approximately half of the errors were off by 2 degrees, and an additional third were off by only 1 degree. They observed few errors that were off by 3 or more degrees.

Other reports on phonetic feature errors show errors made by apraxic patients vary more widely from target sounds. Shankweiler and Harris (1966) observed minimal order in substitution errors. While manner errors were slightly more common than place errors, many of the errors observed bore little resemblance to their targets. LaPointe and Johns (1975) found 38% of their patients' errors were off by two features. While place was the most frequent error, 30%, followed by voicing errors, 26%, combined place and manner errors constituted 20% of the total; place, manner, and voicing

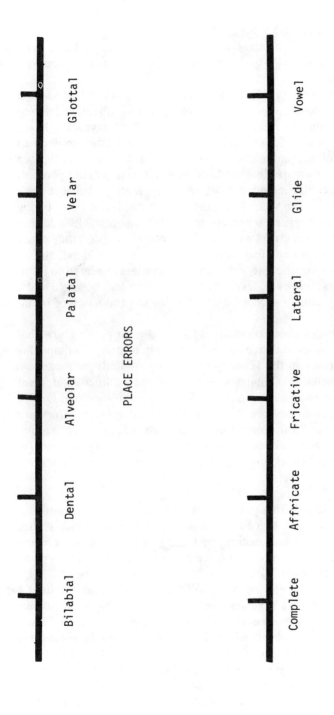

Figure 1. Scales for rating place and manner errors. Place substitutions are rated in the number of degrees the substitution is from the target sound, e.g., a /t/ for /p/ substitution is off 2 degrees. Manner errors are rated on amount of oral articulatory constriction from complete to open, e.g., an /s/ for /p/ substitution would be off 2 degrees. (Adapted from Trost & Canter, 1974.)

contributed 12%; place and voicing, 4%; and manner and voicing, 2%. Manner-only errors, 6%, brought the total to 100%. They agree with Shankweiler and Harris (1966) that many errors have little in common with what was intended.

Finally, Sands et al. (1978) have reported how phonetic dimension errors may change over time. They followed one of Shankweiler and Harris' (1966) patients and compared errors made after ten years of living apraxic with those made close to onset. The early evaluation showed an equal number of voicing and manner errors, 37% each, followed by place errors, 31%; omission errors, 18%; and addition errors, less than 1 percent. Apparently, some errors included more than one feature, because they total more than 100%. Ten years later, the patient displayed 34% voicing errors, 9 percent place errors, 9 percent manner errors, and 34% addition errors. Ten percent of the errors were labelled "other" because they could not be analyzed into phonetic features. Total errors were reduced, and all but additions shrunk significantly. The voicing problem appeared to influence addition errors, however. Over the years, the patient began to add a voiceless fricative, usually perceived as /s/, prior to production of initial sounds.

What do we know about phonetic dimension errors? We know that they are variable. Their incidence varies from study to study. Perhaps this results from variability in the severity of patients studied; perhaps from variability in the methods of analysis. A general, but qualified, statement may be that apraxic patients are in the ballpark, most of the time. One or two phonetic feature errors predominate. Place and manner errors are common. But be ready for the patient or patients who run contrary to most. They have not read the literature, nor has their disorder. They may also sample the phonetic dimensions and provide a smorgasbord of features.

Voiced –Voiceless Errors

Analyses of voicing errors yield one of three results: voiceless consonants are substituted for voiced consonants, voiced consonants are substituted for voiceless consonants, or there is no difference between substitution of one for the other. The literature shows that each type of observation has been made.

Most examinations of voicing errors indicate that the apraxic patient's tendency is to substitute a voiceless consonant for a voiced consonant (Trost & Canter, 1974; Clouzet et al., 1976; Nespoulous et al., 1981). Two-thirds of the voicing errors observed by Trost and Canter involved substitution of a voiceless consonant for a voiced one. However, four of their ten patients made no voicing errors. Clouzet et al. also observed frequent devoicing of voiced consonants. Nespoulous et al., reporting the same observation, commented that when a voiceless target was missed, the error was a voiceless sound produced in another place, e.g., /p/ replaced by /t/.

LaPointe and Johns (1976) found no differences in the direction of voicing errors—voiceless for voiced or vice versa. Similarly, the Sands et al. (1978) patient, followed for ten years, made numerous voicing errors, but both evaluations, early and late, showed no marked difference in the direction of these errors.

Shankweiler and Harris' (1966) results indicate more voiced substitutions for voiceless targets than the reverse. They observed a tendency for their patients to substitute one of three voiced consonants—/b/, /d/, or /g/—for almost every other sound in the inventory.

DeRenzi et al. (1966) apparently join the voiceless-for-voiced group, because they comment, "It is hard to decide if the substitution of voiced consonantal sounds (e.g., b, v, g) by the corresponding voiceless consonants (p, f, k respectively) is due to wrong choice of phonemes (perhaps as a consequence of auditory discrimination defects, . . .) or to lack of synergy of the vocal cords with the muscles of articulation" (p. 55).

We expect apraxic patients to make more substitutions of voiceless consonants for voiced ones rather than the opposite. However, if the patients violate that expectation—show no difference or substitute more voiced consonants for voiceless ones—we do not attempt to convince them that they are wrong, nor do we seriously question our diagnoses.

Anticipatory, Perseverative, and Metathetic Errors

When we were learning to read, we learned that when two vowels went walking the first did the talking and said its name. We were introduced to sound sequences and relationships. When we became students of speech pathology, we experienced how these sequences had to be attended to, usually when we said "larnyx" for "larynx" in Introduction to Anatomy. Some (Lecours & Lhermitte, 1969; Darley, 1969; Johns & Darley, 1970) suggest that sequencing is a particular problem for the apraxic patient. Others have investigated to see if this is so.

LaPointe and Johns (1975) examined three types of sequential errors: anticipatory or prepositioning, where a phoneme is replaced by one that occurs later in the word, e.g., "lelo" for "yellow"; reiterative or postpositioning, where a phoneme is replaced by one that occurs earlier in the word, e.g., "dred" for "dress"; and metathesis, where phonemes switch positions in the word, e.g., "tefalone" for "telephone." All of their subjects produced some sequential errors, but the percent of sequential errors relative to other error types was small. Metathetic errors were just this side of nonexistence: 2 of 13 patients displayed 1 or 3 metathetic errors. Anticipatory errors outnumbered reiterative errors 6 to 1. Every patient made at least one anticipatory error, but only 7 of 13 patients made reiterative errors, and the most for any patient was 3. LaPointe and Johns concluded that sequential errors do exist in apraxia of speech, but they account for a very small percentage of the total errors patients make.

Trost and Canter (1974) also noted a paucity of metathetic errors, 2.8%, in their sample of apraxic patients. Conversely, Sasanuma (1971) reported a patient who displayed 71% metathetic, backward assimilation, or forward assimilation errors. Only 20% of this patient's errors were random substitutions, and 9% were either additions, omissions, or repetitions.

Thus, we expect at least some patients to display anticipatory, perseverative, and metathetic errors. We also expect most of these to be anticipatory. We do not expect these types of errors to abound.

Consonant Errors

Investigators have observed that some words are hard for apraxic patients to say and some words are easy. One thing that contributes to the difficulty appears to be the kinds of sounds contained in the words and how these sounds are combined.

Almost everyone (Darley, 1982; LaPointe & Johns, 1975; Trost & Canter, 1974; Johns & Darley, 1970; Shankweiler & Harris, 1966) agrees that consonant clusters evoke more errors in apraxia of speech patients than singleton consonants. Also, clusters appear to be more difficult in the initial position than in the final position. Certain singleton consonants—affricatives and fricatives—are more difficult than others (plosives, laterals, and nasals); however, difficulty may vary depending upon where consonants reside in the utterance. Certain geographical destinations in the mouth—apicoalveolar and bilabial—are also easier to reach than others.

Table 3 shows the order of difficulty for selected sounds in several investigations. Because stimuli differed, so do results. Nevertheless, clusters are particularly difficult and so are affricatives and fricatives. Plosives, laterals, and nasals are generally easier. Position of the cluster or sound in the utterance has an influence; for example, Shankweiler and Harris observed 75% errors on /Ɵ/ in the initial position but only 62% errors on /Ɵ/ in the final position. Similarly, Trost and Canter report performance on /d/ and /b/ was much better in the initial position than in the final position, and the reverse was seen for /ʃ/, /v/, /tʃ/, /t/, /r/, and /n/.

LaPointe and Johns (1975) ordered the probability of errors according to the place of articulation. Most difficult for their sample of apraxic patients were linguapalatal sounds followed by linguadental, linguavelar, labiodental, glottal, lingua alveolar, and bilabial.

Thus, we expect more errors on clusters than on singletons, and we expect more errors on affricatives and fricatives than on plosives, laterals, and nasals. Sounds produced on the lips or with the tongue tip behind the upper teeth usually are more error-free than sounds produced at other

Table 3.
Order of Difficulty of Selected Sounds for
Apraxia of Speech Patients

Order	Shankweiler and Harris (1966)	Johns and Darley (1970)	Trost and Canter (1974)*	Dunlap and Marquardt (1977)*
D	pl	kl	j	v
I	θ	sl	θ	z
F	kl	spl	dʒ	ʃ
F	sm	skr	ŋ	tʃ
I	z	θ	ʃ	dʒ
C	v	v	v	θ
L	tʃ	l	d	
T	dʒ	dʒ	g	
		z	w	
		ʃ	b	
E	Not	n	m	t
A	Reported	m	n	d
S		k	p	b
Y		b	l	k
		w	r	p
		d	k	n
		h	h	

*Did not report data for clusters.

places. We are not surprised when a given sound is correct in one position in a word but incorrect in another. And we do not wax sore, or even well, amazed when individual patients violate our expectations.

Consonant versus Vowel Errors

Missing from the above discussion was where vowels reside in the hierarchy of difficulty for the apraxic patient. Most (Darley, 1982; Keller, 1978; Clouzet et al., 1976; LaPointe & Johns, 1975; Trost & Canter, 1974; Shankweiler & Harris, 1966) observed more errors on consonants than on vowels. This appears true for groups of patients, but individuals sometimes do not play the game. Vowel errors accounted for only 14% of the total errors LaPointe and Johns observed. However, 1 of their 13 patients made as many vowel errors as he did consonant errors, and 2 patients in their sample made more vowel errors than singleton consonant errors. Similarly, Trost and Canter noted that eight of their ten patients had no difficulty with vowels, but 2 had marked problems. While there was no instance of vowel error being the only error in a monosyllabic word, sometimes the vowel nucleus was distorted, usually by the difficulty patients experienced with the surrounding consonants.

Shankweiler and Harris wondered why their patients had so little difficulty with vowels. They speculated that listeners may be more tolerant with vowels than they are with consonants, and variety in vowel production may be influenced by the speaker's geographic and social environment. Only one of their patients had marked difficulty with vowels, making as many errors as he did on singleton consonants.

Keller (1978) did a detailed analysis of vowel errors in Broca's aphasia patients.He agrees that vowel errors are rare, and he studied only those patients who demonstrated difficulty in producing vowels. Even with this selection criterion, it took 35 hours of tape-recorded samples to obtain 900 vowel errors in 5 patients. Errors were classified as either syntagmatic errors, resulting from the phonological environment and the influence of surrounding sounds, or paradigmatic, not influenced by phonologic environment. Keller's results indicated significantly more paradigmatic errors, 83%, than syntagmatic errors, 17%. This questions Trost and Canter's assumption that vowel errors result from the difficulty of surrounding sounds. His markedness analysis—unmarked = sounds common in the world's languages, learned first, and most resistant to aphasia; marked = uncommon in the world's languages, learned last, and most disrupted by aphasia—revealed no significant differences between marked and unmarked vowel errors. He did note a significant tendency for his patients to substitute low vowels for those produced higher in the mouth.

What we can conclude about consonant versus vowel errors is essentially what is listed in Table 2. Consonant errors are more likely than vowel errors; however some patients may make no more consonant errors than vowel errors. In fact, a rare patient (Lebrun et al., 1973) may make a few more errors on vowels than on consonants.

Phonetic Disintegration

We state in Table 2 that many of the apraxia of speech patient's substitutions appear to be more "difficult" combinations for "easier" ones. Most (Johns & Darley, 1970; Shankweiler & Harris, 1966) agree, but some (Klich et al., 1979) do not. The question has relevance for nosology—is "phonetic disintegration" an appropriate term?—and for theory—is Jakobson's (1961) regression hypothesis (that the loss of speech in a brain-injured adult is the reverse of its acquisition in a child) correct?

Shankweiler and Harris (1966) and DeRenzi et al. (1966) use the term *phonetic disintegration,* but both observed that their patients sometimes uttered difficult strings of consonant clusters as substitutes for intended, easier targets. Thus,there was not a general tendency to simplify by replacing more difficult articulations with easier ones. Furthermore Shankweiler and Harris observed that some of their patients had difficulty with some of the sounds that are difficult for young children, "but there is little reason to assume their difficulty has the same basis" (p. 289).

Johns and Darley (1970) reject the term phonetic disintegration, again, based on their evidence that apraxic patients at times substitute more difficult consonant clusters for easier targets. However, Klich et al. (1979) reported that their patients "systematically reduce linguistic complexity and simplify the production of consonants" (p. 469). They concluded that the substitutions made in apraxia of speech are similar to those made by children.

Our experience indicates that apraxic patients may display a variety of behaviors. Sometimes they substitute more difficult combinations for easier targets, and sometimes they simplify intended productions by uttering easier substitutions or by omitting. Some patients make errors on sounds that are tough for young children, some do not, and some do some of the time but not all of the time. Thus, the sum of the somes does not permit us to support, if we were interested in doing so, the use of the term phonetic disintegration or the validity of the regression hypothesis.

Phonologic Influences on Articulation

Although someone may quarrel with the adjective, we have listed in Table 4 several phonologic influences on articulation by the patient who suffers from apraxia of speech. These include the influence of where the

Table 4.
Phonologic Influences on Articulation in Apraxia of Speech

Initial, medial, and final positions in a word may or may not have an influence on speech sound integrity.

Frequently occurring sounds are more likely to be correct than are infrequently occurring ones.

Articulatory accuracy is better for meaningful than for nonmeaningful utterances.

Errors increase as words increase in length, but this increase is not linear.

Errors increase as the distance between successive points of articulation increases.

Grammatical class, especially when combined with difficult initial phonemes, longer words, and an early position in the utterance, influences the probability of an error.

Adapted from Rosenbek and Wertz, 1976.

sound resides in the word, the frequency of occurrence a sound has in the language, the meaningfulness of the utterance, the length of the word to be uttered, the distance articulators have to travel to produce the next sound in the utterance, and the grammatical class of the word to be uttered. Each influence has a home in the literature, and each has been filtered through our experience with patients. We take time with them because, like the other characteristics, how they are manipulated in appraisal and treatment may influence a patient's probability of success or failure.

Sound Position in Words

Darley (1982) summarized data (Shankweiler & Harris, 1966; Hecaen, 1972a; Trost & Canter, 1974) that indicate that initial sounds in words are more difficult than final sounds. His review shows that this position on position is not unanimous. For example, Johns and Darley (1970), LaPointe and Johns (1975), and Dunlop and Marquardt (1977) found no significant influence exerted by a sound's position in the word to be uttered.

Like most group results, individual patients get lost in general statements about group performance. Trost and Canter (1974) observed more initial errors than final errors, and they found no significant correlation between the two in their sample. Shankweiler and Harris (1966) note a similar result for four of their five patients. However, the Shankweiler et al. (1968) electromyographic investigation also includes a comment on the influence of position in two patients. One made more initial than final errors; the other showed no differences. Johns and Darley (1970) found no significant effect of sound position on the probability of errors; nor did Dunlop and Marquardt (1977). Six of ten patients in the latter study made more final than initial errors; four showed the reverse. LaPointe and Johns (1975) expanded the search to include the influence of the medial position. They report no significant influence exerted by any of the three positions.

We conclude, here and in Table 4, that the position of the sound in a word may or may not have an influence on whether or not it will be produced accurately. As will be seen later when we discuss appraisal and treatment, we believe the influence of position should be probed in individual patients. We are looking for arable treatment targets, and we believe the patient who blows the first sound in "garter" but can say "August" with ease has something to tell us.

Frequency of Occurrence

Trost and Canter (1974) compared their patients' errors with Dewey's data (reported in Fletcher, 1953) on the frequency phonemes occur in the language. Correlations between the difficulty their patients experienced on specific sounds and the frequency these sounds occur in the language were

significant for both initial and final word positions. While other investigations did not make similar comparisons, the similarity of errors between
these and those observed by Trost and Canter lend additional support to
the influence frequency of occurrence has on correct production.

This relationship is fortunate for the apraxic patient because typically,
fewer errors are made on /t/, /n/, and /r/, frequently occurring sounds
(Wood, 1949), and more errors on /j/, /Θ/, and /dʒ/, infrequently occurring
sounds, the overall accuracy is better than it would be if spoken English did
not give him or her a leg up. Patients suffering apraxia of speech are like
most of us; they need all the help they can get.

Meaning and Nonsense

Is it easier for an apraxic patient to say "shed" or "sheb"? Who
cares? Certainly, not everyone. What difference does it make? Some.
Because of constraints in the language that do not permit every sound to
exist in every position in real words, we might go hunting for apraxia of
speech with weird weapons, nonsense words. We also need to know
whether our weapons may have an influence on what we bag. Most of us
want to get some mileage out of the hours we spent in phonetics classes.
What we learned permits us to manipulate sounds skillfully and create all
kinds of combinations. However, these may not make any sense,
especially to apraxic patients. Does nonsense influence their behavior?

Johns and Darley (1970) report that their apraxic patients were significantly better at identifying real words on an auditory–visual perceptual
task than they were in identifying nonsense words. In addition, these
patients made significantly fewer errors repeating real words than they did
nonsense words. Thus, meaning appears to influence accuracy in both
perception and production.

Again, what difference does it make? Perhaps the only difference is
caution. If we load our appraisal and treatment stimuli as some do (Dabul &
Bollier, 1976) with nonsense words, we may evoke more errors than we
would if we used real words. We lean toward the use of real words
whenever possible. However, if we cannot find the sound we want to
appraise in a particular position in a real word, or if we need a few more
treatment stimuli and we have exhausted the supply of real words, we will
make up what we need. We need to remind ourselves of what we are doing,
and remember that it may have an influence on our patient's performance.

Word Length

Shankweiler and Harris (1966) observed that apraxic patients have
difficulty in producing connected speech that is not revealed when producing monosyllables in isolation. Nespoulous et al. (1981) report that their
patients made more errors on multisyllabic words than they did on mono-

syllabic words. Johns and Darley (1970) found apraxic errors increased as words increased in length.

Thus, the longer the word, the greater probability of an apraxic patient making an error. For example, "jab" may be more error-free than "jabber" or "jabbering." We caution that the increase in errors is not linear. And, Johns and Darley (1970) point out that the error in a longer word will occur in the syllable common to all words, e.g., /dʒ/ or /b/ goes awry in "jabber" and "jabbering," not /ɚ/ or /ŋ/.

Articulatory Distance

The longer the trip, the more chance of getting lost. It is easier to go from Madison to Verona than from Madison to Albert Lea. One never attempts to get to Ordway from a distance greater than Sugar City. Similarly, the apraxic patient finds that the further his articulators have to travel from one sound to another, the greater the probability of getting lost.

Trost and Canter (1974) tell us place errors are common. Tongues do not always get to where they were going. Rosenbek et al. (1973a) showed that the series /pʌ, tʌ, kʌ/ was more difficult for their patients than /pʌ, pʌ, pʌ/ or /tʌ, tʌ, tʌ/ or /kʌ, kʌ, kʌ/. While this may support the notion that sequencing is tough for apraxic patients, it also suggests that it is a shorter trip back to /p/ or /t/ or /k/ than it is to a position different from where one started.

We therefore suggest that errors will increase as the distance between successive points of articulation increases. Our patients usually support this assumption by making more errors on "school" than they do on "stool."

Grammatical Class

Grammar resides in the curriculum from the first grade through high school. One of us took a remedial course as a graduate student. Grammar may influence the probability of an error in apraxic patients. However, the data are not consistent.

Dunlop and Marquardt (1977) found no influence of grammatical class—noun, verb, adjective—on errors in their apraxic patients. Deal and Darley (1972) obtained similar results when they manipulated nouns, verbs, adjectives, and adverbs, but when they combined grammatical class with one or more other influences, errors increased. By systematically manipulating grammatical class in combination with either the difficulty of the initial phoneme (affricative, fricative, or consonant cluster), the position of the word in the sentence (one of the first three words), or the length of the word (more than five letters long), errors increased. Combinations of grammatical class and the difficulty of the initial sound and grammatical class and word length were particularly potent in evoking errors.

Nonphonologic Influences on Articulation

Several nonphonologic variables may influence the apraxia of speech patient's probability of success. These are listed in Table 5. They include automatic—reactive versus volitional—purposive speech, stimulus modality, imitative versus spontaneous accuracy, consecutive attempts, motivating instructions, monitoring performance in a mirror, delaying response, binaural masking, and delayed auditory feedback.

Automatic versus Volitional Speech

Darley (1969), as noted in Table 1, suggested that automatic—reactive productions are more error-free in the speech of apraxic patients than volitional—purposive productions. He repeated his belief more recently (Darley, 1982). The Johns and Darley (1970) report contains a similar observation. In addition, Schuell et al. (1964) contend that words and

Table 5.
Nonphonologic Influences on Articulation in
Apraxia of Speech

Within narrow limits, articulatory accuracy is better for automatic—reactive than for volitional—purposive speech.

Articulatory accuracy may be better with auditory—visual stimulation than with auditory or visual (reading) alone.

Watching verbal production in a mirror has no effect on the accuracy of single word production.

Imitative accuracy, unless influenced by the test stimuli, is better than spontaneous accuracy.

Some patients improve if given more than one consecutive attempt at a production.

Motivating instructions, within very narrow limits, have no influence on articulatory accuracy.

Response delay intervals of 0, 3, and 6 seconds do not significantly influence articulatory accuracy.

Binaural masking probably has no facilitating effect on articulation for most patients.

Delayed auditory feedback (DAF) may have a detrimental effect on articulatory accuracy.

Adapted from Rosenbek and Wertz, 1976.

phrases that are highly organized by practice tend to sound more normal than those less practiced.

We have observed that most, not all, of our patients make fewer errors counting, saying the days of the week, and inserting profanity or comments—''I can't say that.''—than they do when conversing, repeating, naming, or describing pictures. However, we do not worry if their performance does not differ or differs only a little between automatic — reactive and volitional — purposive speech. Furthermore, one might argue that this characteristic belongs under phonologic influences. Perhaps it does.

Stimulus Mode

How stimuli are presented to apraxic patients may influence their probability of success, but the data are not consistent. Johns and Darley (1970) report that auditory — visual stimuli (hearing and seeing the clinician produce a word to be repeated) results in better performance than do only auditory (hearing the word) or visual (reading the word) stimuli. Nespoulous et al. (1981) report similar results. Their patients were better at repeating words heard than they were at reading words aloud. Webb and Love (1974), studying the influence of different cues on verbal accuracy by apraxic patients, lend additional support. They observed that whole-word imitation was a better cue than reading.

LaPointe and Horner (1976) studied four stimulus modes, and their results challenge the belief that auditory — visual stimulation results in the best production. Auditory stimulation alone resulted in significantly better production than the other three stimulus modes (auditory and visual, reading, or auditory and reading). In fact, the auditory — visual (watching the clinician) mode resulted in the poorest performance by their patients.

Another type of cue, monitoring one's performance in a mirror, was examined by Deal and Darley (1972). Visual monitoring had no influence on response accuracy. They concluded that their patients were unable to use the information obtained from the mirror, at least without instructions about how or why this information may assist verbal performance.

We believe apraxia of speech patients should be permitted to show the clinician how stimulus modes influence verbal performance. Some appear to profit from combined modes, some do not. Some read stimuli aloud better than they repeat them. We observe, and we let the patients tell us by their performance what helps and what hinders.

Imitation versus Spontaneous Speech

Imitation was believed to be more difficult for apraxic patients than spontaneous speech (Darley, 1969; Johns & Darley, 1970). We had apraxic patients do a lot of imitating, and we loaded the stimuli with sounds that were particularly difficult for our patients to say. However, Trost and Canter (1974) observed that even though their sample displayed a significant correlation between imitative and spontaneous speech (naming), repetition accuracy was significantly better than spontaneous accuracy. Similarly, as noted earlier, Shankweiler and Harris (1966) commented that their patients produced errors in spontaneous speech that were not revealed by having them repeat monosyllables.

Our experience indicates that imitation, unless we influence performance with the stimuli to be repeated, is, generally, better than spontaneous speech. The presence and severity of coexisting aphasia as well as the patient's avoidance of sounds and combinations of sounds that are difficult can, of course, influence comparisons of imitation and spontaneous accuracy.

Repeated Trials

Johns and Darley (1970) report that their patients' performance improved if they were permitted to make several attempts to repeat a stimulus. Repeated production resulted in more accurate speech than repeated stimulus presentations and only one opportunity to produce what was heard. LaPointe and Horner (1976) tested Johns and Darley's observation. Seven apraxic patients were tested in two conditions: one stimulus presentation followed by ten responses versus one stimulation followed by one response. They found no significant differences between accuracy in the two conditions. Four patients ranged from 2% to 7% better on repeated trials, and three patients ranged from 1% to 8% better in the single-response condition. Response variability in the repeated response condition ranged from 23% to 51% when responses were compared to the previous response. While there was a trend toward deterioration of the response in the repeated trial condition, it was not significant.

Warren (1977), in a similar study, compared an immediate imitation condition with one where apraxic patients were permitted to rehearse responses during controlled retention intervals of 5, 15, 30, and 60 seconds. Results varied among his five patients. Two showed no differences between accuracy in the immediate and rehearsal conditions, one was better in the rehearsal condition, and two were better in the immediate condition.

We conclude from the above results and our experience that some patients do improve accuracy if given more than one consecutive attempt to produce a stimulus, and some never reach accuracy no matter how many attempts they make. Of course, what a clinician tells a patient before, during, and after repeated trials may influence the patient's responses. We discuss this later in the treatment chapters.

Motivating Instructions

Stoicheff (1960) demonstrated that a clinician's motivating instructions can influence language performance by aphasic patients. Deal and

Darley (1972) tested the influence of motivating instructions on verbal performance by patients suffering apraxia of speech. Three sets of instructions were used: *positive* (patients were told the stimuli to be read contained easy sounds and words and would be easy to read), *negative* (patients were told the stimuli to be read contained difficult sounds and words and would be difficult to read), and *neutral* (patients were told the difficulty of the material to be read was unknown). Results indicated that the instructions had no influence on oral reading by apraxic subjects.

Therefore, within the limits imposed by the Deal and Darley investigation, we conclude that motivating instructions have no influence on articulatory accuracy in patients suffering apraxia of speech.

Response Delay

Some apraxic patients display obvious latency between the presentation of a stimulus and the repetition of it (Schuell et al., 1964; Johns & Darley, 1970; Trost, 1970). Some treatments for apraxia of speech incorporate a delay between stimulus and response as a step or steps in the treatment hierarchy (Rosenbek et al., 1973a). Deal and Darley (1972) tested the influence of enforced delay on response accuracy. Three intervals were used—zero, no delay between stimulus and response; 3-second delay; and 6-second delay. No significant differences in response accuracy among delay intervals were observed.

Warren's (1977) rehearsal study also incorporated delays into the rehearsal condition. Patients were instructed to respond after 0, 5, 15, 30, and 60 seconds. He found no significant effect of delay on response accuracy. Even when instructed to use the delay interval to rehearse production of the stimulus, as suggested by Deal and Darley (1972), Warren's patients did not improve their accuracy over that in the immediate-response condition.

Auditory Stimulation

Early reports by Birch (1956) and Birch and Lee (1955) suggested that auditory stimulation may improve naming ability in expressive aphasic patients. Replication of their efforts by Weinstein (1959) and Wertz and Porch (1970) produced negative results. Several investigations have explored the influence of a variety of auditory stimulation conditions on response accuracy in apraxic patients.

Deal and Darley (1972) compared performance in two conditions. One required apraxic patients to read a paragraph while being stimulated with 85–95 dB SPL of white noise. The other permitted patients to hear their voices while reading in a no-noise condition. The presence or absence of masking noise had no effect on error production during oral reading.

Shane and Darley (1978) examined the effect of rhythmic auditory stimulation on articulatory accuracy in apraxic patients. Using a metronome, they compared errors in three conditions: the patient's normal, oral reading rate; reading with the metronome set at 75% of the normal rate; and reading with the metronome set at 125% of the normal rate. Articulatory accuracy did not differ significantly among conditions.

Tonkovich and Marquardt (1977) also imposed rhythm on apraxic patients' verbal production. Using Melodic Intonation Therapy (MIT) techniques (Sparks et al., 1974; Sparks & Holland, 1976), melodic intoned performance was compared with normal intonation. Their sample made significantly more errors in the melodic condition than in the normal condition.

Chapin et al. (1981) studied the effects of delayed auditory feedback (DAF) on speech production by Broca's, conduction, Wernicke's, and "posterior' aphasic patients. The Broca's patients were influenced more by DAF than the other types. Compared with performance in a no-delay condition, under DAF the Broca's patients lengthened vowels and made more repetition, substitution, omission, and addition errors.

Thus, auditory stimulation by masking or a metronome appears to have no effect on articulatory accuracy in apraxia of speech. Imposing melodic intonation or delayed auditory feedback seems to erode articulatory performance.

Prosodic Disturbances

Abnormal prosody is apparent in the speech of apraxic patients. Suspected contributions to this are listed in Table 6. They include a tendency toward equal stress, inappropriate intersyllabic pauses, restriction and alteration of normal intonational and loudness contours, effortful groping and repetitive attempts to produce sounds accurately, and slow rate.

Table 6.
Prosodic Disturbances in Apraxia of Speech

Tend toward equal stress.

Use inappropriate intersyllabic pauses.

Exhibit restriction and alteration of normal intonational and loudness contours.

Exhibit effortful, groping, repetitive attempts to produce sounds accurately.

Rate is probably slowed overall.

Prosodic disturbances probably reflect the effects of the primary motor deficit as well as the effort to compensate.

Adapted from Rosenbek and Wertz, 1976.

It is not clear whether the prosodic disturbances reflect the effects of the primary motor disorder or the patient's effort to compensate for it. Darley's (1969) definition suggested compensation. Rosenbek and Wertz (1976) suggest prosodic disturbance, like the articulatory disturbance, results from the motor deficit. Probably both positions are correct. Kent and Rosenbek (1983) discuss this issue at length.

Until recently, prosodic disturbance in apraxia of speech was observed and noted but not studied. Monrad-Krohn's (1947) report of a Norwegian woman who suffered a traumatic Broca's aphasia fascinated us. She recovered language nicely, but a residual prosodic disturbance was mistakenly perceived by listeners as a pronounced foreign accent. Johns and Darley (1970) noted marked prosodic disturbance in their patients. Now, acoustic analysis (Kent and Rosenbek, 1982; Kent and Rosenbek, 1983) is beginning to explain clinicians' perceptions.

Equal Stress

Apraxic speakers sound like they give each syllable in their utterances equal stress. This was observed by Lebrun et al. (1973) and elaborated by Kent and Rosenbek's (1982) acoustic analyses. The former report suggests patients do not produce scanning speech with inappropriate intersyllabic pauses. The latter report, however, provides evidence that inappropriate intersyllabic pauses abound in the apraxic patient's utterances.

The listener's perception of equal stress probably results from the patient's tendency to isolate syllables by separating them in a syllabic series. Syllables are prolonged, and the patient fails to effect syllable reduction when such reduction is appropriate. Thus, the speech pattern is halting because of segment prolongation and inappropriate pauses. Apraxic talkers appear to walk through their utterances by cautiously "tiptonguing" along the syllabic path with fear of falling off what is to be said.

Alteration of Intonational and Loudness Contours

Lebrun et al. (1973) observed that their patients showed syllabic prominence. This, combined with vowel lengthening, frequent insertion of "usually silent letters," and slow articulatory rate, tended to flatten the intonational contour. Kent and Rosenbek (1982) studied the f_0-frequency contour using the Visi-Pitch f_0 display and narrow-band spectrograms. Their patients preserved normal sentence terminal-fall, but the apraxic speakers were so variable that other characteristics could not be identified. In a previous study (Kent and Rosenbek, 1982), they reported the absence of an f_0 contour across syllables. In their view, this absence may be a reflection of "syllable dissociation" (p. 269). Kent and Rosenbek (1983) also studied the intensity envelope in the imitative sentence productions of seven apraxic males. They predicted a flattening of the intensity envelope and tested for it first by measuring peak intensities of the syllables in four sentences. Apraxic speakers and normal controls varied intensity on approximately the same syllables, but the apraxic speakers showed less variation, confirming a flattening of the intensity envelope. Kent and Rosenbek also determined the average intensity for the least intense syllable in each sentence. The apraxic speakers reduced intensity on normally reduced intensity words such as "in" and "on" less than did normal speakers. This also confirms that apraxic speakers flatten the intensity envelope.

Groping

The visible effortful, groping, and repetitive attempts apraxic patients make, apparently in an attempt to produce sounds correctly, work their will on prosody. Kent and Rosenbek (1982, 1983) report that these slow, inaccurate movements disrupt both vowels and consonants. They result in mistiming, and the effect is particularly evident in coordinating voice onset time (Freeman et al., 1978). While groping may occur anywhere in the patient's utterance, it is most obvious as an initiation difficulty and is displayed as false starts and restarts. Kent and Rosenbek (1982) observed incorrecct sound sequences that were linked with their patients' apparent search for intended targets.

Rate

Most researchers, with the possible exception of DiSimoni and Darley (1977), agree that patients suffering apraxia of speech display an overall reduction in rate. Lebrun et al. (1973) comment on their patients' slow rate of articulation. Kent and Rosenbek (1983) also report that the apraxic patient's speech is reduced in rate. They observed that sentence production was two to six times longer than in normal speakers. They also suggest that the slowness results from articulatory prolongation, defined as lengthening of steady-state segments and the intervening transitions, and syllable segregation, in which syllables are isolated sometimes as if each was being produced as a separate entity. Both vowel and consonant sounds are likely to be prolonged.

Vowels, typically given a clean bill of health in perceptual error analysis studies, emerge as culprits in acoustic analyses and explain a portion of the rate disturbance. Shankweiler et al. (1968) noted that apraxic speakers' vowels are prolonged. A similar observation was made by Freeman et al. (1978). They also report that their patient's vowels are significantly longer before voiced final stops than before voiceless final stops Collins et al. (1983) provide evidence that apraxic patients reduce vowel length as words increase in length, but that their word and vowel durations are longer, regardless of word length, than are those of normal speakers.

Durational relationships then seem to be preserved, but absolute durations are increased.

"Foreign Accent"

One of us believes that most apraxic patients sound like the late Ingrid Bergman. Shankweiler and Harris (1966) commented on the dialectical features in their patients' vowels. Monrad-Krohn's (1947) patient sounded like she was speaking here native Norwegian as a second language. Similarly, the Spanish-speaking patient of Clouzet et al. (1976) produced phonemes that resided outside the phonological system of Spanish. Furthermore some of the patient's allophones, even though present in Spanish, were not part of his premorbid dialect. Most clinicians are impressed with the perceptual presence of a "foreign accent" in apraxic patients who spoke English and nothing else prior to onset. The explanation for this, probably, lies in prosodic disturbance.

Kent and Rosenbek's (1982) acoustic analyses of apraxic patients' speech offer some explanations. They suggest that the "foreign accent" sound in apraxia of speech, (frequently described as German or Welsh) results from exaggerated pitch variation, breakdown in rhythm, segmental errors, and a halting style of speech.

Nonarticulatory Characteristics

Over the years, clinicans have noted nonarticulatory behaviors that may coexist with apraxia of speech, explain the nature of the disorder, or assist in differentiating it from other disorders. We list some of these in Table 7. They include the presence or absence of oral, nonverbal apraxia; the ability to anticipate and recognize articulatory errors; the relationship between auditory discrimination and oral production; and the integrity of oral sensation and perception.

Oral, Nonverbal Apraxia

Oral, nonverbal apraxia, problems in making volitional oral, nonverbal movements in the absence of significant paralysis or paresis, may or may not accompany apraxia of speech. Nathan (1947) observed that apraxia of speech and oral, nonverbal apraxia coexist. Goldstein (1948) and Denny-Brown (1958) report that the two conditions can exist independently. De Renzi et al. (1966) found a strong association between the two disorders but observed that they can occur independently. One patient of Lebrun et al. (1973) displayed coexisting oral, nonverbal apraxia, and one did not.

Some investigators have examined the relationship between their severity when the two disorders coexist. De Renzi et al. (1966) found a

Table 7.

Nonarticulatory Characteristics in Apraxia of Speech

May or may not have an accompanying oral, nonverbal apraxia.

Individual patients may anticipate their errors at a level significantly greater than chance.

Patients, as a group, can recognize their errors at a level significantly greater than chance.

Auditory discrimination is usually superior to oral production.

Oral sensation and perception is impaired in some patients.

Adapted from Rosenbek and Wertz, 1976.

significant correlation between the severity of oral, nonverbal apraxia and the severity of articulatory deficit in their patients. LePointe and Wertz (1974) and Bowman et al. (1980) found no significant relationship between severity in the two disorders.

De Renzi et al. (1966) observed that the incidence of oral, nonverbal apraxia was greatest in their Broca's aphasia patients (90%) and their "phonemic jargon" patients (83%). It was less common in conduction aphasia (33%) and Wernicke's aphasia (6%). Fifty percent of their "nonclassifiable" patients displayed oral, nonverbal apraxia. It was absent in their normal and right-hemisphere brain-damaged samples. The presence of limb apraxia was significantly correlated with the presence of oral, nonverbal apraxia, but it was not uncommon to find oral, nonverbal apraxia with no limb apraxia.

LaPointe and Wertz (1974), using tests of isolated oral movement and oral-motor sequencing, found their samples of brain-damaged patients performed worse than normal controls. While not all of the brain-damaged patients had difficulty making oral movements, oral, nonverbal movement deficits were observed in each of their three brain-damaged groups— apraxia of speech, dysarthria, and combined apraxia of speech and dysarthria.

Moore et al. (1976) developed an extensive battery and employed an elaborate scoring system to access oral movement in normals and apraxia of speech, aphasia, and right-hemisphere damage. Oral, nonverbal apraxia was present in all three of the brain-damaged groups, but it was more severe in patients suffering apraxia of speech than in those with aphasia or a right-hemisphere lesion.

Thus, some patients with apraxia of speech may have coexisting oral, nonverbal apraxia, but its absence does not surprise us.

Error Anticipation and Recognition

Deal and Darley (1972) report that apraxic patients are able to predict errors they will make in oral reading at a level significantly greater than chance. However, their patients made many more errors than they predicted they would make. As a group, patients made 72% of the errors they predicted, but they predicted only 45% of the total errors they made. In the same experiment, Deal and Darley (1972) asked their apraxic patients to judge the correctness of their responses. The groups displayed a significant ability to recognize their errors. Again, however, patients made more errors than they recognized.

A related result has been reported by Deal (1974). He examined error consistency and error adaptation in apraxic patients. Upon repeated readings of the same material, his patients displayed a consistency effect; they made errors on the same words from one reading to the next. They also displayed some adaptation; they made fewer errors on successive readings. Reduction in total errors was not great, however, and adaptation varied among patients.

Auditory Discrimination

Darley (1982) summarizes data to support the notion that apraxic patients' speech difficulties cannot be explained by poor auditory perception. Most (Shankweiler & Harris, 1966; Johns & Darley, 1970) tested their apraxic samples' auditory perception of the stimuli used to test speech, and all showed that auditory abilities are superior to oral production.

Some have used difficult auditory tasks to determine the integrity of auditory input in patients who demonstrate apraxia of speech. Aten et al. (1971) administered minimally varied auditory sequences and compared apraxic performance to normal. The apraxic group made significantly more errors thant the normal group; however, three of ten patients performed within the normal range. Aten et al. suggest that the poor performance by the seven impaired patients resulted from coexisting aphasia. Lebrun et al. (1973) report good auditory perception in their patients, demonstrated by the ability to pick out objects whose names begin with the same sound or whose names resembled one another, e.g., "cork" and "fork." Nebes (1975) used rhyming tests to demonstrate that his aphemic patient could form and compare internal auditory images. Shulak (1979) administered pictured and printed words that differed from a spoken stimulus word by only one phoneme to measure "internal speech" in apraxic patients. Her patients performed significantly worse than normals, but performance was quite variable.

Probably the most exhaustive study of auditory ability in apraxic patients was reported by Square et al. (1981). They administered 27 non-speech and speech auditory tests to four groups: pure apraxia of speech, aphasia, apraxia of speech and aphasia, and normal. Pure apraxia of speech patients did not differ significantly from normals, and they performed significantly better on all measures than the aphasia and apraxia of speech and aphasia groups. No significant relationship was found between auditory processing and speech production.

We conclude from the literature and our experience that auditory discrimination is usually better than oral production in patients suffering apraxia of speech. This does not deny the possibility of coexisting aphasia and its influence on auditory ability, or that impaired speech may sometimes result in poor performance on auditory tasks.

Oral Sensation

Investigations of oral sensation and perception in apraxic patients suggest that the disorder may be sensorimotor and not solely motor. Guilford and Hawk (1968) observed that aphasic patients with oral apraxia performed worse on tests of oral sensation than aphasic patients without oral apraxia or normal subjects. Similarly, Larimore (1970) found oral sensory – perceptual deficit in five apraxic patients when he compared their performance on a variety of tests with that of normal subjects.

Rosenbek et al. (1973b) compared performance by apraxic patients, aphasic patients, and normal subjects on three measures of oral sensation and perception—oral form identification, two-point discrimination, and mandibular kinesthesia. Their apraxic group was significantly inferior to the aphasic and normal groups on all three oral sensory – perceptual tests. Apraxia of speech and oral sensory – perceptual deficit were related. The more severe the apraxia of speech, the more profound the oral sensory – perceptual deficit. However, not all patients with apraxia of speech demonstrated impaired oral sensation and perception.

Reports by Deutsch (1981) and Square and Weidner (1976) question those of Rosenbek et al. (1973b). The former found that apraxic patients did not differ from aphasic patients on an oral form identification task, and oral form performance was not related to severity of apraxia of speech. The latter observed that apraxic patients had more difficulty than normals in oral form identification but not on a test of mandibular kinesthesia. Square and Weidner, like Deutsch, found no relationship between oral form identification and severity of apraxia.

Thus some, not all, patients who suffer apraxia of speech appear to have impaired oral sensation and perception. The oral sensory deficity may or may not be related to the severity of apraxia of speech.

THIRD GENERATION CHARACTERISTICS

What we have called first generation characteristics flowed from clinical observations and early behavioral studies. Our second generation characteristics were drawn from perceptual and acoustic studies spurred by early reports. Recently, investigators have taken the apraxic patient's behavior into the laboratory in attempts to see what clinical researchers have heard. These constitute our third generation characteristics.

Acoustic Characteristics

Some of the acoustic data discussed here were included in our earlier discussion on prosody. Most of what we know about the acoustic characteristics of apraxic speakers' productions come from wide-band and narrow-band spectrographic analysis. While rivulets of disagreement flow into the stream of emerging evidence, we are able to state some general acoustic correlates of apraxic speech. These have been adapted from Kent and Rosenbek (1983) and are listed in Table 8.

General Characteristics

Kent and Rosenbek (1983) observed that apraxic talkers have a slow speaking rate when their performance is compared with normal speakers. Sentence duration in apraxia of speech is two to six times longer than in normal speech. This results from articulatory prolongation and syllable segregation. In addition, their apraxic patients displayed less variation in

Table 8.
Acoustic Characteristics of Apraxia of Speech

Slow speaking rate with prolongations of transitions and steady states as well as intersyllabic pauses.

Restricted variations in relative peak intensity across syllables.

Slow and inaccurate movements of the articulators to spatial targets for both consonants and vowels.

Frequent mistiming or dyscoordinations of voicing with other articulatory movements.

Occasional errors of segment selection or sequencing including intrusion, metathesis, and omission.

Initiation difficulties often characterized by false starts and restarts.

Complex sound sequences associated with an apparent search for the intended targets.

Adapted from Kent and Rosenbek, 1983.

relative peak intensity across syllables. This tended to flatten the intensity envelope. Voicing errors were frequent, and there was wide variability in voicing errors both within and among apraxic speakers. Acoustic analyses revealed what perceptual studies have not, the presence of vowel errors. These include both substitutions and distortions. Spectrograms also revealed slow, inaccurate movements in the production of both vowels and consonants; frequent mistiming and dyscoordination of voicing; occasional errors in segment selection and sequencing; initiation difficulties characterized by false starts and restarts; and the presence of complex sound sequences apparently related to a search for the intended target. Kent and Rosenbek (1982) noted flagrant prosodic disturbance in apraxia of speech and labelled this "dysprosody." While it differs from prosodic disturbance in some of the dysarthrias, they comment that it shares some features seen in ataxic dysarthria.

Voice Onset Time

The poor coordination of voicing with other articulatory movement noted by Kent and Rosenbek (1983) was also observed by Blumstein et al. (1977) and Freeman et al. (1978). The latter group studied one patient who displayed an abundance of voicing errors. They detected marked difference in voice onset time (VOT) when compared with normal speakers' productions. One-third of their patient's voicing errors occurred on initial stops. Voiceless stops were perceived as being voiced. Spectrographic analysis revealed that the patient's lag time for voiced stops was longer than normal, and his lag time for voiceless stops was shorter than normal. This resulted in compression of lag time and a marked overlap in VOT for voiced and voiceless stop production. Freeman et al. report a significant relationship between spectrographically determined VOT and listeners' perceptions.

Durational Characteristics

There is ample evidence to indicate that apraxic speakers have difficulty in programming durational control of speech segments. However, reports disagree on whether durations are longer or shorter than normal production and whether or not vowels are affected differently than consonants. All agree that durational characteristics in apraxic talkers are more variable than in normal talkers.

Bauman et al. (1975) report that vowel durations in their apraxic patients were significantly shorter than vowel durations in normals. Consonant durations were extremely variable compared with consonant duration in normals. DiSimoni and Darley (1977) observed durations of target consonants that were significantly shorter in their patients than in normal speakers. Fager and Deutsch (1981) obtained similar results. Freeman et al.

(1978) and Collins et al. (1983) observed that vowel durations were longer in apraxic speakers. Freeman et al. elaborated that vowels were significantly longer before voiced final stops than before voiceless final stops. Collins et al. found significantly longer vowels in apraxic patients than in normals and, in another investigation (Collins et al., 1979), observed significantly longer vowel durations in apraxic patients than in aphasic patients who did not suffer apraxia of speech.

Two investigations (Fager & Deutsch, 1981; Collins et al., 1983) studied progressive shortening of vowels as syllables are added to a base word. Both observed that apraxic patients follow the rule of progressively shortening the vowel as syllables are added; however, their vowels are longer than those of normals in all forms of the word.

Are apraxic talkers slower or faster than normals? Kent and Rosenbek (1983) and Itoh et al. (1980) suggest the former. DiSimoni and Darley (1977) suggest the latter. Disagreement may result from the methods used to measure rate. Kent and Rosenbek (1983) observe that DiSimoni and Darley (1977) base their conclusion on the assumption that a shorter segmental duration of /p/ reflects a more rapid articulatory movement. However, DiSimoni and Darley measured the interval of voicelessness and not the stop gap for /p/. Because apraxic speakers may display dyscoordination between laryngeal and supralaryngeal movements, what DiSimoni and Darley demostrated was that their apraxic speaker had shorter intervals of voicelessness than their normal speaker, and their results are not directly related to the rates of movement of the oral articulators.

Acoustic analyses of apraxia of speech are beginning to let us see some of what we have been hearing. To some extent, acoustic analyses are indicating that our golden cochleas are not as precise as the sonographic stylus. What sounds one way may look another. Acoustic studies are also verifying perceptual suspicions. For years we have suspected that apraxic patients, even when correct (no substitutions, distortions, omission, etc.), were not *quite* correct. The acoustic data confirm our suspicions. We welcome these contributions.

Physiologic Characteristics

Shankweiler et al. (1968) comment, "A good deal can be inferred indirectly about articulatory movements by listening to speech under controlled conditions. One ought, however, to be able to learn much more by studying the motor processes directly" (p. 4). Well, some have, and their results support the faith of Shankweiler et al. in physiologic investigation of apraxia of speech. In recent years, apraxic patients have been coupled to EMG, movement transducers, accelerometers, X-ray microbeams, and

Table 9.
Physiologic Characteristics in Apraxia of Speech

Presence of antagonistic muscle co-contraction.

Produce continuous, undifferentiated EMG activity.

Instances of a shutdown in muscle activity.

Instances of movement without appropriate voicing.

Dyscoordinated, added, and groping movements.

Reduced peak expiratory flow in some patients.

pulmonary function equipment. Results emerging from these studies permit us to formulate the physiologic characteristics listed in Table 9.

Physiologic abnormalities in apraxia of speech patients, culled from several reports, include antagonistic muscle co-contraction; continuous, undifferentiated EMG activity; movement not accompanied by appropriate voicing; dyscoordinated, added, and groping movements; and reduction in peak expiratory flow.

EMG Evidence

Shankweiler et al. (1968) recorded EMG activity from surface electrodes placed on the lips, tongue, and hyoid in two apraxic patients. They observed grossly abnormal EMG traces in both. Repeated utterances of the same word revealed rampant variablity in the timing of sequential movements. Simultaneous peaks from all electrode locations showed a marked reduction in the ability to move articulators independently. Fromm et al. (1982) report similar observations in their EMG investigation using hooked wire electrodes in the lip and facial muscles of three apraxic patients. Both reports indicate EMG yields good agreement with other methods of investigation; in addition, it provides information about the temporal and spatial organization of apraxic speech that cannot be seen or heard in the acoustic end product.

Movement Data

A variety of movement devices have been used to study the apraxic patient. Itoh et al. (1979) used a fiberscopic system to observe velar movement during speech in an apraxic patient. Repeated utterances of the same word revealed marked variability in the pattern of velar movement among productions. However, in spite of the variability, the patient approximated the normal pattern of velar movement for a given phonetic context.

In a second study, Itoh et al. (1980) employed an X-ray microbeam system to obtain simultaneous observation of an apraxic patient's movement of several articulators—lips, tongue, and velum. They observed that the temporal organization of articulatory movements differed from that of a normal subject and two dysarthric patients. Velar movement was not always coordinated with tongue movement, and inconsistency in this coordination may explain inconsistency in apraxic errors. In addition, the apraxic patient's pattern and velocity of articulatory movements differed from normal.

Fromm et al. (1982) made multiple observations of three apraxic patients and three normal subjects. They used a movement transduction system to monitor movement of the lips and jaw; EMG electrodes in the lip musculature and the mentalis; and an accelerometer attached over the thyroid cartilage to monitor onset of voicing. Their results indicate marked differences between their apraxic and normal subjects, and the abnormalities seen in the apraxic patients differed from those they had observed in previous investigations with dysarthric patients. The muscle control and movement abnormalities detected in their apraxic patients are included in Table 9. Fromm et al. conclude that there is a need to redefine apraxia of speech and include the presence of substantial dyscoordination among multiple speech muscles and speech movements. They also stress the need to study apraxia of speech with direct observations of the underlying pathophysiology. Many of the aberrations are either silent or may be perceived as normal because of transient compensatory behaviors that, at times, overcome the neuromuscular abnormality.

Respiration

Keatley and Pike (1976) obtained 13 measures of pulmonary function on 5 apraxic patients. The measures included a variety of flows and volumes that can be tapped by an Automated Pulmonary Function Laboratory apparatus. The most sensitive was peak expiratory flow, the largest flow achieved during forced expiration, measured in liters per minute. Four of the patients displayed peak expiratory flow that was lower than normal. Pulmonary function was related to the severity of apraxia of speech. The most severe patient displayed abnormal values on 10 of the 13 measures, and the mildest patient was within normal limits on all measures.

What do the physiologic data on apraxia of speech tell us? They provide evidence of the underlying neuropathology that may escape the ear. In addition, they explain some of what the ear can hear. Because they identify and amplify, they should be included in the research and clinical armamentarium.

A SUMMARY

Unless one's preferred activity is analytic digression, it is time to end our discussion of apraxia of speech's characteristics. There is a danger in saying more than one wants to know and, of course, saying more than we know. We take time with the preceding because, we believe, knowing what may typify apraxia of speech is useful. It is useful in understanding the nature of the disorder and in managing it. When we go looking for apraxia of speech, we use its characteristics to identify what we find. We remain alert, and we remind ourselves that individual apraxic patients will not meet all of the characteristics identified in group studies. Failure to do so does not, necessarily, cast a patient out of his ilk.

In the identification and understanding of any disorder, clinicians search for the fundamental issue, the one called bedrock. Bedrock has one great virtue—its stability. When you have reached it, you know where you are. Because of conflicting reports and because not all patients display all characteristics, one might conclude that bedrock, at the present time, in the understanding and management of apraxia of speech is variability. There is, however, sufficient consistency in what we know to use it in identifying most patients who suffer apraxia of speech. For those we cannot label during our first hour together, time and additional probing find them out.

Today, we can condense all we have discussed into the following four salient, clinical characteristics of apraxia of speech:

1. Effortful, trial and error, groping articulatory movements and attempts at self-correction.
2. Dysprosody unrelieved by extended periods of normal rhythm, stress, and intonation.
3. Articulatory inconsistency on repeated productions of the same utterance.
4. Obvious difficulty initiating utterances.

Those patients whose spontaneous and imitative speech reveal the above, we call apraxic.

We use our perceptual talents, and we add the emerging use of acoustic and physiologic instrumentation. We are careful not to interpret acoustic and physiologic data as theodicies that refute, entirely, the misspent youth of the ear. We use these to challenge, to explain, to amplify, to improve what we know and what we do. For now, and probably forever, these tools will mainly supplement. In the hands of skilled researchers, they may firm theory, and, more importantly, they may improve practice.

5

Appraisal and Diagnosis

Looking for apraxia of speech should not resemble a search for the last passenger pigeon—listening for that sound of distant thunder one has not heard, looking for that certain flash of color one has never seen. Like tales of the passenger pigeon, the literature is filled with phrases that catch and hang on the mind. When looking for apraxia of speech, one wants to make sure one finds it and not a mourning dove. This chapter is about the looking and the finding.

We spent the previous chapter listing and discussing characteristics that typify the patient who suffers apraxia of speech. Now, we turn to how one identifies these characteristics and labels what is found. The process is as old as speech pathology. It is called appraisal and diagnosis.

Appraisal is the looking. It requires data collection. Its purposes are to provide sufficient information to make a diagnosis; and, if appropriate, focus treatment. Diagnosis is the finding. It is an exercise in affixing the appropriate label. Its purpose is to rule out inappropriate labels and to ensure that what one has is one thing and not another.

We believe clinicians are supposed to know everything they can figure out. We do not believe we should make up answers just because we cannot tolerate unanswered questions. Appraisal is a means for figuring things out to make a diagnosis; it is a search for something we can name if we find it. The naming, that is diagnosis.

APPRAISAL

Appraising apraxia of speech is like getting to know a city. It requires views from different perspectives. Having apraxic patients only repeat consonant clusters gives no indication of their use of syntax or semantics, or their reading, writing, or auditory comprehension. Even after these are sampled on appraisal's afternoon Greyline Tour, there is a need to stand back and see the pattern provided by the pieces. Like exploring cities, one is less likely to get lost appraising apraxia of speech if one has a map.

One should also avoid confusing the symptoms observed with the method of analysis. Give anything with two legs a test for aphasia, and there is a strong probability of finding aphasia. Test only repetition of plosives, and if you find any errors at all, they are likely to be errors on plosives. While there is a multitude of evaluation tools for digging into apraxia of speech, few exist commercially. That is good and as things should be. One samples with several measures; examines the interaction among methods, stimuli, and symptoms; and knows or does not know whether the person is apraxic. A test does not make the decision; a clinician does.

Finally, enough appraisal is enough appraisal. Proper appraisal avoids the Three Bear's dilemma. Too much is too hot, too little is too cold. One seeks the "just right." On the one hand, appraisal must be repeated for verification. We must be careful not to make a future and a world out of a single day. On the other, we seek adequate but not exhaustive appraisal. One trades the demands of time with those of thoroughness. For example, enough appraisal to focus some treatment is enough appraisal. One may continue with additional appraisal to answer unanswered questions, but one need not complete appraisal prior to initiating treatment. Treatment should not await appraisal's exhaustion. There is always more to explore. But delve too deeply or look too long and what has been seen early may have vanished. The patient is no longer being managed; he is being observed.

Therefore we stop our appraisal short of indulgence, a healthy distance this side of a metaphysical experience. We insist that each piece of an appraisal have a purpose. We do not seek a mystique, a mythos. We remind ourselves that apraxia of speech bears no resemblance to motherhood. We get on with it.

Generally, we appraise apraxic patients much the same as we appraise all brain-damaged patients, because initially we do not know that they are apraxic. We collect three types of data: biographical, medical, and behavioral. Each assists in serving appraisal's purposes.

Biographical Data

We want to know as much as we need to know about our patients. Basic biographical data—name, residence, marital status, etc.—tell us how patients prefer to be addressed, where they live, whether where they live puts them within treatment's reach, and whether there will be anyone at home when they get there.

Some biographical data may have prognostic significance. For example, age, education, premorbid handedness, highest occupational level achieved, occupational status at onset, and premorbid intelligence have surfaced in the prognostic literature as possible predictors of improvement. Other biographical facts may explain articulatory and language errors. Knowing the number and kinds of languages spoken prior to onset may, for example, explain a part of linguistic deficit not attributable to brain damage, a /Θ/ for /s/ substitution that results from having spoken Spanish and not from being apraxic. Some biographic information may influence treatment's focus, content, and methods. For example, patients who live alone or in an institutional environment will not have an available ear to monitor and correct apraxic productions. Taciturn talkers prior to becoming brain damaged do not become verbose after. Hobbies, interests, and passions make better treatment stimuli than nonsense syllables.

Finally, the collection of biographic data does not end after appraisal's first day. Throughout management we monitor biographical facts that may change over time, e.g., handedness, marital status, language usage, living environment, or occupational status.

Medical Data

We remind ourselves that our patients are not our patients. They are on loan from the primary care physician—the neurologist, physiatrist, internist, or general practitioner. We should seek these sources for data that may assist our management. Some of the information that might prove useful is listed in Table 1.

Certain pieces of medical information assist in making a diagnosis. Visual and auditory acuity assist in explaining reading and auditory comprehension deficits. The presence of right hemiplegia suggests the possibility of aphasia and/or apraxia of speech. Localization of brain damage that includes the third frontal convolution also suggests the possibility of apraxia of speech. Other pieces of medical data assist in formulating a prognosis. For example, patients with a single episode, a small lesion confined to Broca's area, close to onset, and in good health are believed to have better potential for improvement than those with multiple episodes, large or bilateral lesions, long duration of symptoms, and major coexisting medical problems.

Benson (1979) advises the neurologist to remain "on line" after medical diagnosis and assist in rehabilitation. We agree, and we welcome this collaborative effort. We also initiate contact early when we collect and discuss a patient's medical data.

Table 1.
Medical Data Collected to Assist Management of Patients Suspected of Suffering
Apraxia of Speech

Vision	Acuity, corrected and uncorrected; field abnormalities
Auditory	Acuity, aided and unaided; ear pathologies
Limb involvement	Upper and lower; spasticity, weakness, coordination
Brain stem signs	Facial weakness, facial sensory loss, nystagmus, ocular movement (EOM) and/or gaze impairment, dysphagia, other bulbar signs
Etiology	Type (CVA, trauma, infection, etc.); onset
Previous CNS involvement	Type, onset
Localization	Current episode and any previous episodes; source (clinical, EEG, C-T, etc.)
Specific, complete diagnosis	For example, thrombosis of middle cerebral artery, with right hemiparesis, hemisensory defect, hemianopsia, and expressive aphasia
Other major medical diagnoses	For example, diabetes, chronic cardiac arrythmia, etc.
Medications	Number, types, and side effects

Behavioral Data

Appraising apraxia of speech requires letting patients tell you about
their problem. We ask, the patients respond if they can, and we probe with
a variety of tools and techniques. We try to stay out of the patient's way as
much as we can to avoid finding only what we permit to appear. When we
do intervene, we do so with a variety of measures designed to satisfy
appraisal's purposes. A basic battery for appraising apraxia of speech is
listed in Table 2. This is descriptive, not prescriptive. Time and the patient
dictate which and how many of the measures will be administered. Usually,
we attempt to sample language, speech, nonverbal oral movements, limb
gestures, and intelligence. The results from administering one measure
may suggest the need to administer another. Again, we avoid letting our
patients soak in our psychometric marinade too long.

Table 2.
Appraisal Battery for Patients Suspected of Suffering Apraxia of Speech

Behavior	Measures
Language	Porch Index of Communicative Ability (Porch, 1967)
	Boston Diagnostic Aphasia Examination (Goodglass and Kaplan, 1972)
"Functional" communication	Communicative Abilities in Daily Living (Holland, 1980)
Speech	Motor speech evaluation
	Sound-by-position tests
	A Deep Test of Articulation (McDonald, 1964)
	Templin-Darley Tests of Articulation (Templin & Darley, 1960)
Oral, nonverbal movements	Oral peripheral examination
	Tests of isolated oral movement
	Tests of oral-motor sequencing
Intelligence	Coloured Progressive Matrices (Raven, 1962)
Supplementary tests	
Auditory comprehension	Token Test (DeRenzi & Vignolo, 1962)
Reading	Reading Comprehension Battery for Aphasia (LaPointe & Horner, 1979)

Language Measures

We want to know whether our apraxic patients have coexisting language deficits, and if they do, what these language deficits are. Most have a coexisting language deficit, and that deficit usually is aphasia.

The Porch Index of Communicative Ability (PICA) (Porch, 1967) provides a quantified measure of language. An overall percentile can be computed as well as percentiles for gestural, verbal, and graphic performance. In addition to giving a picture of the patient's language deficits, the PICA provides two measures of limb gestures that may indicate the presence of limb apraxia and four measures of speech that may reveal apraxic errors. PICA profiles, especially the Modality Response Summary, may show a pattern of performance that suggests the presence of apraxia of speech. For example, inordinately low verbal performance coexisting with much better gestural and graphic performance may signal apraxia of speech. However, the best clues to the presence of apraxia yielded by the PICA come from what the patient does on the verbal subtests. Wertz, Rosenbek, and Collins (1978) demonstrated that PICA verbal subtests permitted clinicians to identify 71% of a sample of apraxic patients correctly. Figure 1 shows PICA Modality Response Summaries for three patients who were eventually diagnosed as displaying apraxia of speech. The patients differ in severity, and each displays coexisting aphasia.

P.M. was mild, both in aphasia and in apraxia of speech. He performed at the 91st percentile overall on the PICA. Modality performance was 97th percentile, gestural; 81st percentile, verbal; and 90th percentile, graphic. In conversation, one had to ask P.M. if he was aphasic. He admitted he must be, because his language was not as good as it was prior to his stroke. Mild apraxic errors surfaced on PICA verbal subtests. These included consistent prosodic disturbance; substitutions of sounds which he attempted to correct, usually successfully; and infrequent groping prior to initiating the first sound of words. His speech and language did not prevent him from returning to employment as a pipe fitter in an oil refinery. Persisting right hemiparesis required some modification of his duties.

J.D. was moderate, both in aphasia and apraxia of speech. He performed at the 69th percentile overall on the PICA. Modality performance was 85th percentile, gestural; 53rd percentile, verbal; and 71st percentile, graphic. Language deficits were present in all modalities—auditory comprehension, reading, oral expressive language, and writing. He had sufficient speech to permit prosodic disturbance, articulatory errors, and oral groping to emerge out of his agrammatic productions. A year of treatment resulted in significant improvement in both aphasia and apraxia but not enough to permit J.D. to return to his weekly runs as a railroad conductor. Currently, he spends his days as an active participant in a recreational vehicle club and growing the best zucchini in Alameda County.

B.S. was severely aphasic, and (we suspected) severely apraxic. He performed at the 24th percentile overall on the PICA. Modality performance was 17th percentile, gestural; 33rd percentile, verbal; and 37th percentile, graphic. He understood some of what he heard, read an occasional word, repeated a few words, and copied a few. While most attempts at volitional speech were stifled, his efforts to repeat suggested apraxia of speech was submerged in his dense aphasia. Coexisting significant auditory comprehension deficit rendered the conviction that he was also apraxic tentative. Fourteen months of treatment and spontaneous recovery resulted in sufficient resolution of his aphasia to permit confirmation of our early suspicion he was also apraxic. Currently, his PICA overall percentile has reached the 50th. He continues in treatment designed to combat both his aphasic and apraxic deficits.

The other language measure listed in Table 1 is the Boston Diagnostic

Porch Index of Communicative Ability

MODALITY RESPONSE SUMMARY

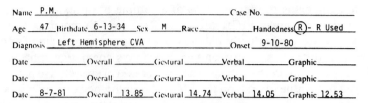

Name __P.M._____ Case No. _____

Age __47__ Birthdate _6-13-34_ Sex __M__ Race_____ Handedness Ⓡ - R Used

Diagnosis __Left Hemisphere CVA_____ Onset __9-10-80__

Date _____ Overall _____ Gestural _____ Verbal _____ Graphic_____

Date _____ Overall _____ Gestural _____ Verbal _____ Graphic_____

Date __8-7-81__ Overall _13.85_ Gestural _14.74_ Verbal _14.05_ Graphic _12.53_

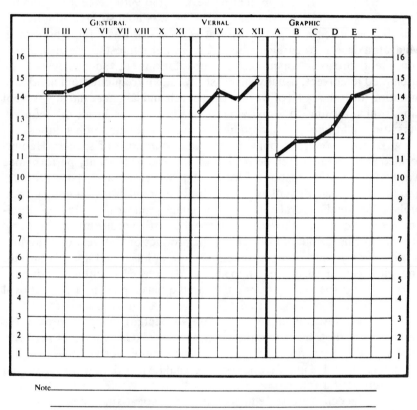

Note_____

Published by
CONSULTING PSYCHOLOGISTS PRESS
577 College Avenue   Palo Alto, California

Figure 1. PICA Modality Response Summaries for three patients displaying coexisting apraxia of speech and aphasia.

Porch Index of Communicative Ability

MODALITY RESPONSE SUMMARY

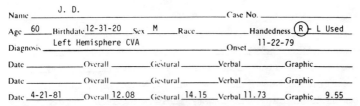

Name _____ J. D. _____ Case No. _____

Age __60__ Birthdate _12-31-20_ Sex _M_ Race _____ Handedness (R) L Used

Diagnosis ___Left Hemisphere CVA_____ Onset __11-22-79_____

Date _____ Overall _____ Gestural _____ Verbal _____ Graphic _____

Date _____ Overall _____ Gestural _____ Verbal _____ Graphic _____

Date _4-21-81____ Overall _12.08__ Gestural _14.15__ Verbal _11.73____ Graphic__9.55__

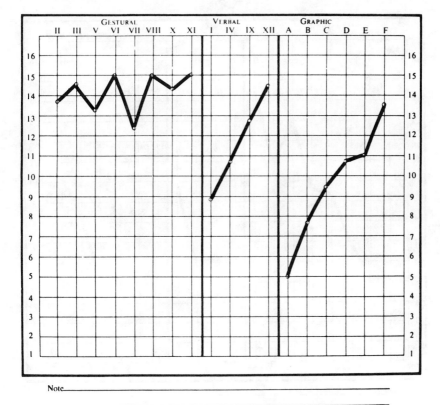

Note_____

Published by
CONSULTING PSYCHOLOGISTS PRESS
577 College Avenue   Palo Alto, California

Figure 1. *(continued)*.

Porch Index of Communicative Ability

MODALITY RESPONSE SUMMARY

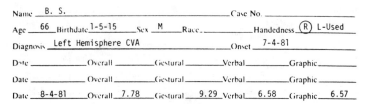

Name __B. S._____ Case No. _____

Age __66__ Birthdate __1-5-15__ Sex __M__ Race _____ Handedness (R) L-Used

Diagnosis __Left Hemisphere CVA_____ Onset __7-4-81__

Date _____ Overall _____ Gestural _____ Verbal _____ Graphic _____

Date _____ Overall _____ Gestural _____ Verbal _____ Graphic _____

Date __8-4-81__ Overall __7.78__ Gestural __9.29__ Verbal __6.58__ Graphic __6.57__

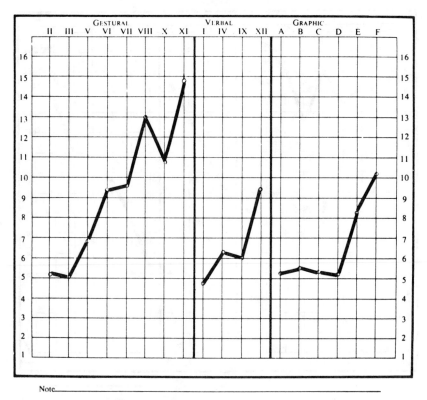

Note_____

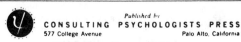

Published by
CONSULTING PSYCHOLOGISTS PRESS
577 College Avenue   Palo Alto, California

Figure 1. (*continued*).

Aphasia Examination (BDAE) (Goodglass & Kaplan, 1972). It provides samples of language behavior untapped by the PICA, and it permits classifying the type of aphasia if one is present. Measures of conversation, picture description, repetition, and naming also provide a sufficient speech sample to indicate the presence of apraxia of speech.

Many, probably most, of the apraxic patients we see fall within the tolerance limits of Broca's aphasia, shown in Figure 2, on the BDAE Rating Scale Profile of Speech Characteristics. Severity of aphasia can be rated on the Aphasia Severity Rating Scale from 0, "No useable speech or auditory comprehension," to 5, "Minimal descernible speech handicaps." Typically, the severity of Broca's aphasia ranges between 1 and 4. Seven behaviors are ranked on a 7-point scale on the Rating Scale Profile of Speech Characteristics. Tolerance limits for Broca's aphasia range from 1 to 4 ratings of melodic line, phrase length, articulatory agility, and grammatical form; must be 7, "absent," on paraphasias in running speech; and range from 5 to 7 on ratings of word finding and auditory comprehension. One need not administer the entire BDAE to complete the rating scale and attempt to type the aphasia. Performance on the Conversational and Expository Speech measures, including picture description auditory comprehension subtests, and repetition subtests is sufficient to complete the rating scale and attempt to type patients. However, administering the complete BDAE provides additional information about a patient's language ability, including reading and writing, and expands the samples of language obtained on the PICA.

Not all of the patients we label apraxic will profile as Broca's aphasia on the BDAE. Some are unclassifiable in that they do not fit into the traditional BDAE types; some are "mixed," while melodic line, phrase length, articulatory agility, and grammatical form fit the Broca's profile, auditory comprehension is more severely involved than is typical in Broca's aphasia; and some are "global," all modalities are severely involved. Figure 3 shows BDAE profiles for the patients we discussed previously.

P.M. had essentially normal phrase length, grammatical from, word finding, and auditory comprehension. He displayed no paraphasias in running speech. His prosodic disturbance was represented by a mildly abnormal melodic line, and his apraxic errors appear as moderately impaired articulatory agility. His BDAE profile is unclassifiable in the Boston system.

J.D. falls nicely into the Broca's aphasia range. Melodic line, phrase length, articulatory agility, and grammatical form are impaired. He displayed no paraphasias in running speech. Word finding leaned toward exclusive use of content words. Auditory comprehension, while not normal, was close to it.

B.S. was severely aphasic and probably apraxic. His melodic line,

Patient's Name _____ Date of rating _____

                                                          Rated by _____

APHASIA SEVERITY RATING SCALE

0. No usable speech or auditory comprehension.

1. All communication is through fragmentary expression; great need for inference,
    questioning and guessing by the listener. The range of information which can be
    exchanged is limited, and the listener carries the burden of communication.

2. Conversation about familiar subjects is possible with help from the listener. There are
    frequent failures to convey the idea, but patient shares the burden of communication
    with the examiner.

3. The patient can discuss almost all everyday problems with little or no assistance.
    However, reduction of speech and/or comprehension make conversation about certain
    material difficult or impossible.

4. Some obvious loss of fluency in speech or facility of comprehension, without significant
    limitation on ideas expressed or form of expression.

5. Minimal discernible speech handicaps; patient may have subjective difficulties which are
    not apparent to listener.

RATING SCALE PROFILE OF SPEECH CHARACTERISTICS

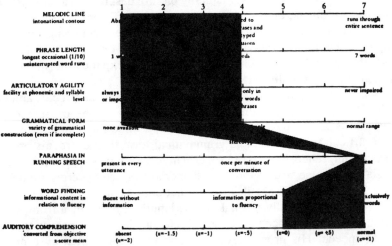

Figure 2.   BDAE profile showing the range of Broca's aphasia (after Goodglass &
Kaplan, 1972).

phrase length, articulatory agility, grammatical form, and auditory comprehension were grossly abnormal. He rendered no paraphasias in running
speech. In fact, he gave no running speech. The few words he uttered were
content words; thus he was rated 7 in word finding. His profile was that of
global aphasia. Currently, time and treatment have permitted him to evolve
into a Broca's profile at 15 months postonset.

We have discussed two of the language measures we use. There

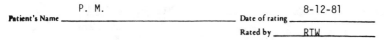

Patient's Name ____P. M._____ Date of rating ___8-12-81_____

Rated by _____RTW_____

APHASIA SEVERITY RATING SCALE

0. No usable speech or auditory comprehension.

1. All communication is through fragmentary expression; great need for inference, questioning and guessing by the listener. The range of information which can be exchanged is limited, and the listener carries the burden of communication.

2. Conversation about familiar subjects is possible with help from the listener. There are frequent failures to convey the idea, but patient shares the burden of communication with the examiner.

3. The patient can discuss almost all everyday problems with little or no assistance. However, reduction of speech and/or comprehension make conversation about certain material difficult or impossible.

4. Some obvious loss of fluency in speech or facility of comprehension, without significant limitation on ideas expressed or form of expression.

⑤ Minimal discernible speech handicaps; patient may have subjective difficulties which are not apparent to listener.

RATING SCALE PROFILE OF SPEECH CHARACTERISTICS

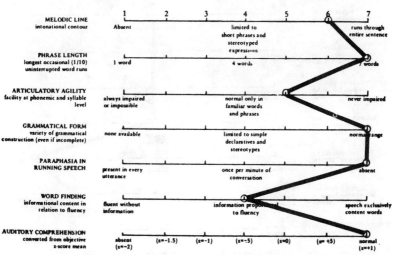

Figure 3. BDAE profiles on three patients displaying coexisting apraxia of speech and aphasia. (Other two profiles appear on pp 94–95.)

certainly are others that provide similar information. The Western Aphasia Battery (Kertesz, 1982) samples all language modalities and permits typing of aphasia according to the traditional taxonomy. The Aphasia Language Performance Scales (Keenan & Brassell, 1975); Examining for Aphasia (Eisenson, 1954); Language Modalities Test for Aphasia (Wepman & Jones, 1961); Minnesota Test for Differential Diagnosis of Aphasia

Patient's Name _____ J. D. _____ Date of rating ___ 4-14-81 ___
                                                    Rated by _____ RTW _____

APHASIA SEVERITY RATING SCALE

0. No usable speech or auditory comprehension.

1. All communication is through fragmentary expression; great need for inference,
    questioning and guessing by the listener. The range of information which can be
    exchanged is limited, and the listener carries the burden of communication.

2. Conversation about familiar subjects is possible with help from the listener. There are
    frequent failures to convey the idea, but patient shares the burden of communication
    with the examiner.

③. The patient can discuss <u>almost all everyday problems</u> with little or no assistance.
    However, reduction of speech and/or comprehension make conversation about certain
    material difficult or impossible.

4. Some obvious loss of fluency in speech or facility of comprehension, without significant
    limitation on ideas expressed or form of expression.

5. Minimal discernible speech handicaps; patient may have subjective difficulties which are
    not apparent to listener.

RATING SCALE PROFILE OF SPEECH CHARACTERISTICS

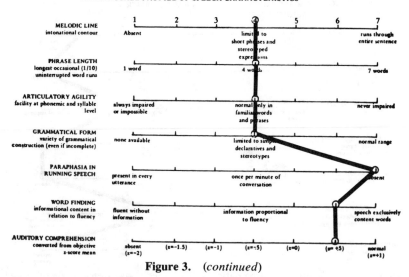

Figure 3. (*continued*)

(Schuell, 1965b); and the Neurosensory Center Comprehensive Examination for Aphasia (Spreen & Benton, 1969) all provide a comprehensive look
at language. We do not argue which measure or measures be administered.
We do advocate that a language measure be administered to patients suspected of suffering apraxia of speech. Appraisal's purposes demand that
we detect or rule out coexisting aphasia, and if it is present, that we
determine its severity. Besides providing samples of speech behavior that
may assist in determining the presence of apraxia of speech, aphasia tests

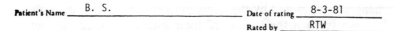

Patient's Name ___ B. S. _____ Date of rating ___ 8-3-81 ___
                                                              Rated by ___ RTW ___

APHASIA SEVERITY RATING SCALE

0. No usable speech or auditory comprehension.

1. All communication is through fragmentary expression; great need for inference, questioning and guessing by the listener. The range of information which can be exchanged is limited, and the listener carries the burden of communication.

2. Conversation about familiar subjects is possible with help from the listener. There are frequent failures to convey the idea, but patient shares the burden of communication with the examiner.

3. The patient can discuss almost all everyday problems with little or no assistance. However, reduction of speech and/or comprehension make conversation about certain material difficult or impossible.

4. Some obvious loss of fluency in speech or facility of comprehension, without significant limitation on ideas expressed or form of expression.

5. Minimal discernible speech handicaps; patient may have subjective difficulties which are not apparent to listener.

RATING SCALE PROFILE OF SPEECH CHARACTERISTICS

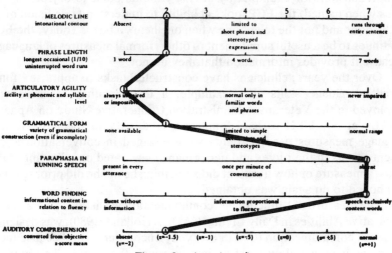

Figure 3. (*continued*)

tell us which modalities may be best to stimulate in therapy designed to combat apraxia, how much language a patient has to drive some of the demands we make in apraxia treatment, and whether treatment should focus on both the apraxia and the aphasia.

"Functional" Communication Measures

In the 1970s, clinicians who managed brain-damaged adults began to explore language context as well as language content. Impetus for this movement was prompted by the many patients who appeared to function better or worse than the results of their traditional language appraisal suggested they should. Fiftieth pecentile performers on the PICA returned to work. Family and friends of significantly impaired aphasic and apraxic patients reported minimal disruption in daily routines and social activities. Conversely, patients with less involvement failed on errands to the store even though performance on the language tests suggested that they should succeed. Why? Some patients used residual speech and language skills in everyday encounters better than others, and the language measures available, administered in the confines of the clinic, did not assess what happened in communicative attempts in the world beyond the clinical cubicle.

An early attempt to tap "functional" communication was provided by the Functional Communication Profile (FCP) (Sarno, 1969). Its purpose was to quantify communicative behavior a patient uses when interacting with other persons and events, not communicative behavior when interacting with test stimuli and a clinician. Forty-five behaviors in 5 categories—movement, speaking, understanding, reading, and miscellaneous—are rated on a 9-point scale. Unlike the traditional tests that measure auditory comprehension (for example, by having patients point to objects or pictures when named) the FCP looks at ability to understand television or go to the door and not the telephone when one hears a buzz. Today, the FCP continues to be a useful supplement to other, formal measures of language, because it provides information that they do not.

Over the years, clinicians have constructed tasks to appraise "functional" language skills. For example, a Conversation Measure was employed in the Veterans Administration Cooperative Study on Aphasia (Wertz, et al., 1981) to lend functional credibility to the more formal language measures used. Patients were engaged in conversation about recent events in their lives and performance was rated on a 7-point scale. Thus, a measure of how a patient did something he or she did prior to onset and hoped to do again was obtained.

The measure of "functional" communication we list in Table 2, Communicative Abilities in Daily Living (CADL) (Holland, 1980), was designed to assess communication used in everyday encounters. But because most clinicians cannot follow most patients through the worlds they explore every day, the CADL permits this assessment to take place in the clinic. Sixty-eight items are scored on a 3-point scale, 0–2. These range across ten categories—reading, writing, and using numbers to estimate, calculate, and judge time; speech acts; utilizing verbal and nonverbal context; role playing; sequence and relationship-dependent communicative behavior; social conventions; divergences, the ability to generate logical possibilities; nonverbal symbolic communication; deixis, movement-related or movement-dependent communicative behavior; and humor, absurdity, or metaphor. The clinical measure was validated by comparing CADL clinical performance by a sample of patients with what they were observed to do when followed through their daily routines and environments. It provides a pretty good notion of how patients communicate in the portions of their lives spent out of our site.

While no norms are available for patients demonstrating apraxia of speech, we can compare our patients' CADL performance to normative data provided for normals and five types of aphasia—global, mixed, Wernicke's, Broca's, and anomic. For the rare apraxic patient who displays no coexisting language deficit, we can compare his or her CADL performance with that of normals to determine how his apraxic errors may influence "functional" communication. For those patients who have coexisting aphasic deficits, we can utilize the CADL norms for the appropriate type of aphasia, usually global, mixed, or Broca's, to estimate "functional" communication.

The three patients discussed earlier received a CADL. P.M. obtained a CADL score of 132 out of the possible 136. His performance placed him above the normal mean and implied his communicative ability was "functional." It was. He lived alone, kept a checking account with no assistance, and returned to work. J.D. obtained a CADL score of 104, slightly below the mean for Broca's aphasia patients. He lived at home with his wife, relied on her to pay the bills and transact family business, and maintained an active social life in his retirement. When he went to the store, he came home with the requested items and the correct change. B.S. obtained a CADL score of 64, about 1 standard deviation above the mean for Global aphasic patients. He lived at home with his wife, she took care of the family business, and he was present in social situations but not much of a participant. He assisted around the house and yard, but he avoided contacts with tradesmen and the telephone.

Thus, we obtain a "functional" communication measure on our patients, usually the CADL, to estimate how well they might do in daily communicative encounters. As Holland (1980) observed, CADL performance correlates positively and significantly with performance on the traditional language measures. It also amplifies and extends these by showing us what a patient can and cannot do to solve problems posed by some of the situations that may be faced in environments other than ours.

Speech Measures

Few standardized measures are available for appraising apraxia of speech. Most clinicians utilize what they have collected in graduate classes, clinical practicum, suggestions in texts (Darley et al., 1975), and occasional reports (Wertz and Rosenbek, 1971). There is a similarity in these sources. Almost all suggest the use of rapid alternating articulation tasks, repetition of monosyllabic and multisyllabic words, repetition of sentences, conversation, picture description, and oral reading. An attempt to trace the sources and give credit to originators is futile. Too many have contributed. The traditional tasks, depending upon how they are used, provide a good look at a patient's speech.

One commercially available measure exists. Dabul (1979) developed the Apraxia Battery for Adults. Its purpose is to verify the presence of apraxia in adults and to give a rough estimate of its severity. Six subtests—diadochokinetic rate, increasing word length, limb apraxia and oral apraxia, latency and utterance time for polysyllabic words, repeated trials test, and inventory of articulation characteristics of apraxia—are administered. Performance is rated on a checklist of apraxic features to verify the presence or absence of apraxia of speech. Severity comes from ratings on each subtest—mild to moderate or severe to profound.

Motor speech evaluation. We use the Motor Speech Evaluation shown in Table 3. Its origins are spread throughout the literature. Our contribution, at most, was to pull a variety of tasks together and provide some general instructions. Its purpose is to identify patients we want to probe more thoroughly with oral, nonverbal tests, and articulation tests. It is a screening tool, and it usually takes less than 20 minutes to administer. We stress the need for useful data. Three steps may be required to obtain these. If a patient does not make a response that provides diagnostic information, e.g. suggests either aphasia, apraxia, or dysarthria, after the first request, we repeat. If the second response is still ambiguous, we cue, e.g., "Listen, watch me, and do what I do." Completion of the Motor Speech Evaluation should indicate what to do next, and that decision comes from useable data, not a bundle of ambiguous responses.

Scoring the Motor Speech Evaluation can be descriptive—we use "A" for apraxic productions, "P" for paraphasias, "D" for dysarthria, "U" for nondiagnostic errors, "O" for other errors, and "N" for normal responses. It can be multidimensional, e.g., utilize the PICA 16-point scale. Or, it can employ narrow or broad phonetic transcription. We are not after a score; we seek an impression about the pattern of behavior we witness.

The tasks are traditional: conversation, vowel prolongation; repetition of monosyllables /pʌ/, /tʌ/, /kʌ/; repetition of a sequence of monsyllables /pʌ-tʌ-kʌ/; repetition of multisyllabic words; multiple trials with the same word; repetition of words that increase in length; repetition of monosyllabic words that contain the same initial and final sound; repetition of sentences; counting forward and backward; picture description; repetition of sentences used volitionally to determine consistency of production; and oral reading.

Table 3.
Motor Speech Evaluation

Instructions:

These stimuli are to be recorded for patients suspected of demonstrating a motor speech disorder. Recording should be done with a standard loudness level and distance from microphone to patient. In each instance, elicit as adequate an attempt as the patient is capable of producing. Repeat ("Try it again. Say ____") and cue ("Watch me and do what I do.") all ambiguous responses. The cue for spontaneous speech is to continue asking questions. The cue for sentence imitation is to have the patient repeat one word at a time. The cue for the reading passage is to select one sentence, it does not matter which, and have the patient read each word as you point to it.

Scoring can be completed on the spot or from the tape and, depending on the purpose, can take a variety of forms:

A. *A* if apraxic, *P* if paraphasic; *D* if dysarthric; *U* if nondiagnostic error is observed; *O* if the error is other than above and specify what it seems to be, e.g., hearing. Score *N* if normal.

B. *Multidimensional.* Use the PICA multidimensional system which is appropriate for all responses except for picture description and reading.

C. *Transcription.* Broad or narrow phonetic transcription at time of sample or after.

   I. Elicit five minutes of conversational speech according to the Boston Diagnostic Aphasia Examination method (pp. 4–5 of Goodglass and Kaplan, 1972, *The Assessment of Aphasia and Related Disorders*). Be sure to ask questions about illness, hospital stay, and speech and nonspeech symptoms.

   II. "I want you to say /ɑ/ as long and evenly as you can. Like this—/ɑ/" ____.

   III. "Now, I want you to say some other sounds as long, as fast, and as evenly as you can."

     (a) "Say /pʌ-pʌ-pʌ/ as long, etc."

     _____

     (b) "Say /tʌ-tʌ-tʌ/ as long, etc."

     _____

     (c) "Say /kʌ-kʌ-kʌ/ as long, etc."

     _____

   IV. "Now, I want you to put three sounds—/pʌ/, /tʌ/, and /kʌ/—together and say /pʌ-tʌ-kʌ/ as long, as fast, and as evenly as you can. Like this, /pʌ-tʌ-kʌ, pʌ-tʌ-kʌ, pʌ-tʌ-kʌ/" etc._____"

Table 3.
(Continued)

V. "Say these words for me as well as you can. You only have to say them once."

1. gingerbread _____
2. artillery _____
3. snowman _____
4. responsibility _____
5. catastrophe _____
6. television _____
7. several _____
8. tornado _____
9. statistical analysis _____
10. Methodist Episcopal Church _____

VI. "Now I want you to say these words after I say them. Repeat each word five times." (Score each production of each word.)

1. artillery: _____ _____ _____
_____ _____ _____

2. impossibility: _____ _____ _____
_____ _____ _____

3. catastrophe: _____ _____ _____
_____ _____ _____

VII. "Now, say these words after I say them."

1. thick: _____
thicken: _____
thickening: _____
2. jab: _____
jabber: _____
jabbering: _____
3. zip: _____
zipper: _____
zippering: _____
4. please: _____
pleasing: _____
pleasingly: _____
5. flat: _____
flatter: _____
flattering: _____

VIII. "Now, these."

1. mom _____
2. judge _____
3. peep _____
4. bib _____

Table 3.
(*Continued*)

5. nine ———————————
6. tote ———————————
7. dad ———————————
8. coke ———————————
9. gag ———————————
10. fife ———————————
11. sis ———————————
12. zoos ———————————
13. church ———————————
14. lull ———————————
15. shush ———————————
16. roar ———————————

IX. "Say these sentences after me." (Cue is to give one word at a time with strong visual cue.)

1. The valuable watch was missing. ———————————

2. In the summer they sell vegetables. ———————————

3. The shipwreck washed up on the shore. ———————————

4. Please put the groceries in the refrigerator. ———————————

X. "Count from one to twenty."

1. ————	8. ————	15. ————
2. ————	9. ————	16. ————
3. ————	10. ————	17. ————
4. ————	11. ————	18. ————
5. ————	12. ————	19. ————
6. ————	13. ————	20. ————
7. ————	14. ————	

"Now, backwards, twenty down to one."

20. ————	13. ————	6. ————
19. ————	12. ————	5. ————
18. ————	11. ————	4. ————
17. ————	10. ————	3. ————
16. ————	9. ————	2. ————
15. ————	8. ————	1. ————
14. ————	7. ————	

XI. "Tell me what is happening in this picture." (Elicit at least one minute of picture description from the *Boston Diagnostic Aphasia Examination* "Cookie Thief" picture).

Table 3.
(*Continued*)

XII. "Repeat these sentences after me." (Use any four sentences the patient
     used spontaneously at any point in the evaluation. Write or transcribe the
     original (O) and the repetition (R).)

   1. O: _____
      R: _____
   2. O: _____
      R: _____
   3. O: _____
      R: _____
   4. O: _____
      R: _____

XIII. "Now, read this passage out loud." (Have the patient read the "Grandfather
      Passage." Write or transcribe errors that may have diagnositc importance.)

Summary

Diagnosis	Absent	Present	Suspected	Undetermined
Normal				
Aphasia				
Apraxia of speech				
Dysarthria (specify type)				
Language of confusion				
Language of generalized intellectual impairment				
Voice disorder (specify)				
Other (specify)				

Adapted from Rosenbek & Wertz, 1976.

Generally, we expect apraxic patients to reveal their deficit in conversation by producing apraxic articulatory errors and abnormal prosody.
Unless patients have an apraxia for phonation or are extremely severe,
they should have little difficulty with vowel prolongation and repeating
single monosyllables. When required to produce the sequence /pʌ-tʌ-kʌ/,

their apraxia of speech should show itself by initiation difficulty; substitution, omission, or rearrangement of the syllables; slow rate; equal and even stress; and stops, starts, and reattempts to produce the sequence. The multisyllabic words and short phrases should reveal apraxia of speech if it is present, because they are multisyllabic and contain sounds and clusters that are difficult for apraxic patients. Repeated trials on the same word may show inconsistent articulatory errors and a combination of correct and incorrect productions among the five attempts. Words of increasing length may show more errors on longer words than shorter words. Monosyllabic words that begin and end with the same sound may show more errors in the initial position than in the final position; however, some apraxic patients make more errors in the final position and others show no difference. Sentences are loaded with multisyllabic words and sounds believed to be difficult for apraxic patients. In addition, abnormal prosody not seen on single words may surface in sentence repetition. Having the patient count forward and backward contrasts automatic speech, counting forward, with volitional speech, counting backward. Apraxic patients should display more errors on the latter, but this task can be contaminated by coexisting aphasia or cognitive impairment. Picture description, like conversation, requires volitional speech and can be contrasted with repetition tasks. Apraxic patients should reveal articulatory and prosodic disturbance when describing pictures. Having the patient repeat sentences he produced volitionally sometime during the evaluation checks consistency. We expect apraxic patients to be inconsistent, and this task may separate the apraxic patient from the one with conduction aphasia. In addition, oral reading of phonetically balanced material, such as the "Grandfather Passage," taps most of the sounds contained in English and permits comparison of speech in oral reading with speech on repetition tasks and more volitional, purposive tasks.

We summarize performance by checking the absent, present, suspected, and undetermined boxes for the possible diagnoses—normal language, aphasia, apraxia, dysarthria, language of confusion, language of generalized intellectual deficit, voice disorder, or other. Our summary should suggest the next step in appraisal.

If the Motor Speech Evaluation confirms or increases our suspicion that the patient is apraxic, we employ one or more of the articulation tests listed in Table 2 to collect an inventory of which sounds are most often produced incorrectly and in which contexts. Doing this begins to satisfy one of appraisal's purposes, focusing treatment. If we elect to treat, we want to know where to begin. Articulation tests assist in developing a hierarchy of difficulty.

Sound by position tests.   Articulation errors revealed on the Motor Speech Evaluation and the articulation tests are probed further by the Sound by Position Test suggested by Rosenbek (1978). Table 4 shows how

Table 4.
Sound-by-Position Tests. Selected Stimuli are Evaluated By Having the Patient
Repeat Consonants in Initial, Medial, and Final Positions

Initial	Final	Medial
pæt	tæp	ʌ pæt
pɑd	dɑp	ʌ pɑd
pik	kip	ʌ pik
bæt	tæb	ʌ bæt
bɛd	dɛb	ʌ bɛd
bɪf	fɪb	ʌ bɪf
tɪn	nɪt	ʌ tɪn
tʌb	bʌt	ʌ tʌb
teɪm	meɪt	ʌ teɪm
dip	pid	ʌ dip
dɛn	nɛd	ʌ dɛn
dɑk	kɑd	ʌ dɑk
kʌm	mʌk	ʌ kʌm
koUt	toUk	ʌ koUt
kɑn	nɑk	ʌ kɑn
guf	fug	ʌ guf
gʌt	tʌg	ʌ gʌt
gɑt	tɑg	ʌ gɑt

Adapted from Rosenbek, 1978.

selected stimuli are placed in the initial, medical, and final positions in real
and nonsense words to determine accuracy and consistency. We are looking for possible treatment targets. The patient who produces a sound
correctly in at least one position in a word, we believe, is telling us that
sound is more amenable to treatment than one that is not produced correctly in any context. Table 4 shows manipulation of stop-consonants.
These are examples; other sounds or clusters can be evaluated in a similar
manner.

Stimulus modes. Evaluating the influence of stimulus modes may be
a part of appraisal, or it may wait until diagnosis is made and treatment is
about to begin. It does not matter when the influence of stimulus mode is
determined, but it needs to be done sometime.

We look to see whether our patients' productions are better or worse
when the same words are produced in a variety of conditions. We have

them name pictures, repeat the names after we say them, and read the names. Apraxic patients may vary. Some may read better than they repeat or name. Others are skilled repeaters and lousy namers and readers. We want to know what a patient does best, and what is more difficult. It assists in focusing treatment. It tells us how one stimulus mode can evoke success, and how another can make the task more difficult when the patient is ready to be pushed.

Collins et al. (1980) used four conditions—masking, reading, silent rehearsal, and aloud rehearsal—in an attempt to differentiate among three patients with similar but not identical motor speech programming disorders. Their results suggest that the use of different stimulus modes may be diagnostic and may assist in differentiating among apraxic patients to sort the "for sures" from the "kind ofs" and the "who knows."

Determining severity.   One of appraisal's purposes is to determine severity. This must be separated from diagnosis. We do not know of an appraisal measure that yields a score that indicates that one patient is apraxic and another is not. Diagnosis comes from observing whether a pattern of behavior is present or not. Nevertheless, we do want to estimate severity, because it may have prognostic importance, and it provides a baseline for evaluating efficacy if we elect to treat.

We have mentioned several approaches for estimating the severity of apraxia of speech. Dabul (1979) uses a 3-point system—0, 1, 2—and a summary to rate apraxia as mild to moderate or severe to profound. The PICA 16-point multidimensional system was listed as an alternative in the Motor Speech Evaluation. However, the PICA system may not differentiate between aphasic and apraxic errors, e.g., a self-correction (10) could be "fork, no knife" or "knipe, no knife" in a patient's attempt to say "knife." Similarly, we do not know whether a related response (7) on the same task results from saying "fork" or "knipe."

Collins et al. (1980) have developed a 14-point multidimensional system, shown in Table 5, that eliminates ambiguity. They offer it as a "scale of goodness" for rating severity in apraxic patients. It has the virtue of elaborating responses with descriptive anchors, and thus preserves information lost in a plus or minus system or a numerical rating scale. It differentiates apraxic errors from paraphasic errors. It also taps a variety of behaviors that typify apraxia of speech—delay; prosodic disturbance; distortion; self-correction; groping; and articulatory errors, including substitutions, omissions, and additions. Its refinement may provide one of our unmet needs.

The traditional 7-point severity scale has been popular in rating the overall severity of apraxia of speech (Rosenbek & Merson, 1971; Wertz et al., 1978; Wertz et al., 1981). Using 1 to indicate mild and 7 to indicate severe has resulted in reliable inter- and intrajudge agreement. Sometimes,

Table 5.
Multidimensional Scoring System to Determine Severity in Apraxic Patients

Score	Description
14	Normal
13	Normal, except slow because of changes in articulation and/or pause time
12	Normal, except for prosodic disturbance (pitch, loudness, stress, effort)
11	Distortion
10	Distortion and prosodic disturbance
9	Self-correction
8	Self-correction except for prosodic disturbance
7	Self-correction except for distortion
6	Groping which does not cross phoneme boundaries and which is followed by the correct response
5	Sound substitution(s), omission(s), or addition(s), without sound distortion(s) or prosodic disturbances, but may have mild to moderate changes in articulation and/or pause time. Word remains recognizable
4	Sound substitution(s), omission(s), or addition(s) with distortion(s) or prosodic disturbances. Word remains recognizable
3	As in 5 above except word is unrecognizable
2	As in 4 above except word is unrecognizable
1	No response; or rejection; or unintelligible, undifferentiated response

Adapted from Collins et al., 1980.

the ends of the scale are expanded, and 0 is used to signify no deficit, 8 to indicate no scorable response, and 9 to state undetermined.

Rosenbek and Merson (1971) reported that the use of a 7-point severity scale correlated significantly with the total number of articulation errors made by apraxic patients. They used six imitative and three spontaneous tasks and rated "phonemic" errors—additions, omissions, substitutions, distortions, repetitions, prolongations—and "nonphonemic" errors—pause, audible groping, unintelligible, totally off target, rejections. Combined nonphonemic errors correlated +.76 with overall severity rated on the 7-point scale and yielded a coefficient for predicting severity of .57. Adding phonemic errors increased the correlation to +.94 and the coefficient of prediction to .89. Rosenbek and Merson suggest that a patient's total nonphonemic errors are the best predictor of overall severity, and that repeating polysyllabic words and sentences are the most useful tasks.

Patient data. Table 6 summarizes performance on the Motor Speech Evaluation for our three patients. P.M. and J.D. reveal the presence of apraxia of speech. B.S.'s performance increased our suspicion that he was apraxic.

P.M. had no difficulty with vowel prolongation, repeating monosyllables, or repeating monosyllabic words. His conversation, picture description, and oral reading revealed frequent articulation errors, usually substitutions he was able to correct, and abnormal prosody. Repeating the monosyllabic sequence /pʌ-tʌ-kʌ/ he was slow, and he moved cautiously across the syllables in the sequence. Similar behavior was seen in counting backward. Multisyllabic word and sentence repetition evoked substitution errors and abnormal prosody. The Templin–Darley Sentence Test of Articulation (Templin & Darley, 1960) revealed correct production of all singleton consonants in all positions tested except /dʒ/ and /j/. Clusters, /pr/, /pl/, /sk/, /spl/, /str/, and /skw/, were incorrect. Tested in the sound-by-position format, all were produced correctly at least once in at least one position. P.M. repeated better than he read aloud or spoke spontaneously. His overall severity was rated 2 on the 7-point scale.

J.D. carried the additional burden of significant aphasia along with his load of apraxia of speech. Vowel prolongation and repeating monosyllables were normal except for a slow rate on /kʌ/. Attempts at /pʌ-tʌ-kʌ/ yielded inconsistent sequencing errors across trials. Conversation, picture description, and oral reading were agrammatic and included a wealth of substitution errors and flagrant prosodic disturbances. Repeating multisyllabic words and sentences showed articulatory and prosodic deficits. Monosyllabic word repetition was better, and infrequent errors were self-corrected. Repeated trials were inconsistent in the errors produced, and none of the words tested was correct in any of the repeated attempts. Counting forward was correct, but slow. Counting backward required prompting to keep things moving. Repeating words of increasing length yielded more errors on longer words, and repeating sentences produced spontaneously showed consistent agrammatism but inconsistent articulatory errors. Because of reading deficits, we had J.D. repeat the Templin–Darley Articulation Test stimuli. Inconsistent errors were seen on /k/, /g/, /f/, /Θ/, /ʃ/, and /j/. Consistent errors were seen on /tʃ/, /dʒ/, and all blends. Plosives placed in the sound-by-position format revealed inconsistent errors across positions, but each sound tested was produced correctly, at least once, in some position. He repeated better than he read aloud or spoke volitionally. J.D. was rated 4 on the 7-point severity scale.

B.S. was globally aphasic as well as (we suspected) severely apraxic.

Table 6.

Results of the Motor Speech Evaluation on Three Patients Suspected of Suffering Apraxia of Speech

Measure	Patient Performance		
	P.M.	J.D.	B.S.
Conversation	Articulation errors; prosodic deficit	Articulation errors; prosodic deficit; agrammatic	No conversation elicited
Vowel prolongation	Normal	Normal	Normal
Repeating monosyllables	Normal	Normal, but slow on /kʌ/	Initiation difficulty
Repeating monosyllabic sequence	Slow	Slow, inconsistent errors in sequencing	Rejected
Repeating multisyllabic words	Self-corrected errors	Frequent articulatory errors	Rejected
Multiple trials	Inconsistent errors, self-corrected	Inconsistent errors, no correct productions	Rejected
Words of increasing length	More errors on longer words, most were self-corrected	More errors on longer words	Errors on monosyllabic words, longer words rejected
Repeating monosyllabic words	Normal	Infrequent errors, self-corrected	Frequent articulatory errors
Repeating sentences	Errors self-corrected; prosodic deficits	Frequent errors; words omitted	Rejected
Counting forward and backward	Normal forward, slow backward	Slow forward, backward required prompts	Prompts necessary forward, backward rejected
Picture description	Normal syntax; self-corrected errors; prosodic deficit	Sparse; agrammatism; frequent articulatory errors; prosodic deficit	Rejected

Table 6.
(*Continued*)

Measure	Patient Performance		
	P.M.	J.D.	B.S.
Repeating sentences produced	Prosodic deficit; inconsistent errors, self-corrected	Inconsistent errors; prosodic disturbance	Not tested, no sentences produced
Oral reading	Prosodic deficit; most articulatory errors self-corrected	Numerous reading and articulatory errors; omission of words; prosodic deficit	Rejected
SUMMARY	Apraxia of Speech	Aphasia and Apraxia of Speech	Severe Aphasia; Severe Apraxia of Speech Suspected

Most tasks on the Motor Speech Evaluation were rejected. Vowel prolongation was normal. We got a few /pʌ/s with repeated trials and a /tʌ/ or two. He repeated a few monosyllabic words correctly, but most were produced with substitutions in the initial position. He counted forward with so many prompts that it became a repetition task. Repetition of the Templin-Darley Articulation Test words indicated that vowels were intact if we were liberal on rating distortions; all clusters were incorrect; and accuracy was inconsistent on most singletons. Not one was error-free on repeated trials. B.S. repeated better than he read aloud or spoke volitionally, and he did not do the former with much accuracy. Sound-by-position testing with plosives showed errors on all sounds in one of the positions. Bilabials were more robust than alveolars and palatals, and medial and final positions yielded more success than the initial position. We rated B.S. 6 on the 7-point severity scale.

Oral, Nonverbal Movement

We appraise our patient's ability to make oral nonverbal movements to determine the presence of significant paralysis, paresis, or oral apraxia. The measures include an oral, peripheral examination; a test of isolated oral movements; and a test of oral motor sequencing.

Significant weakness, slowness, and dyscoordination can affect articulation. The result is usually one of the dysarthrias. However, slowness characterizes some movements of some apraxic speakers. Fromm et al. (1982) observed dyscoordination in their instrumental evaluation of apraxia of speech. Research, we hope, will eventually tell us if slowness and dyscoordination in apraxia and dysarthria differ. In an attempt to differentiate apraxia of speech from dysarthria, we lay on the hands, make requests to move structures, and observe. Facial, mandibular, tongue, palatopharyngeal, and laryngeal muscles are assessed. If we detect significant slowness, weakness, or dyscoordination, we probe further to determine whether these result from apraxia or dysarthria.

Sources for oral, nonverbal movement tasks are several. Dabul (1979) offers a few. DeRenzi et al. (1966) list their battery. The BDAE (Goodglass & Kaplan, 1972), Western Aphasia Battery (Kertesz, 1982), and Minnesota Test for Differential Diagnosis of Aphasia (Schuell, 1956b) contain tasks for assessing oral agility. Probably the most complete evaluation of oral, nonverbal movement was offered by Moore et al. (1976). Fourteen oral gestures were appraised in four stimulus conditions and two response modes. Performance was rated with two evaluation systems. We have listed some of their tasks plus a few of our favorites in Table 7.

We use the same three-step approach suggested in the Motor Speech Evaluation in an attempt to collect useful data—request; repeat; cue, "Listen, watch me, do what I do." Performance can be rated right or wrong or with any number of scales or scoring systems. Usually, the former suffices, especially if the need for a repeat or cue is indicated. We note whether the patient uses a hand to assist in making the oral gestures, e.g., guides his tongue with his fingers; verbalizes the request rather than making the response, e.g., says "cough" when requested to produce a cough; or displays groping movements in his effort to comply. We look for signs of weakness, slowness, and dyscoordination that may have escaped notice on the oral peripheral examination, and we look for the presence of oral, nonverbal apraxia. The former may have diagnostic importance, and the latter may have prognostic and therapeutic implications.

Added to the test of isolated oral movement is one of oral motor sequencing. Some patients may show no difficulty in making a single movement, but when required to put two or more oral, nonverbal movements together in a sequence, they omit, substitute, or rearrange the sequence. The oral motor sequencing tasks shown in Table 7 are taken from LaPointe and Wertz (1974). They constitute a sufficient sample to search for what we seek. The format (request, repeat, cue) and scoring system can be similar to that used for testing isolated oral movements; however, one might want to note which and how many movements were made and whether the sequence was complete but rearranged.

None of our three example patients displayed significant paralysis or paresis of the oral musculature. P.M. had no difficulty on the isolated oral movements tasks. He completed all oral motor sequencing tasks, but he required repeats for the two 5-step sequences. We concluded that he did not display oral, nonverbal apraxia. J.D. made all of the movements required in the isolated oral movement tasks, but he requested repeated

Table 7.
Tests of Isolated Oral Movement* and Oral Motor Sequencing†

Isolated Oral Movement

Instructions: I want you to make some movements with your lips, tongue, and jaw. Listen carefully and do just what I ask.

1. Stick out your tongue.
2. Try to touch your nose with your tongue.
3. Try to touch your chin with your tongue.
4. Bite your lower lip.
5. Pucker your lips.
6. Puff out your cheeks.
7. Show me your teeth.
8. Click your teeth together.
9. Wag your tongue from side to side.
10. Clear your throat.
11. Cough.
12. Whistle.
13. Show that you are cold by making your teeth chatter.
14. Smile.
15. Show me how you would kiss a baby.
16. Lick your lips.

Oral Motor Sequencing

Instructions: Now, I want you to put some movements together. Watch me and do what I do.

1. Tongue (touch upper lip center)—Jaw (lower and raise)
2. Teeth (click once)—Lips (pucker)

Table 7.
(*Continued*)

---

3. Jaw (lower and raise)—Teeth (bite lower lip)—Lips (show teeth)

4. Tongue (touch lower lip center)—Lips (pucker)—Tongue (lick lips)

5. Lips (show teeth)—Teeth (bite lower lip)—Jaw (lower and raise)—
   Tongue (lick lips)

6. Cheeks (puff out)—Lips (pucker)—Jaw (lower and raise)—Tongue (lick
   lips)

7. Teeth (click once)—Lips (pucker)—Jaw (lower and raise)—Tongue
   (lick lips)—Teeth (bite lower lip)

8. Lips (pucker)—Tongue (lick lips)—Teeth (click once)—Cheeks (puff
   out)—Tongue (touch upper lip center)

---

*Adapted from Moore et al., 1976.
†Adapted from Lapointe & Wertz, 1974.

instructions on five of these. He produced both of the three-step oral motor sequences, but he could not produce any of the four- and five-step sequences after five trials on each. We think we exceeded his memory and not his oral motor sequential ability. We concluded that he had no significant oral, nonverbal apraxia. B.S. required a repeat and cue on every isolated oral movement task. Even with the additional help, he produced only four oral gestures correctly. Oral groping, use of his fingers to guide his tongue and lips, and aborted attempts at the task implied that we were seeing inability to make volitional oral movements and not a lack of auditory comprehension of our requests. We stopped oral motor sequencing testing after five failures on each of the two-step sequences. We concluded that B.S. displayed moderate to severe oral, nonverbal apraxia.

Limb Movements

We appraise our patients' ability to make volitional limb gestures to detect the presence of limb apraxia and to determine candidacy for a treatment we call intersystemic reorganization—the use of meaningful gestures to improve verbal performance. Again, tests of limb apraxia can be found in a variety of sources (Dabul, 1979; Goodglass & Kaplan, 1972; Kertesz, 1982).

Our patients are appraised with the gestures listed in Table 8. These are taken from the Mayo Clinic Procedures for Language Evaluation (unpublished). We use the same three-step procedure, if necessary (request; repeat; cue, "Listen. Watch me and do what I do.") to collect

Table 8.
Tests to Determine the Presence of Limb Apraxia.

Instructions: I want to see how you use your hands and arms to make some gestures. Listen carefully and do just what I ask.

1. Show how an accordian works.

2. Show me how you salute.

3. Wave goodbye.

4. Threaten someone with your hand.

5. Show that you are hungry.

6. Thumb your nose at someone.

7. Snap your fingers.

8. Show how you would play a piano.

9. Indicate that someone is crazy.

10. Make the letter "O" with your fingers.

Adapted from the Mayo Clinic Procedures for Language Evaluation, unpublished.

useful data. Scoring can be pass–fail, multidimensional, or on a rating scale. A 3-point scale, e.g., 2 for accurate and immediate gestures; 1 for accurate but delayed gestures or an acceptable overall pattern with defective amplitude, accuracy, force, or speed; 0 for partial, perseverative, irrelevant, or no gesture, is useful. We test the patient's preferred hand or, if there is hemiplegia, the noninvolved hand.

P.M. produced all gestures correctly, and we concluded that he was free of limb apraxia. J.D. produced all gestures correctly, but he required repeated instructions on two of the ten tasks. His performance suggested no limb apraxia. B.S. required repeats and cues on all tasks. Given these, he performed correctly, and we did not suspect the presence of significant limb apraxia.

Intelligence

We want some indication of our patients' intellectual level. Our sources are the patient's family—their estimate of his premorbid intelligence and whether or not that has changed since onset; the measures collected by psychology or neuropsychology; and those that we administer. Our purpose is to determine whether a patient can assist in solving some of the problems brought about by the brain damage; develop strategies; develop alternative solutions when one attempt fails; reduce uncertainty when faced with ambiguity; or learn.

In Table 2, we list the Coloured Progressive Matrices (CPM) (Raven, 1962) as a suggested measure of intelligence. It has the advantage of being, for the most part, nonverbal; thus a brain-damaged-patient's performance is not contaminated too much by his or her language deficit. Raven (1962) describes the CPM as a test of nonverbal visual thinking. The patient is required to select one of six alternatives to complete a pattern that has a piece missing. Three sets of 12 problems permit a possible total score of 36. Comparision of CPM performance with language or apraxic deficits seldom yields a significant correlation. We think it is a measure of premorbid intellect filtered through the restrictions imposed by brain damage.

P.M. was correct on 26 of the 36 CPM problems. This placed him at the 30th percentile for normals and the 60th percentile for aphasic patients on norms developed by Wertz and Lemme (1972). His performance was consistent with his family's estimate of normal premorbid intelligence. J.D. obtained a total score of 29. This placed him between the 40th and 50th percentiles for normals and between the 70th and 80th percentiles for aphasic patients. His performance matched his wife's estimate of normal premorbid intelligence. B.S., the most severely aphasic and apraxic of the three patients, obtained the best score on the CPM. His total score of 31 placed him between the 50th and 60th percentiles for normals and at the 80th percentile for aphasic patients. His performance corresponds with his wife's estimate of average to above average premorbid intelligence.

Supplementary Tests

If time permits, we administer the Token Test (DeRenzi & Vignolo, 1962) to obtain additional information about our patient's auditory comprehension and the Reading Comprehension Battery for Aphasia (LaPointe & Horner, 1979) to tell us more about reading strengths and deficits.

The Token Test exists in a variety of forms. It was developed by DeRenzi and Vignolo (1962) as a sensitive test for aphasia to detect auditory comprehension deficits that may be missed on the more comprehensive language tests. Twenty tokens that differ in three dimensions—color, shape, size—are used to test a patient's comprehension of auditory stimuli that gradually increase in length and complexity. The DeRenzi and Vignolo version contains five parts. The first four use ten commands in each part to increase the length of the auditory stimulus. Part V contains 21 commands that manipulate the grammatical complexity of the auditory stimulus. Thus, a total possible score is 61. Performance is rated correct or incorrect on each item. Wertz and Lemme (1972) have provided normative data.

Other versions of the token test exist. Spreen and Benton (1969) have included a modified Token Test in the Neurosensory Center Comprehensive Examination for Aphasia. Thirty-nine items, adapted from the DeRenzi and Vignolo test, are scored to give credit for each part of a command a patient performs correctly. A total score of 163 is possible. Norms for normal and aphasic performance are provided. McNeil and Prescott (1978) developed the Revised Token Test to provide a more systematic appraisal of auditory comprehension than is contained in earlier versions. Length and complexity are systematically manipulated across ten subtests. Performance is scored on a 15-point multidimensional scale.

Our three patients were tested with the DeRenzi and Vignolo (1962) Token Test. P.M. made no errors on the 61-item test. His performance placed him above the 90th percentile for both normal adults and aphasic patients. J.D. was correct on 45 items. His performance placed him at the 80th percentile for aphasic patients and below the 10th percentile for normals. B.S. was correct on 12 items. His performance placed him between the 20th and 30th percentiles for aphasic patients and below the 10th percentile for normals.

LaPointe and Horner's (1979) Reading Comprehension Battery for Aphasia (RCBA) provides a systematic evaluation of reading behavior in brain-damaged adults. Ten subtests sample visual, auditory, and semantic confusions in reading single words; functional reading; synonyms; sentence comprehension; short paragraph comprehension; factual and inferential comprehension of paragraphs; and morpho-syntactic reading. Scoring for the 100 items is plus or minus. The test amplifies reading subtests contained in comprehensive measures of language.

P.M. obtained a total score of 99, indicating that his reading ability was within normal limits. J.D.'s total score was 80. The most difficult subtests for him were paragraph reading and morpho-syntax. B.S. obtained a total score of 40. Beyond the single-word level, he found reading close to impossible.

Other Measures

There are other things one might do to appraise apraxia of speech. Some depend upon the resources available and the training of the appraiser. Patients' utterances can be recorded and submitted to acoustic analysis. Spectrograms can be made and analyzed. Kent and Rosenbek (1982, 1983) have demonstrated that spectrographic analyses of apraxic speech show what the ear captures, explain some of what the ear finds confusing, and reveal some of what the ear misses. Similarly, utilization of physiologic instrumentation—EMGs; measures of respiration; movement transducers, accelerometers, etc.—provide a look at behavior that may be apraxic. Presently, both acoustic and physiologic appraisal of patients reside in the realm of research and are not commonly employed in most clinics. As we learn more and more about what they can provide, their use will probably migrate from the laboratory into the clinic.

Most clinicians can, and some do (Deutsch, 1981; Rosenbek et al., 1973b) appraise oral sensation and perception. These measures, usually oral form identification and 2-point discrimination, require a minimum of training and equipment. Because they are quite expensive in terms of clinician and patient time, we do not employ them routinely. Seldom do they provide the missing piece of evidence that tells us whether a patient is apraxic or not.

Finally, there are behaviors that are noted but not measured. One can look for signs of a patient's awareness, motivation, frustration, and coping strategies. These may have prognostic relevance. The patient who is aware of errors and hungry to do something about them, uses frustration to seek solutions rather than blue the air, and develops coping strategies to solve problems rather than create them will find prognosis smiles rather than frowns. When English reveals itself to patients in all of its unutterable irrelevances, it helps if they can view their efforts as risible, at least at times, and not revolting.

Some have become enamored with apraxia of speech and find it in every patient appraised. We caution against this, because it is incorrect. All brain-damaged patients are not apraxic. One of appraisal's purposes is to segregate. Another is to determine what coexists. For example, aphasia does not live on a separate planet that does not share the same orbit with apraxia of speech. Being spoony about apraxia of speech should not influence appraisal, because, if it does, it will influence diagnosis. Appraisal should be designed to reveal and not conceal.

DIAGNOSIS

Appraisal provides the data, but as Rosenbek and LaPointe (1981) have observed, "the data are not the diagnosis" (p. 168). Apraxia of speech is not recognized by a single test or a battery of tests. Diagnosis comes from identifying a specific pattern of speech behavior that meets criteria established to recognize its presence.

One cannot wish a diagnosis. If you only say the word, you are destined to listen to the silence of nothing happening. Thus, diagnosis is not magical. Calling it that amounts to admitting that you do not know how it is done. Diagnosis takes effort, experience, and knowledge. To be good at it, the clinician needs to say, "I like to diagnose!" with the same conviction and dedication as he or she might muster when saying, "I like to breathe."

Not all patients receive a diagnosis, at least not right away. Some are easy. They bite you on the nose and make you see their diagnosis. In others, diagnosis is made with comfort but not total conviction. Yet others do not reveal the missing link; the one that perhaps is there within reach but not quite identifiable. It is like looking for your glasses when they are on the tip of your nose. To find the link, one may begin with diagnostic therapy. Sometimes, there is a decision, but it is just that the clinician does not make it. Treatment gradually evolves into that most appropriate for apraxia of speech, because that is what is most appropriate for the patient. We try to avoid wandering this path, but it does happen.

Diagnosis has a single purpose: put a label on the problem. One attempts to differentiate what the patient has from other disorders he or she might have but does not have. Or, one attempts to identify the presence of coexisting disorders. Because diagnosis implies prognosis and the appropriate management, we attempt to be specific. We avoid statements that resemble those that flow from some bureaucratic minds, "proposed possible preliminary outline of suggested alternative considerations for a conceivable tentative recommendation." We use the biographical, medical, and behavioral data collected; compare threse with what we know constitutes apraxia of speech; and state our conclusion. In most patients, the statement will be, "no evidence of apraxia of speech," or "apraxia of speech," modified with an adjective—mild, moderate, marked, severe—indicating severity, "coexisting with" (insert the appropriate adjective indicating severity) "aphasia."

Differentiating Apraxia of Speech From What It May Masquerade As

The errors one can make in diagnosing apraxia of speech are, of course, two, saying that it is present when it is not or saying that it is not present when it is. Typically, the probability of an error increases when distinguishing between apraxia and aphasia or apraxia and dysarthria. But, because some (Hornstein, 1971) identify apraxia in demented patients or those suffering the language of confusion, these disorders must be either ruled out or identified as coexisting.

Apraxia versus Language of Confusion

The language of confusion has been described by Darley (1969) as reduced recognition and understanding of and responsiveness to the environment, faulty memory, unclear thinking, and disorientation in time and space. Structured language tests usually evoke normal syntax and word finding. But, if the patient is permitted to wander, he may confabulate and provide irrelevant responses. Confusion often results from trauma. The brain damage is typically diffuse and bilateral, and the duration of symptoms is transient. If confusion persists, one may suspect dementia.

Thus, the language of confusion separates itself from apraxia of speech by its localization—bilateral and diffuse as opposed to unilateral and focal—and its duration—transient as opposed to persisting. Furthermore, as shown in Table 9 and Figure 4, Halpern et al. (1973) demostrated that apraxic patients and language of confusion patients can be differentiated on the basis of fluency and relevance errors. Apraxic patients make a large number of fluency errors and few relevance errors. The reverse is seen in the language of confusion: few fluency errors and an abundance of relevance errors. Additional characteristics that differentiate between the two disorders are syntax, frequent errors in apraxia compared with performance on other tasks, and few errors in confusion compared with performance on other tasks, and reading comprehension and writing to dictation, fewer errors in apraxia than in confusion. Based upon the performance of the two groups on speech and language measures, we can separate one from the other, and we seldom confuse apraxia of speech with the language of confusion.

Apraxia versus Language of Generalized Intellectual Impairment

The language of generalized intellectual impairment, seen in dementia, has been described by Darley (1969) as deterioration of performance on more difficult language tasks; reduced efficiency in all language modalities; and greater impairment on language tasks requiring better retention, closer attention, and powers of abstraction and generalization. The severity of language impairment is approximately the same as the severity of impairment in other mental functions. Brain damage usually results from cortical atrophy, as seen in Alzheimer's disease, or from multiple cerebral infarcts. Thus, localization is bilateral and diffuse.

Like the language of confusion, the language of generalized intellectual impairment can be differentiated from apraxia of speech by its localization—bilateral and diffuse. In addition, it has a different rapidity of onset. Dementia evolves slowly, and the exact date of onset is difficult to determine. Conversely, apraxia of speech has a rapid onset, and the date can be set with precision—whenever the CVA, trauma, or surgery occurred.

Behavioral deficits differ in the two disorders. Table 10 and Figure 5 show the salient characteristics to be fluency, syntax, and reading comprehension. Compared with performance on other tasks, apraxic patients make a large number of fluency and syntax errors. Patients with the language of generalized intellectual impairment make very few. Reading comprehension is difficult for the intellectually impaired. It is less difficult for the apraxic patient. Differentiating apraxia of speech from the language of generalized intellectual impairment, usually, is not difficult. Bayles (1982) reports that disruption of phonology is seen only in the very severely demented patient. It is the primary problem in apraxia of speech, regardless of severity.

Table 9.
Rank Order of the Percentage of Impairment on Ten Measures of Speech, Language, and Arithmetic for Language of Confusion Patients and Apraxia of Speech Patients*

Rank Order	Language of Confusion†		Apraxia of Speech†	
	Task	%	Task	%
1	Arithmetic	54	Adequacy	30
2	READING COMPREHENSION	47	FLUENCY	22
3	WRITING TO DICTATION	44	Arithmetic	21
4	RELEVANCE	40	SYNTAX	20
5	Adequacy	28		
5½			Auditory Comprehension	13
			WRITING TO DICTATION	13
6	Auditory Comprehension	24		
7	SYNTAX	21	Auditory Retention	11
8	Naming	19	Naming	7
9	Auditory Retention	17	READING COMPREHENSION	6
10	FLUENCY	14	RELEVANCE	2
Mean		28		14

*Adapted from Halpern et al., 1973.
†Measures in capital letters tend to differentiate the two groups.

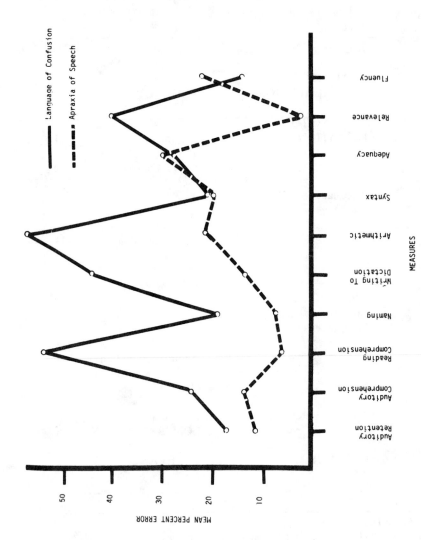

Figure 4. Comparison of language of confusion patients and apraxia of speech patients on ten measures of speech, language, and arithmetic. Overall mean percent error for language of confusion patients is 28% and for apraxia of speech patients is 14%. (Adapted from Halpern et al, 1973.)

Table 10.
Rank Order of the Percentage of Impairment on Ten Measures of Speech, Language, and Arithmetic for Generalized Intellectual Impairment and Apraxia of Speech Patients*

Rank Order	Generalized Intellectual Impairment†		Apraxia of Speech†	
	Task	%	Task	%
1	Adequacy	45	Adequacy	30
2	READING COMPREHENSION	41	FLUENCY	22
3	Arithmetic	40	Arithmetic	21
4	Auditory Comprehension	29	SYNTAX	20
5	Auditory Retention	18		
5½			Auditory Comprehension	13
			Writing to Dictation	13
6	Naming	16		
7	SYNTAX	11	Auditory Retention	11
8			Naming	7
8½	Relevance	10		
	Writing to Dictation	10		
9			READING COMPREHENSION	6
10	FLUENCY	9	Relevance	2
Mean		22		14

*Adapted from Halpern et al., 1973.
†Measures in capital letters tend to differentiate the two groups.

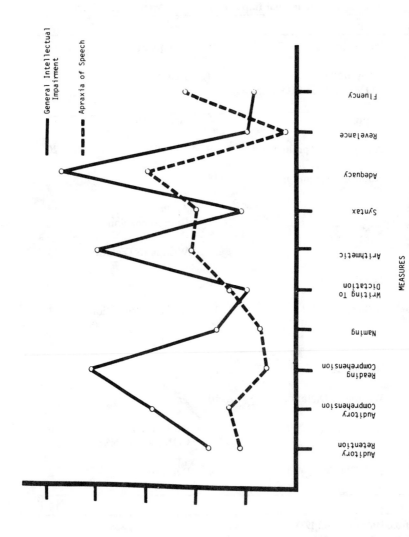

Figure 5. Comparison of generalized intellectual impairment patients and apraxia of speech patients on ten measures of speech, language, and arithmetic. Overall mean percent error for generalized intellectual impairment patients is 22% and for apraxia of speech patients is 14%. (Adapted from Halpern et al., 1973.)

Apraxia versus Aphasia

The task in differentiating apraxia of speech from aphasia is twofold. First, there is a need to determine whether apraxia is present or absent. Second, when the two coexist, there is a need to identify the presence of both and determine how the symptoms of each interact. Apraxia of speech is not more or less aphasia. It is other than aphasia. There is also a mutually inhibitive relationship between apraxia of speech and aphasia. The association is harmful to one or the other or both.

As shown in Table 11 and Figure 6, Halpern et al. (1973) have listed characteristics that may differentiate apraxia of speech from aphasia. The salient characteristics are auditory retention, fluency, syntax, writing to dictation, and naming. Their sample of aphasic patients made an abundance of errors on auditory retention tasks. Their sample of apraxic patients made very few. Similarly, naming was more difficult for aphasic patients than for apraxic patients. The other three characteristics must be examined on the basis of their rank order of difficulty. Apraxic patients made fewer errors than aphasic patients on fluency, syntax, and writing to dictation. However, fluency and syntax accounted for more of the total errors in apraxic patients' performance than in the aphasic patients' performance. Thus, fluency and syntax errors typified performance in apraxia of speech but not in aphasia. Similarly, while errors in writing to dictation were fewer in apraxic patients, they were ranked fifth in severity and characterized apraxic performance more than they characterized aphasia, where they ranked ninth.

Using the above approach permitted Halpern et al. to differentiate between aphasia and apraxia of speech. However, severity in their apraxic patients, 14%, was much milder than in their aphasic group, 31%. In addition, little attention was given to coexisting aphasia in their apraxic sample. Errors in adequacy, auditory comprehension, writing to dictation, auditory retention, naming, and reading comprehension imply that the Halpern et al. apraxic patients were also aphasic. Differentiating between apraxic patients and aphasic patients, therefore, may be difficult when coexisting aphasia in an apraxic patient is more pronounced. Rosenbek (1978) has observed that any time severe aphasia is present, apraxia will be difficult to diagnose. The best one can do is hypothesize about the presence of apraxia. However, the diagnosis may not be crucial, because the therapy will probably be to reduce the aphasia. Nevertheless, there are a few things one might do to strengthen the hypothesis when apraxia coexists with severe aphasia and to tease out the presence of apraxia when aphasia is less severe.

Kent (1976b) has listed neuropathologic, neuropsychologic, and associated disturbances and speech characteristics that assist in differentiating apraxia of speech from literal paraphasia. Localization of brain damage in

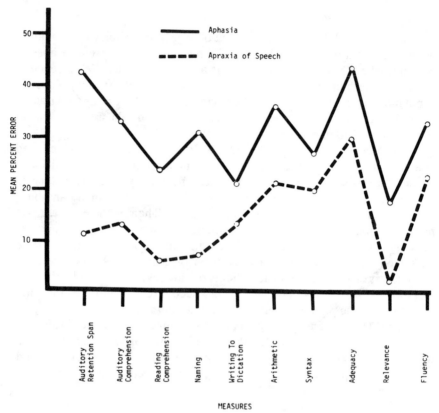

Figure 6. Comparison of aphasic patients and apraxia of speech patients on ten measures of speech, language, and arithmetic. Overall mean percent error for aphasic patients is 31% and for apraxia of speech patients is 14%. (Adapted from Halpern et al., 1973.)

both is usually unilateral; however, in apraxia of speech the lesion is typically anterior, while in literal paraphasia the lesion is typically posterior, temporal and/or parietal. In apraxia of speech, one sees disturbed motor programming due to impairment of motor association systems. The disturbance is manifested in difficulty in initiating, selecting, and sequencing articulatory gestures. Conversely, disturbed motor programming in literal paraphasia is secondary to impairment of sensory association systems or their frontal projections. Right hemiplegia is common in the apraxic patient, and if he or she is also aphasic, the language deficits usually profile as Broca's aphasia. The patient who displays literal paraphasia, usually shows no hemiplegia. The language deficits profile as Wernicke's or conduction aphasia. The speech characteristics of the apraxic patient are

Table 11.

Rank Order of the Percentage of Impairment on Ten Measures of Speech, Language, and Arithmetic for Aphasic Patients and Apraxia of Speech Patients*†

Rank Order	Aphasia†		Apraxia of Speech†	
	Task	%	Task	%
1	Adequacy	43	Adequacy	30
2	AUDITORY RETENTION	42	FLUENCY	22
3	Arithmetic	36	Arithmetic	21
4			SYNTAX	20
4½	Auditory Comprehension	33		
	FLUENCY	33		
5				
5½			Auditory Comprehension	13
			WRITING TO DICTATION	13
6	NAMING	31		
7	SYNTAX	27	AUDITORY RETENTION	11
8	Reading Comprehension	24	NAMING	7
9	WRITING TO DICTATION	21	Reading Comprehension	6
10	Relevance	18	Relevance	2
Mean		31		14

*Adapted from Halpern et al., 1973.
†Measures in capital letters tend to differentiate the two groups.

125

errors of phoneme substitution, altered prosody, and difficulty in initating speech. Similarly, the literal paraphasic patient also makes susbstitution errors, but these are much less predictable than in apraxia of speech. Phonemic additions and errors in phoneme sequence are common in literal paraphasia, but prosody is normal, as is fluency. Finally, one must remember that apraxia of speech is a symptom complex, and literal paraphasia is only a symptom.

Our clinical experience agrees with Kent's observations. The apraxic patients we see produce a high number of errors that are only slightly off target. Patients with literal paraphasia produce errors that are way off target. Apraxic patients may produce non-English speech sounds, but paraphasic patients confine themselves to English speech sounds. Substitution errors in apraxia are usually predictable. Not so in literal paraphasia. Apraxic patients may make a few more errors on initial sounds, and literal paraphasic patients may make more errors on final sounds. Also, apraxic patients distort suprasegmentals, but patients with literal paraphasia preserve suprasegmentals. Of course, not everyone [for example, Blumstein (1973) and Buckingham (1979)] agrees with our observations.

Blumstein (1973) contends that apraxia of speech cannot be differentiated from Wernicke's aphasia with traditional articulation analyses. Halpern et al. (1976) disagree. Twenty-eight of the 30 aphasic patients without apraxia of speech they studied made no phonetic errors in spontaneous speech. Seventy-five percent of the errors they observed were semantic or syntactic errors or failure to respond. Burns and Canter (1977), studying conduction and Wernicke's aphasic patients, observed more errors on final consonants than on initial consonants. Furthermore, they tallied more errors in phoneme sequencing than Trost and Canter (1974) and LaPointe and Johns (1975) found in apraxic patients. Nespoulous et al. (1981), comparing Broca's and conduction aphasic patients, noted differences that differentiated the two types. Conduction patients made more sequencing errors than Broca's patients. Broca's patients were more lawful in their substitutions; for example, they made voicing errors that remained within class for manner and place. Conduction patients were lawless. But, if traditional articulation analysis should fail, Kent and Rosenbek (1982) have deomonstrated that prosodic analysis will differentiate apraxic patients from aphasic patients.

Therefore we believe that apraxia of speech can be diagnosed even when it coexists with aphasia. It usually does. Wertz et al. (1970) reviewed 228 cases, and apraxia resided in combination with aphasia and/or dysarthria in 88%. Rose et al. (1976), examining patients referred for treatment and those who were not, reported 68% of the patients referred for treatment had a mixed problem, aphasia combined with apraxia and/or dysarthria.

Interestingly, all of the patients not referred had a single disorder. Diagnosis is more difficult when the severity of coexisting aphasia mounts, but it is possible. In the patients whose severity of coexisting aphasia permits only a paucity of oral expression, one hypothesizes, as Rosenbek (1978) suggests, and waits for time and treatment to expose apraxia's presence or absence.

Apraxia versus Dysarthria

Differentiating apraxia of speech from dysarthria requires separation of two motor speech disorders. Again, the two may coexist, and in these cases the need is to detect the presence of both and determine how the two interact. As we have mentioned, we expect apraxic patients to have coexisting aphasia. The dysarthric patient may also display a coexisting language deficit, depending upon where the damage to his nervous system occurred and what caused it. Darley (1969) describes dysarthria as a group of speech disorders resulting from disturbances in muscular control—weakness, slowness, or incoordination—of the speech mechanism due to damage to the central or peripheral nervous system or both. The term encompasses coexisting neurogenic disorders of several or all the basic processes of speech—respiration, phonation, resonance, articulation, and prosody.

Halpern et al. (1973) did not study dysarthric patients. Therefore, we do not have comparative data similar to those discussed for aphasia, confusion, and generalized intellectual impairment. However, Kent (1976b) has provided a set of characteristics for differentiating apraxia of speech from dysarthria. The neuropathology differs. In apraxia of speech, damage is usually unilateral and anterior. In dysarthria, it is usually bilateral if cerebral but typically it is subcortical. As stated earlier, apraxia of speech results from disturbed motor programming because motor association systems are involved. Initiation, selection, and sequencing of articulatory gestures are disrupted. Conversely, in dysarthria, there is disturbed execution of movement due to impairment of motor projection systems, e.g., upper and/or lower motor neuron systems. One sees paralysis, weakness, ataxia, and/or involuntary movement. The apraxic patient is often right hemiplegic, and if language is impaired, it reveals itself as Broca's aphasia. Dysarthric patients will probably display analogous impariment of the non-speech musculature—paralysis, weakness, ataxia, involuntary movement, but lexical and syntactic language usage is usually intact. Speech characteristics in apraxia are errors of phoneme substitution, abnormal prosody, and initiation difficulty. In dysarthria, distortion errors predominate; articulation tends to be imprecise; and phonation, resonation and respiration are altered.

Our clinical experience confirms Kent's observations and those of Johns and Darley (1970) and others who have differentiated apraxia of speech from dysarthria. Substitution errors appear to predominate in apraxia; distortion errors are most frequent in dysarthria. Nonphonologic variables have an effect on the apraxic patient's speech. They have less of an effect on the dysarthric patient. Apraxic patients produce resonance that is normal or, at least, near normal. Resonance balance in dysarthria is frequently disturbed. Seldom do we see consistent dysphonia in apraxia. There is a frequent presence of dysphonia in many dysarthrias. Cranial nerves function near their normal limits in apraxia, but they are involved in dysarthria. Additional differences between the two disorders can be elaborated by touring the different levels and processes of speech.

Respiration is essentially normal in apraxia of speech; however, some patients may show difficulty in initiating quiet exhalation on request, and severely apraxic patients may display reduced forced expiratory flow. Depending upon the type, dysarthric patients may have reduced respiration for speech because of muscle weakness or rigidity, coordination of respiration and other speech processes, reduced overall loudness, tendency toward monoloudness, and inappropriate and irregular changes in loudness.

Phonation is essentially normal in the apraxic patient. Voiced—voiceless substitutions are articulatory problems, not laryngeal abnormalities. Phonatory deficit in dysarthria is influenced by the type present. It may take the form of reduced range, speed, and strength of laryngeal movements; impaired coordination of phonation and other speech processes; dysphonia that includes breathiness, harshness, or a strained or strangled quality; or pitch abnormalities including a tendency toward monopitch or inappropriate pitch changes.

Resonance in apraxia of speech is essentially normal. If nasal –oral substitutions occur, and they are rare, they reflect articulation abnormality rather than velopharyngeal incompetence. Resonance abnormality in dysarthria, depending upon the type, may be revealed as reduced range, speed, and strength of velopharyngeal movements; impaired coordination of resonance with other speech processes; or resonance imbalance which includes nasal emission or consistent or inconsistent hypernasality.

Articulatory behavior in apraxic patients includes a high proportion of substitution, addition, repetition, and, dependeing upon severity, omission errors; a few metathetic errors; a significant influence by other variables, such as word length; and a tendency toward error inconsistency. Articulation in dysarthric patients, depending upon type, includes a high proportion of distortion errors; few, if any, metathetic errors; a lesser influence by other variables, such as word length; and a tendency toward error consistency. On rapid, alternating, articulatory tasks, apraxic patients, depending upon severity, will show adequate range of movement and strength. However, again depending upon severity, they may substitute sounds, perseverate on sounds, or produce recurring utterances. Dysarthric patients, depending upon type and severity, may display reduced range, speed, and strength. Timing may be impaired. Errors will most likely be distortions.

Prosodic disturbance abounds in both apraxia of speech and dysarthria. In apraxia, the patient's effortful, trial-and-error groping may disrupt stress, intonation, and rhythm. There is some constriction of intonational contours, abnormalities in articulation time and sound durations, and an inappropriate distribution and length of pause time. Loudness and pitch are adequate, but they may not be used appropriately to produce normal prosody. Dysarthric patients do not produce trial and error groping behavior, but, depending upon type, they display abnormal prosody. Some constrict intonational contours. Some produce abnormalities in articulation time and sound durations. In hypokinetic, hyperkinetic, and ataxic dysarthria, there is inappropriate distribution and length of pause time, but for different reasons than in apraxia. Involvement of pitch and loudness also works its will on the dysarthric patient's prosody.

Finally, apraxia of speech and dysarthria differ in nonspeech symptoms. Oral, nonverbal apraxia may be present in apraxia of speech. It is absent in dysarthria. Primary function is intact in apraxia, but it is often involved in dysarthria. Peripheral paralysis or paresis, if present at all in apraxia, is usually confined to the face or hemiplegic limbs. It is impossible to generalize about peripheral symptoms in dysarthria because of the variability of diseases that result in dysarthria. Possibilities include rigidity, flaccidity, spasticity, incoordination, and abnormal movements.

Thus, we can and do differentiate apraxia of speech from dysarthria. The task is more difficult when the two disorders coexist. However, use of the characteristics and contrasts discussed above and the presence or absence of significant paralysis or paresis in muscles used for speech permit application of the appropriate label.

CASE EXAMPLES

P.M. received a diagnosis of mild apraxia of speech coexisting with mild aphasia. Appraisal told us that his language deficits were mild in all modalities; he was fluent; and his apraxia was represented by infrequent, inconsistent articulatory errors and prosodic disturbance. No significant paralysis or paresis of the oral musculature was detected. None of his communication deficits prevented his returning to work. He indicated that he would rather spend his time on the job than in the clinic. His condition and his desires suggested that treatment, if done at all, be limited to counseling and explanation of what may affect his speech. That was what was done, and P.M. picked up his life only slightly altered from the way it was prior to suffering a left hemisphere CVA. He is not a normal talker, but he approaches being one.

J.D.'s diagnosis was moderate apraxia of speech coexisting with moderate aphasia. Our appraisal tasks revealed what his problems were and how they might be treated. His language and speech deficits plus a coexisting cardiac condition prompted J.D. to elect early retirement. He lived at home and came to see us for outpatient treatment. His therapy was divided, about equally, into that designed to combat apraxia and that designed to reduce aphasia. Time and that treatment rolled back the severity of both. Unfortunately, a heart attack, a second CVA, and a fall that broke his hip erased his gains, and we are beginning again.

B.S.'s initial diagnosis was severe aphasia and suspected severe apraxia of speech. Our appraisal tasks indicated that his limited verbal output contained more than semantic and syntactic errors. However, its paucity and the marked auditory comprehension and reading deficits clouded our conclusion about the presence of apraxia. So, we followed Rosenbek's (1978) suggestions. We treated his aphasia and hypothesized apraxia of speech would surface as aphasic deficits retreated. It did. At three months postonset, B.S.'s profile had changed from global to Broca's aphasia and frequent, inconsistent articulatory errors; groping behavior; and initiation difficulty; and prosodic disturbance confirmed our early suspicion that he was apraxic. Treatment split its focus, part on continued efforts to reduce aphasia and part designed to combat apraxia of speech. Today, at 16 months postonset, treatment continues. Aphasia has improved more than apraxia, and change in both has slowed. Now, more of our time together is spent in tangling with B.S.'s apraxia of speech.

Biographical data on these three patients told us that they were literate and normally intelligent prior to onset. All three had a home to reside in that was within treatment's reach and someone there or nearby to assist. Medical data localized each patient's lesion in the left hemisphere, showed a lack of previous CNS involvement, and an absence of brain stem signs. Our behavioral measures revealed the presence and severity of language deficits and the presence and severity of apraxia of speech. For B.S, we had to wait to confirm the latter, and our patience was rewarded. Medical data and examination of oral peripheral function ruled out significant dysarthria. What the patients did on language and motor speech tasks permitted focusing treatment for each, a diagnosis, and a good guess at prognosis. The collabroative effort—the physician's, our's, and the patient's—met appraisal's and diagnosis' purposes and permitted us to provide management.

SUMMARY

While appraisal and diagnosis have their purposes, so do clinicians and patients. Not all of the patients we see are pushed through every piece of appraisal listed in this chapter. Our purposes differ for different patients. Some seek only our opinions, not our efforts. For these, we probe until we have something to say about what a patient has and what can or cannot be done about it. The patients and their families sift what we have to say through their circumstances and their plans for the future. Acceptance or rejection is theirs. Our identification of a fine treatment candidate does not automatically cast a patient in that role. One must elect to play the part. Most do. For those who do not, we respect their wishes, leave the door open, and wish them well. Some of life's decisions are too important to be influenced by our facts.

Some patients do not get an immediate diagnosis. We exhaust our appraisal measures and find that we are still searching for a label. We counsel patience and perseverance. We continue to probe with diagnostic therapy, and usually patients, in time, teach us what they should be called and how to manage them best.

Appraisal and diagnosis of patients who may suffer apraxia of speech are miniature lessons in life. The exercise can impart such wisdom as no pleasure is purchased without some risk and disappointment. If we are systematic in our appraisal and permit our patients to reveal what they have, the risks are reduced and the disappointments diminished.

6

Prognosis

Prognosis is an exercise in augury. Like all attempts to predict the future, forecasting for the patient who suffers apraxia of speech has resulted in a variety of views. Apraxia of speech and its lessening have received a mixed blessing. Compare the following.

> There are hints that anarthria has a significant retarding effect on recovery of expression (Vignolo, 1964, p. 367).

> A person whose infarction is confined to the Broca area experiences an initial period of mutism with some disturbance in language function, followed quickly thereafter by the emergence of speech which is remarkably free of agrammatism . . . the person rapidly recovers the ability to write well, and in the months and years that follow, may show only a residual facial–lingual–palatal–pharyngeal paresis, mild ideomotor facial dyspraxia for skilled movements, and only slight hesitance in speech, taking the form of speech dysprosody or speech dyspraxia (Mohr, 1980, pp. 2–3).

Vignolo's anarthria is characterized by severe reduction in the flow of speech, marked phonemic disorders of expression—elisions or substitutions of phonemes—and articulatory difficulties, usually accompanied by oral apraxia. It qualifies as kin to what we call apraxia of speech. Its bleak future was repeated by Basso and Vignolo (1969): "Other things being equal, the presence of phonemic articulatory disorders has a poor prognostic significance." However, as Darley (1982) observed, the dire prediction was not supported by the data in the Basso, Capitani, and Vignolo (1979) treatment study. These patients resided in their nonfluent groups, and nonfluency had no significant influence on recovery in their treated and untreated samples.

Mohr's observations flow from his own patients (Mohr, 1973, 1980; Mohr et al., 1978) and his review of the historical and contemporary literature. While he separates minor or "baby" Broca syndrome, a lesion confined to Broca's area, from Broca's aphasia, a lesion involving a larger area, patients with either experience improvement. The primary difference, he believes, is that some language deficit persists in the latter but not the former. Tompkins et al. (1981) quarrel with Mohr's conclusion. They report a case of minor Broca syndrome with mild language deficit at ten months postonset.

Our experience agrees with both Vignolo and Mohr. Some of our apraxic patients have experienced amazing improvement. Others remained severe despite our and their prolonged and best efferts. What we cannot agree with is that patients with apraxia of speech return to normal speech. If one does, that journey is accomplished in a matter of hours, or at the most a week, postonset. These patients seldom become our patients. Apraxia of speech that persists for more than a week is apraxia of speech that will persist. Like alcoholism and drug addiction, there are, in our experience, no ex-apraxic patients. But, for treated patients, we believe that apraxia of speech retreats, in varying amounts, and that the prognosis for some improvement is excellent.

Figure 1 shows a variety of responses to treatment in patients who represent a range of initial severities. L.D. suffered bilateral CVAs. He was aphasic, apraxic, and dysarthric when we met him. While he was functionally literate before his strokes, his four years of education did not qualify him as a strong reader and writer. One year of treatment and spontaneous recovery resulted in a significant retreat in L.D.'s aphasia, but his motor speech deficits remained severe. Today, he communicates with gesture, some verbalization (usually unintelligible) and an individually designed communication board. He drives, he participates in family functions, and he fills his day. He is a walker but not a talker. His combined dysarthria and apraxia of speech devastate most attempts at oral expression. W.B.'s left-hemisphere CVA left him with mild aphasia, moderate apraxia of speech, and mild right hemiplegia. Three months of daily, in-patient treatment may have boosted the return provided by spontanious recovery. At four months postonset, W.B. returned to work full time in his plumbing business. He continues to run it today with help from his wife and business partner. D.J. was an auto mechanic when a stroke pulled him out of his shop and into the hospital. He was markedly aphasic and severely apraxic. His dense right hemiplegia at onset improved enough in the lower extremity to permit him to walk and drive. His aphasia and apraxia improved during three years of treatment—daily for one year, three times a

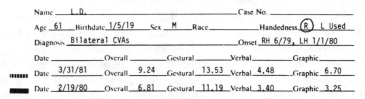

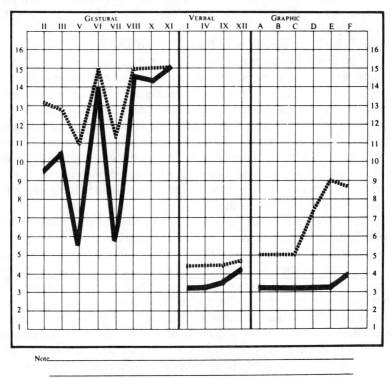

Figure 1.   PICA Modality Response Summaries showing pre- and posttreatment performance by four patients displaying apraxia of speech and coexisting aphasia.

week for two years. Currently, he attends a maintenance group once a week and spends the rest of his days assisting his son in running a used car business. His speech, though not normal, is sufficiently adequate to prompt us to buy a car from him. W.G. is a lesson in tenacity. We met him when he was three months shy of nine years postonset. He had received six months of treatment during the first year following his stroke. He was

Porch Index of Communicative Ability

MODALITY RESPONSE SUMMARY

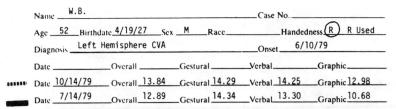

Name ___W.B._____ Case No._____

Age __52__ Birthdate_4/19/27__ Sex __M__ Race_____ Handedness (R) R Used

Diagnosis ___Left Hemisphere CVA_____ Onset ___6/10/79_____

Date _____Overall _____Gestural_____Verbal_____Graphic_____

••••••• Date _10/14/79_____ Overall_13.84__ Gestural_14.29__ Verbal_14.25___Graphic_12.98___

▬▬▬ Date _7/14/79_____Overall_12.89__ Gestural_14.34__ Verbal_13.30___Graphic_10.68___

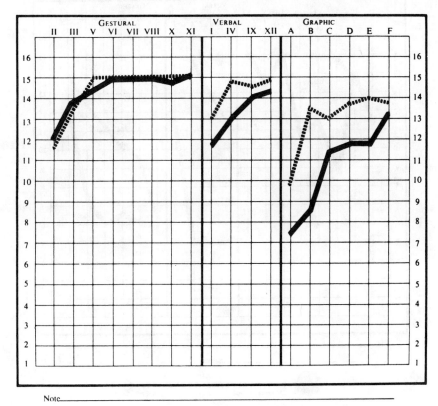

Note_____

Published by
CONSULTING PSYCHOLOGISTS PRESS
577 College Avenue   Palo Alto, California

Figure 1. (*continued*).

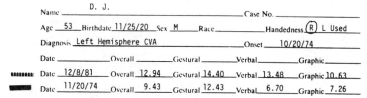

*P*orch *I*ndex *of* *C*ommunicative *A*bility

MODALITY RESPONSE SUMMARY

Name _____ D. J. _____ Case No. _____

Age __53__ Birthdate _11/25/20_ Sex _M_ ____Race_____Handedness (R) L Used

Diagnosis _Left Hemisphere CVA_____Onset ____10/20/74_____

Date _____Overall _____Gestural_____Verbal_____Graphic_____

Date _12/8/81_ Overall _12.94_ Gestural _14.40_ Verbal _13.48_ Graphic _10.63_

Date _11/20/74_ Overall_9.43_ Gestural _12.43_ Verbal_6.70_ Graphic_7.26_

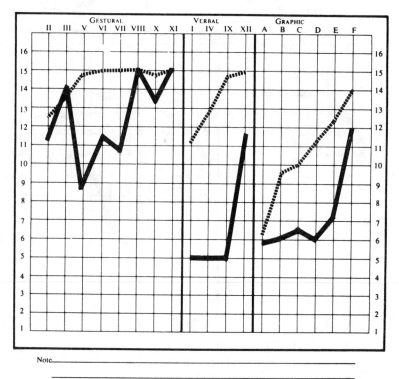

Note_____

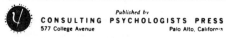

Published by
CONSULTING PSYCHOLOGISTS PRESS
577 College Avenue   Palo Alto, California

Figure 1. *(continued).*

moderately aphasic and moderately apraxic. His day was filled with hospital volunteer service and odd jobs to supplement his disability income. We
treated him three days a week for a little over two years. He improved.
Toward the end of that treatment, he decided he wanted to reenter the
world of work. He did. A functional, midly apraxic talker sees that the
hospital laundry gets done and is back on time.

When each of these patients entered our clinics, we gave him a prog-

P*orch* I*ndex of* C*ommunicative* A*bility*

MODALITY RESPONSE SUMMARY

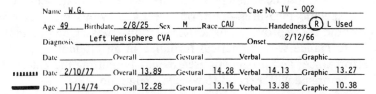

Name W.G.   Case No. IV - 002

Age 49   Birthdate 2/8/25 Sex M   Race CAU   Handedness (R) L Used

Diagnosis Left Hemisphere CVA   Onset 2/12/66

Date _____ Overall _____ Gestural _____ Verbal _____ Graphic _____

⊞⊞⊞⊞⊞⊞ Date 2/10/77   Overall 13.89 Gestural 14.28 Verbal 14.13 Graphic 13.27

▬▬▬▬ Date 11/14/74 Overall 12.28 Gestural 13.16 Verbal 13.38 Graphic 10.38

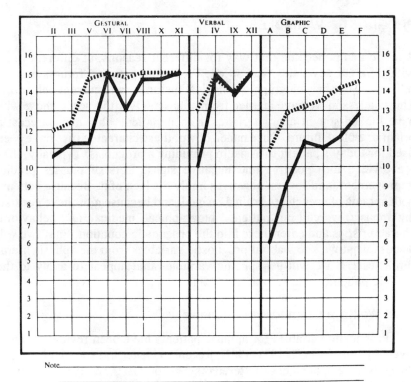

Note_____

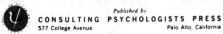

Published by
CONSULTING PSYCHOLOGISTS PRESS
577 College Avenue   Palo Alto, California

Figure 1. (*continued*).

nosis. We applied an adjective—good, guarded, poor, or grave—and we attempted a best guess at "prognosis for what" to make our prediction meaningful. The "for what" is crucial, and, unfortunately, it is what we do least well. The "for what" eschews "for normal speech." That does not happen. The "for what" ranges from being able to make one's point in most situations, although speech may retreat completely at the appearance of a policeman or an irate spouse, to returning to one's chair behind the loan desk in the local savings and loan. We used some of the methods that are discussed below. They include culling prognostic variables—what others have observed to influence change in patients or the lack of it; behavioral profiles on specific measures—performance by previous patients who improved or did not improve; statistical prediction—massaging a patient's current performance with numerical formulae in an attempt to predict future performance; and prognostic treatment—permitting the patient to tell us how he or she will respond to what we might do.

PROGNOSTIC VARIABLES

Apraxic adults become that way for different reasons, at different ages, with different severities, and so on. Predicting patients' futures may be influenced by their biographies, medical histories, and current behaviors. This is a lesson we have learned from aphasia. Over the years, those who have looked sought characteristics in their patients that may forecast a bright or a bleak future. Once nailed down, these characteristics have been used for today's patient to assist in providing a prognosis. Typically, they are divided into positive and negative signs. Lots of plusses predict improvement, and several negatives imply the lack of it. Because patients with apraxia of speech are brain damaged, and because most have coexisting aphasia, we cull our patients' biographical, medical, and behavioral characteristics and enter these into the prognostic equation. First, we will discuss what we know about prognostic variables from the aphasia literature. Second, we will list specific variables that appear to apply to the apraxic patient.

What We Have Learned From Aphasia

Prognostic variables for aphasic patients have been reviewed extensively by Darley (1972, 1975, 1982). Recent evidence has solidified some of the early beliefs, but it has shattered others. Some of the early "facts" have fallen. Some of what we thought we knew we have found was wrong or not worth knowing. Let us examine a few of the facts.

Biographical Variables

Age, some say, is an important prognostic sign. Younger patients are expected to improve more than older patients (Eisenson, 1949; Wepman, 1951; Vignolo, 1964; Sands et al., 1969). Not so, say others (Culton, 1969; Sarno & Levita, 1971; Smith, 1972; Keenan & Brassell, 1974; Deal & Deal, 1978; Basso et al., 1979; Hartman, 1981). Does age have an influence on the patient's future? Probably not, if age is the single negative factor in the patient's prognostic equation.

A similar set of conflicting answers exists for the influence of premorbid intelligence. Eisenson (1949) listed premorbid high intelligence as a negative sign for patients who became aphasic. Smarter patients were aware of how far they had fallen and awareness of this loss led to depression. Conversely, Wepman (1951) and Messerli et al. (1976) suggest that patients with higher premorbid intelligence have a better outcome than those who were not as bright before onset. Our experience is that premorbid intellect, when it can be ascertained—usually it cannot—may or may not influence a patient's future. When it surfaces, it influences the ability to create and use strategies (usually ones we have not thought of) to compensate for persisting deficits; for example, gathering test items in a pile to one side to ensure that, if wrong, the same mistake is not made twice. As important as premorbid intellect, we believe, is a persisting tenacity to achieve. Just as effort can elevate classroom performance, it can work its will in treatment. We like to see patients come bright and hungry.

Another biographical variable that has received some interest is occupational status. Most (Sarno et al., 1970; Keenan & Brassell, 1974) agree that how a patient earned his or her living prior to onset has no significant influence on the prognosis for improvement once that patient becomes aphasic. However, there is disagreement about the influence of employment at the time of onset. Sarno and Levita (1971) report that patients who were working when they became aphasic improved more than those not employed at onset. Conversely, Marshall et al. (1982) found no influence on improvement postonset exerted by employment at the onset of aphasia. Our experience dictates that the kind of work a patient did and whether or not he or she was working upon becoming aphasic and apraxic has little influence upon whether that patient gets better. The kind of work a patient did and the demands it makes on speech may dictate whether or not he or she will return to that job. We have known a bank loan officer who made fine improvement and attained functional speech, but he and his former colleagues agreed that his gains were insufficient for him to return to his desk. Similarly, one of us is treating a patient whose speech is quite adequate for most situations but not up to the demands of driving a morning and evening commute for the local transit company. On the other hand, we have treated a salesman who remains moderately apraxic, but with the help of his spouse, he maintains his premorbid volume. In addition, there is a 50th percentile overall on the PICA patient who left our clinic to resume his rural mail route.

Medical Variables

What causes the aphasia and apraxia may have an influence on whether and how much either improve. Patients who suffer closed head trauma are reported to have a better prognosis than those who suffer a CVA or penetrating head trauma (Alajouanine et al., 1957; Eisenson, 1964; Luria, 1963). Kertesz and McCabe (1977) observed six of seven traumatic cases who displayed significant recovery within the first three months postonset. Their vascular cases made less gain and took longer to attain it. Eisenson (1964) also points out that aphasia following multiple CVAs results in a poorer prognosis than aphasia following a single CVA.

Where the damage occurs and the extent of that damage appears to influence improvement. Yarnell et al. (1976) summarize data that indicate that size, location, and number of lesions correlate with the amount of recovery. A large lesion, many small lesions combined with one large lesion, and bilateral lesions all forecast a poor prognosis for recovery. Eisenson (1964) agrees, and he observes that single lesions that spare the temporal–parietal region forecast the best future for language improvement. Glosser et al. (1982) report that aphasia resulting from a subcortical hemorrhage takes longer to abate than aphasia subsequent to cortical involvement.

Most observers (Eisenson, 1949, 1964; Anderson et al., 1970) agree that patients in better physical condition with no sensory deficits have a more favorable prognosis for improved language than those who are ill and display significant sensory involvement.

The bulk of our experience is with patients who have suffered a CVA. We have seen our share of patients with other etiologies, but the number of these do not tempt us to prognosticate confidently using only etiology as the best clue to unravel the future. Most of our patients have suffered frontal lobe damage combined with injury to the surrounding territory. Again, however, our experience and access to precise localization data do not prompt us to predict. Generally, we view multiple CVAs as a warning that the patient's future may be cloudy. We like to see healthy, bright individuals with the stamina to combat the rigors of intensive treatment and sufficient auditory, visual, and tactile acuity to permit us to explore a variety of stimulus modes.

Behavioral Variables

Behavior is, of course, linked to medical variables. For example, severity, type of aphasia, and the presence of apraxia of speech probably relate to the size and location of the lesion. However, because behavioral influences do not surface until the patient is immersed in a psychometric marinade, and because they change over time, we consider them separately.

Severity of aphasia forecasts the future. Almost everyone agrees that the less severe patient has more potential for ultimate recovery (Basso et al., 1979; Butfield & Zangwill, 1946; Gloning et al., 1976; Hartman, 1981; Keenan & Brassell, 1974; Kertesz & McCabe, 1977; Messerli et al., 1976; Sands et al., 1969; Sarno & Levita, 1971, 1979; Schuell et al., 1964; Wepman, 1951). Kertesz (1979) cautions that one must separate amount of improvement from final outcome. For example, severe patients may improve more than milder patients, but the severe patient does not attain the eventual skills that the milder patient does.

Type of aphasia and what it predicts about improvement is controversial. Kertesz and McCabe (1977) reported that anomic and conduction types have the best prognosis for achieving recovery. However, Broca's and Wernicke's types also make significant gains. Their global patients, while experiencing a lot of change, never attained very useful language skills. Lomas and Kertesz (1978) report similar observations. Conversely, Prins et al. (1978) found no difference in recovery among types. And Basso et al. (1979), comparing fluent and nonfluent patients, found no significant effect of type on recovery in their treatment study. Thus, the influence of type of aphasia on improvement or the lack of it remains debatable. Probably, a part of the controversy is fueled by the different typing systems employed and when the patient is typed. For example, a fluent versus nonfluent dichotomy collapses the types contained in the system employed by Goodglass and Kaplan (1972) and Kertesz (1979). That collapsing is confounded by severity. Global patients, the most severe, are put in the nonfluent bin and may exaggerate severity in nonfluent aphasia. Furthermore, Kertesz and McCabe (1977) observed a good deal of migration among types—some patients who were one type close to onset evolved into other types as time passed. Therefore, the Broca's aphasic patient who has evolved from global aphasia may not have the same potential for improvement as that of a patient who begins as a Broca's aphasic patient. Time and type may interact.

Finally, how long postonset a patient is seen is believed to influence how much change there will be. The rule is that the closer to onset, the more likely improvement will occur with or without treatment. Differences of opinion exist regarding how close to onset. Culton (1969) pulls the curtain on significant spontaneous recovery at two months postonset. Others (Deal & Deal, 1978; Butfield & Zangwill, 1946; Vignolo, 1964; Basso et al., 1979; Kertesz & McCabe, 1977) believe that potential for change is greater prior to six months postonset than later. Wepman (1951) extends the period to one year, and Marks et al. (1957) noted improvement in some patients after a year postonset. Furthermore, some personal accounts of aphasia (Moss, 1972; Dahlberg & Jaffee, 1977) describe changes that occur well into the future. Nevertheless, most patients seem to experience the majority of their return of language skills within the first six months postonset.

Summary

Other variables that influence improvement in aphasia probably exist—premorbid handedness, sex, social milieu, motivation, etc. Those discussed above are listed in Table 1 along with what the literature implies about their potencies. The problem with using these variables for predic-

Table 1.
Selected Variables Suggested To Have An Influence on
Improvement in Aphasia.

Variable	Status*
Age	?
Education	?
Premorbid intelligence	?
Occupational status	?
Etiology	+
Size of lesion	+
Localization	+
Health	+
Severity	+
Type of aphasia	?
Time postonset	+

*+ = agreement; ? = conflicting reports.

tion, as Vignolo (1964) observed, is that variables do not simply exist, they coexist. The potency of one may be mediated or negated by the presence of one or more others. Marshall et al. (1982) point out that no single variable can predict improvement or the lack of it. Therefore, if one is using prognostic variables as a ticket into treatment, Darley's (1979) advice should be considered: "No single negative factor is so uniformly potent as to justify excluding a patient from at least a trial of therapy" (p. 629).

We caution that prognostic variables useful for predicting change in aphasia may or may not be useful for predicting change in apraxia of speech. Aphasia is not apraxia. Nevertheless, because most of our apraxic patients also display some degree of aphasia, what we know about aphasia may be useful.

Prognostic Variables in Apraxia of Speech

What do we know about the influence of biographical, medical, and behavioral variables on improvement in patients suffering apraxia of speech? We know less than we do about their influence on recovery from aphasia. Typically, the presence of apraxia of speech is submerged in aphasia in the prognosis literature. However, a few observations have surfaced.

We can begin with the influence of apraxia on the recovery of oral expression. Opinion varies. Keenan and Brassell (1974) report that all of their patients who began and ended with poor speech exhibited a severe motor speech impairment, primarily apraxia or dysarthria. Gloning and Quatember (1964) and Goldstein (1948) offer similar observations. Conversely, Rosenbek (1978) suggests that, with help form therapy, the apraxic patient's prognosis is probably better than that of the patient with aphasia. Marks et al. (1957) support this view. However, Lecours and Lhermitte (1976) followed one patient for ten years who displayed no dramatic change in speech. Unfortunately, it is difficult to predict the influence apraxia of speech has on the recovery of functional communication. Apraxia of speech typically resides in a bog of aphasia, and its severity varies as does that of the coexisting aphasia. Attempts to extract apraxia of speech from this morass and demonstrate its influence on improvement are difficult if not impossible.

The most comprehensive statement about the influence of biographical, medical, and behavioral variables has come from Mohr et al. (1978). Handedness, age, sex, education, occupation, and associated sensory and motor deficits, they observed, were not helpful in predicting the rate and extent of improvement. Some of these and other prognostic signs have been given, at least, brief attention. Specifically, location of the lesion; type of aphasia; mutism; presence of oral, nonverbal apraxia; and severity of coexisting aphasia have attracted comments about their influence on improvement.

Mohr and his colleagues (1980, 1978) forecast a promising future for the patient whose lesion is confined to Broca's area. Larger lesions, they report, result in more severe symptoms and bring the burden of coexisting language deficit that is classified as big Broca's aphasia. Penfield and Roberts (1961) suggest that involvement of Broca's area results in less severe aphasia than involvement of other areas that produce aphasia. Kertesz (1979) and Kertesz and McCabe (1977) agree that Broca's aphasia is bound to get better. While they gave it an "intermediate" prognosis, compared with other types, their Broca's patients joined conduction aphasic patients in achieving the largest amount of recovery. The improvement that occurred was greatest in the first three months, slowed after six months, and plateaued after a year from onset. Thus, because most of the patients we see who demonstrate apraxia of speech profile as Broca's aphasia, we can use what we know about Broca's aphasia to predict change in apraxic patients. What we know is that improvement will occur, and that the improvement will be substantial. If a patient was fortunate and suffered damage confined to Broca's area, Mohr (1980) predicts a fine future.

Apraxia of phonation has been examined as an influence on the future. Mohr (1980) acknowledges that patients with Broca's area damage, baby and big, may be mute in the early days postonset. This appears to wane, however. Darley et al. (1975) have made the same observation and reached the same conclusion. Rosenbek (1978) is more pessimistic. If sound cannot be evoked with explanation, manual minipulation, etc., he suggests that one should frown. The patient may be severely aphasic as well as severely apraxic. If he or she remains mute beyond a few days, one should worry. Mutism that persists is likely to be mutism that will continue to persist.

Fascination with oral, nonverbal apraxia waxes and wanes. It has waxed enough to provide a variety of opinion. Some researchers (Butfield, 1958; Vignolo, 1964; Webb & Love, 1974) caution that the presence of oral, nonverbal apraxia is a negative prognostic sign and will interfere with improvement in speech. Others (De Renzi et al., 1966) observed that the severity of oral, nonverbal apraxia is significantly correlated with the severity of articulatory disturbance; however, some patients display severe oral apraxia coexisting with only mild articulation deficit. Yet others (Bowman et al., 1980; La Pointe & Wertz, 1974) found no significant relationship between the severity or oral, nonverbal apraxia and the severity of articulation deficit. We believe that oral, nonverbal apraxia needs to be identified, and that it needs to be watched. Its prognostic significance resides in its influence on treatment tasks that require patients to make movements and assume articulatory positions. It may erode one's supply of treatment techniques.

How aphasic a patient is may influence how much the coexisting apraxia improves. Helm (1978) lists global aphasia and auditory comprehension scores below −1 on the BDAE as criteria to exclude patients from a trial of Melodic Intonation Therapy, an effective treatment for some patients with apraxia of speech. Wepman (1958) suggests that the ability to self-correct is a favorable prognostic sign in aphasia. Because we expect our apraxic patients eventually to assume responsibility for correcting their errors along the path to becoming their own therapists, severe aphasia that restricts self-correction will impede progress. As Rosenbek (1978) also observed, the presence of severe aphasia may delay attacking apraxia of speech, because the therapy will probably be to reduce the aphasia. Given a choice, we prefer our apraxic patients to have sufficiently intact language to make them candidates for a variety of treatments for apraxia of speech. Thus, we prefer the coexisting aphasia be mild to, at most, moderate.

In a search for prognostic indicants in patients with apraxia of speech, Wertz (in press) tested relationships among a variety of variables for apraxic patients who participated in the Veterans Administration Cooperative Study on Aphasia (Wertz et al., 1981). Initial severity of apraxia of speech and improvement in apraxia of speech were correlated with age, education, PICA performance, Token Test performance, a conversational rating, and performance on the Coloured Progressive Matrices (Raven, 1962). No significant relationships were found between the initial severity of apraxia of speech or change in apraxia of speech and age or years of education. Initial severity of apraxia of speech was significantly related to the initial severity of the PICA Verbal percentile ($p < 0.05$), initial severity on the conversation rating ($p < 0.05$), and change in apraxia of speech ($p < 0.05$). The later correlation was negative, indicating that milder patients made more change than severe patients. Change in apraxia of speech was significantly related ($p < 0.05$) to initial severity on the Coloured Progressive Matrices. Thus, patients with higher nonverbal intelligence at one month postonset changed more than patients with lower nonverbal intelligence. All other comparisons were not significant ($p < 0.05$).

What are the variables that influence prognosis in apraxia of speech? None that have withstood rigorous examination. Nevertheless, our experience and the literature permit us to describe the patient we believe to have a bright future. He or she is the one who is less than a month postonset; who suffered a small lesion confined to Broca's area; has minimal coexisting aphasia; does not display significant oral, nonverbal apraxia; is in good health; and who has the stamina to outlast us in intensive treatment. These patients are rare, and because they are, predicting for most of the patients we see on the basis of prognostic variables is difficult.

BEHAVIORAL PROFILES

The use of neuropsychological tests to predict a brain-injured patient's future is popular (Heaton & Pendleton, 1981). For aphasia and apraxia of speech, this approach was pioneered by Schuell (1965a). It involves evaluating patients with a variety of tasks, constructing profiles of their performance, and predicting improvement based on change in performance by previous patients who had similar profiles. Keenan and Brassell (1974) used this method to predict the recovery of verbal skills, and Porch (1981) uses it to predict potential performance on the PICA. J. Sarno et al. (1971), however, caution that predictions based on tests for aphasia may not be realized as functional gain.

Schuell (1965a) developed five major prognostic groups and two minor syndromes based on her retrospective look at the initial *Minnesota Test for Differential Diagnosis of Aphasia* (MTDDA) (Schuell, 1965b) performance by patients whose change, or the lack of it, was documented. Initial profiles for patients who showed good recovery were used to forecast a positive prognosis, and initial profiles for patients who displayed limited recovery were used to predict a poor prognosis. Her early reports (Schuell et al.,

1964; Schuell, 1965a) identified a Group 3, aphasia with sensorimotor involvement. Although Schuell did not use the phrase apraxia of speech, her description of these patients identifies them as those we call apraxic with coexisting aphasia. The revision of Schuell's groups by Sefer (Schuell, 1973) maintains the former Group 3 and redefines one of the previous minor syndromes. Thus, today we have two prognostic groups that, we believe, include patients with apraxia of speech.

The previous minor syndrome is now called mild aphasia with persisting dysfluency. It is described as resembling Schuell's simple aphasia, except for the accompaniment of persisting dysfluency. The speech signs—articulatory errors, slow and nonfluent speech, and more articulation errors on less common and longer words—implies the presence of apraxia of speech coexisting with simple aphasia. Prognosis for this group is reported to be excellent for recovery of language. While normal articulation can be attained at times, it disintegrates when conscious control lapses. Automaticity and fluency are not regained, and dysfluency may persist in the presence or the absence of aphasia.

The former Group 3, aphasia with sensorimotor involvement, is defined as severe reduction of language in all modalities accompanied by difficulty in discriminating, producing, and sequencing phonemes. Prognosis for these patients is reported to be limited, but some functional recovery of language skills is attained. Patients are able to communicate their needs in intelligible speech; however, their verbal responses are slow and labored. Some language modalities remain impaired to some extent.

Schuell's behavioral profile method permits making an early, data-based prediction for patients who suffer apraxia of speech and coexisting aphasia. Difficulties arise, however, when a patient's performance indicates apraxia of speech coexisting with aphasia, but his MTDDA performance cannot be classified as mild aphasia with persisting dysfluency or aphasia with sensorimotor involvement. Even when the patient can be classified, the prognosis is limited to descriptive adjectives.

Porch (1981) has offered three methods for predicting future performance on the PICA. They are High-OA Prediction (HOAP), High-OA Prediction Slopes, and Intrasubtest Variability. He lists these as "best guesses" of future performance derived from what the patient reveals in his or her current performance. The theory is that a patient's current, best performance will predict overall performance in the future.

The High-OA Prediction (HOAP) method involves administering a PICA, computing the overall and nine high (mean of the nine best subtests) scores, and utilizing the percentile tables in the PICA Manual to predict future performance. For example, the patient, W.T., shown in Figure 2, performed at the 36th percentile overall on the PICA at one month postonset. The mean of his nine high subtests was 12.69. By entering the

P*orch* I*ndex of* C*ommunicative* A*bility*

SCORE SHEET

Name __W. T._____ Onset __8/4/81__ No. _____

Date __9/15/81__ By __RTW_____ Time __2:27__ to __3:46__ Total Time __79 MIN__

Test Conditions __STANDARD_____

Patient Conditions __GOOD, COOPERATIVE_____

Glasses: __YES____ Hearing aid: __NO____ Dentures: __NO_____ Hand Used: __L____

ITEM	I	II	III	IV	V	VI	VII	VIII	IX	X	XI	XII	A	B	C	D	E	F
1. Tb	5	9	11	14	12	13	12	15	4	15	15	11			⑤	5	7	14
2. Cg	4	7	11	4	8	13	12	10	7	9	15	4	⑤	⑤	⑤	5	6	14
3. Pn	4	11	11	⑤	12	15	12	15	⑤	15	15	8			⑤	6	13	14
4. Kf	5	7	7	7	7	15	11	15	7	10	13	15			⑤	7	6	14
5. Fk	8	11	12	4	7	10	12	15	9	15	15	15	⑤	⑤		6	6	14
6. Qt	⑤	7	7	⑤	12	15	12	15	12	15	15	15				5	6	11
7. Pl	4	11	12	4	12	13	12	15	⑤	15	15	13				5	13	11
8. Mt	4	7	7	11	11	15	12	15	8	15	15	9			⑤	6		11
9. Ky	4	13	12	12	12	15	11	13	⑤	15	15	15				5	13	13
10. Cb	7	12	11	⑤	12	15	12	15	⑤	15	15	15	⑤	⑤		7	10	13
TIME	2:34	2:39	2:43	2:48	2:51	2:53	2:55	2:56	3:02	3:04	3:06	3:08	3:11	3:16	3:21	3:28	3:41	3:46
MINUTES	7	5	4	5	3	2	2	1	6	2	2	2	3	5	5	7	13	5
MODALITY	VRB	PTM	PTM	VRB	RDG	AUD	RDG	VIS	VRB	AUD	VIS	VRB	WRT	WRT	WRT	WRT	CPY	CPY
MEAN SCORE	5.0	9.5	10.1	7.1	10.5	3.9	11.8	14.3	6.7	13.9	4.8	12.0	5.0	5.0	5.0	5.6	8.6	12.9
%ILE	9	38	32	37	41	46	44	15	33	40	17	34	52	38	32	34	35	49
VARIAB.	30	35	19	69	15	11	2	7	23	11	2	30	0	0	0	14	44	11

MPO	OVERALL	WRITING	COPYING	READING	PANTOMIME	VERBAL	AUDITORY	VISUAL
1	9.53	5.15	10.75	11.15	9.80	7.70	13.90	14.55
%ile	36	33	38	41	34	34	44	15
Variab.	323	14	55	17	54	152	22	9
Mean Var.	17.9	3.5	27.5	8.5	27.0	38	11.0	4.5

	Gestural	Verbal	Graphic	9 HI	9 LO	HOAP	Correction	Target
Score	12.35	7.70	7.02	12.69	6.39	12.54	0	
%ile	38	34	36	37	34	70	0	70 %

CONSULTING PSYCHOLOGISTS PRESS
577 College Avenue   Palo Alto, California

Figure 2. PICA score sheet and Aphasia Recovery Curve showing data for PICA prognostic prediction. (Figure 2 continues on page 148.)

overall percentile column in the PICA Manual and moving upward to an overall score of 12.69, one can establish target performance at the 70th percentile. The patient is expected to attain the target at six months postonset. W.T. was at the 63rd percentile at six months postonset. He was treated three times a week and continued on that schedule at one year postonset. Twelve months after onset, he performed at the 68th percentile.

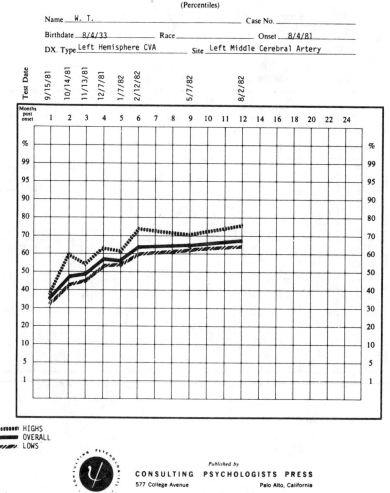

Figure 2. *(continued)*.

Porch's High-Overall Prediction Slopes (HOAP Slopes), he suggests, are more appropriate for predicting performance when the patient is more than one month but less than six months postonset. HOAP Slopes, provided in the PICA Manual, permit using a patient's current overall performance, selecting the coordinates where the current overall percentile and time postonset intersect, and traveling up the slope to find predicted performance at six months postonset. For example, W.T. performed at the 49th percentile overall at three months postonset. This lies between the 40th and 50th percentile HOAP slopes at three months postonset. Traveling upward on the HOAP Slope graph, one would predict performance between the 70th and 80th percentile at six months postonset. Again, W.T. was at the 63rd percentile, overall, at six months postonset.

The third method, intrasubtest variability, utilizes Porch's concept of the Peak Mean Difference (PMD). It is consistent with his belief that a patient's best performance predicts potential overall performance at a future date. While the High-OA Prediction (HOAP) and the High-Overall Prediction Slopes (HOAP Slopes) use early performance on the nine high subtests, the PMD uses item performance within individual subtests to predict the future. In Figure 2 the row labelled "Variab." shows the results of computing the PMD for each of W.T.'s 18 PICA subtests. The mean for a subtest is subtracted from the best score on that subtest. For example, in Subtest I, W.T.'s best score was 8, his "peak" performance. His mean for that subtest, 5.0, subtracted from his peak score yields a Variab. of 30. Decimal points, apparently, are ignored. Variability on the subtests is summed to obtain the overall and modality Variab. shown at the bottom of the score sheet. Porch suggests, "If the PMD is high (+400), the patient is demonstrating a large discrepancy between his potential level of functioning and his actual performance, and therefore he has the capacity for improvement" (Porch, 1981, p. 104). Conversely, a low PMD, (−200), indicates little variability and a poor capacity for change. W.T.'s overall variability at one month postonset was 323. His overall PICA performance improved from the 36th percentile, at that time, to the 63rd percentile at six months postonset.

Two empirical tests of Porch's predictive methods have been conducted. Wertz et al. (1980) evaluated the predictive precision in the High-OA Prediction (HOAP) and the High-Overall Prediction Slopes (HOAP Slopes) methods with 85 patients who had sustained a single, left-hemisphere CVA and had been tested with the PICA at least twice within the first six months postonset. Their correlations betweeen predicted performance and performance obtained were significant ($p < 0.01$). However, analysis of individual patient performance revealed that neither method placed more than 67% of their patients within plus or minus 10 percentile units of the PICA score obtained. Aten and Lyon (1978) tested the PMD method for predicting change in 72 patients who were followed from one month to nine months postonset. They concluded that variability in performance within a task did not predict later improvement or the lack of it. Porch and Callaghan (1981) have suggested that both tests of the predictive methods contain "some methodological and interpretive limitations" (p. 188).

What is the contribution of the behavioral profile methods for predicting change in apraxia of speech? Schuell's (1973) prognostic groups, we believe, tell us about the future for patients who display apraxia of speech coexisting with aphasia. If a patient can be classified into one of the two groups, the clinician has some data-based evidence on which to hang a prognosis. Porch's (1981) methods do not speak specifically about the future for patients with apraxia of speech. They were designed to predict change in PICA performance for patients who are aphasic and may or may not display coexisting apraxia of speech. He does suggest (Porch, 1981) that patients with "middle cerebral lesions often retain high PMD levels well into the chronic stages of recovery and with treatment continue to have a slowly rising OA level" (p. 104). The behavioral profiles do, at least, add a piece of information that may assist in unraveling the prognostic riddle.

STATISTICAL PREDICTION

Use of multiple regression techniques by Porch et al. (1973, 1974, 1980); Marshall and Phillips (in press); and Marshall et al. (1982) employed prognostic variables to predict change in aphasia. While group results are promising, the application by Deal et al. (1979) of the formulae generated indicates that the technique is not ready for application with individual patients.

The technique involves generating an equation that emplqyes a priori measures collected during an initial evaluation to predict future performance. For example, listening, reading, speaking, and writing abilities at one month postonset may be used to predict overall communicative ability at 12 months postonset. The analysis may involve one or more steps. In Step One, a prediction is attempted using the predictor (e.g., auditory comprehension at one month postonset) having the highest correlation with the criterion variable (e.g., severity of aphasia at 12 months postonset). An analysis of variance is performed on all other predictors to determine whether their inclusion in the predictive equation significantly increases predictive precision. If including an additional variable increases prediction, Step Two is performed by adding the second predictor (e.g., naming ability at one month postonset) to the predictive equation. The stepwise procedure is continued until no new predictor significantly increases predictive precision or all a priori predictors have been included.

Porch et al. (1980) used four predictors—PICA Gestural, Verbal, and Graphic scores and age—collected at one month postonset to predict PICA Overall performance at 3, 6, and 12 months postonset. The predicted scores for their sample of patients correlated significantly ($p < 0.001$) with the scores the patients actually obtained at the different points in time postonset. Marshall and Phillips (in press) used a stepwise discriminant function procedure to predict conversational ability in aphasic patients following a period of treatment. Their results indicate that patients likely to regain verbal communication are younger, healthy, close to onset, not severely aphasic, and fluent. Marshall et al. (1982) utilized a stepwise multiple regression procedure to examine the predictive value 11 prognostic variables had on forecasting response to treatment in 110 aphasic patients. The most potent variables were age, months postonset when treatment began, and the number of treatment sessions. Finally, Deal et al. (1979) utilized the predictive equation generated by Porch et al. (1980) to predict for 90 aphasic patients. Correlations between predicted PICA performance and the performance actually obtained were significant ($p <$ 0.001); however, less than half of their sample attained PICA overall scores that were within plus or minus 5 percentile units of the score predicted.

Thus, statistical prediction of improvement in aphasic and apraxic patients appears to be more promising than practical or precise. Its potential is worth pursuing. For example, application of stepwise multiple regression techniques that employ variables believed to influence change (initial severity; presence and severity or oral, nonverbal apraxia; severity of coexisting aphasia; etc.) may test the potency of these for predicting change in apraxia of speech and, eventually, generate predictive equations that are applicable with individual patients. The effort required to move this approach from interest to use is enormous. Large samples of apraxic patients must be identified and evaluated. followed over time, and reevaluated. Then, retrospectively, one looks for early predictors of eventual performance. The path to making statistical prediction clinically applicable, though long and laborious, is probably worth the plodding.

PROGNOSTIC TREATMENT

The more precise one wants to be about prognosis, the more it costs in time, both patient's and clinician's. Mohr (1980) observed that apraxic patients improve even if we do nothing. If we bring them into the clinic room and set the contingencies for good performance correctly, however, their improvement is faster and goes further. We call this exercise prognostic treatment. We see if we can accelerate change by creating the right environment with testing and treatment to show the patient the way. Within 20 treatment sessions, sometimes less, we let patients tell us their prognoses for improvement. We rely on four determinants: improved performance on treated tasks, generalization, retention, and willingness to practice. If the patient learns; generalizes what is learned on one task by displaying improved performance on another, untreated task; retains what has been learned; and is willing to practice, practice, and practice, we believe that the prognosis for improvement, with treatment, is great.

The first three determinants—learning, generalization, and retention—are measured according to the demands of the single-subject design (Hersen & Barlow, 1976). As an aid in reading the figures that display multiple-baseline, single-subject design data, the reader is reminded that baseline, pretreatment performance, is to the left of the first dotted line; performance during treatment is shown between the dotted lines; and performance posttreatment is to the right of the second dotted line. To be convincing, performance should improve only after treatment has begun. Unfortunately for the researcher but fortunately for the patient, speech does not know this. It has not read Herson and Barlow (1976), and it is as willing to respond to physiologic recovery as it is to the clinician. This muddies waters if one is attempting to demonstrate the efficacy of a treatment. For prognosis, however, it is a good sign indicating that speech is ready to move if given the opportunity and a bit of help from a clinical chum.

Ability to Learn

Regardless of what you call your method of treatment—facilitation, stimulation, reorganization, education, or Harold—you expect your patient to learn when it is applied. If he or she does not, the method is wrong or the patient has a bleak future. We expect our patients to learn, and the rapidity that they display in doing so is prognostic.

We select, from our appraisal data, a behavior that is arable. We baseline it in at least three sessions, and then we intervene with treatment. If performance improves in a limited number of sessions, we smile and search for adjectives that describe a favorable prognosis.

Figure 3 shows response to prognostic treatment by D.J. on the vowels /i/ and /u/. We began during the first week we met him, which was his fifth week postonset. Performance on both stimuli were baselined by having D.J. produce 20 repetitions of each vowel in three sessions. In the fourth session, we began to treat /i/ with massed practice using auditory and visual stimulation and some laying on of the hands to get D.J. into the correct articulatory posture. At the end of the fourth session and for the next ten sessions we ran a daily criterion performance on /i/ with the 20 repetitions. /u/ was baselined through session seven, and in session eight, we began to treat it. The vowel /i/ began to improve, perhaps under spontaneous recovery's gentle prodding, perhaps from treatment, or from both. The /u/ moved only when we intervened with treatment. Perhaps spontaneous recovery got on board, perhaps treatment of /i/ generalized to /u/. The whys are not important. D.J. learned when prodded, and that learning led us to predict a bright future for return of speech.

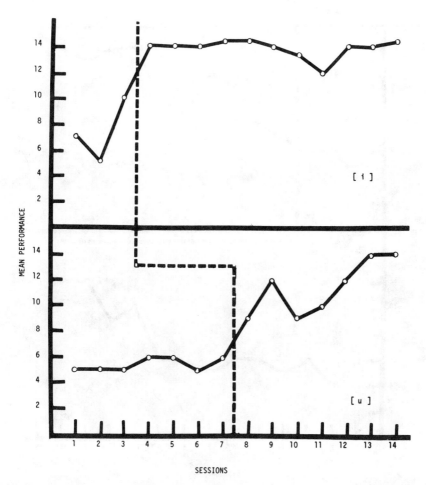

Figure 3. Response to prognostic treatment by D.J. showing ability to learn the production of two vowels, /i/ and /u/. Performance is shown as the mean of 20 productions scored with the PICA multidimensional scoring system.

Generalization

No one has the time to relearn each and every articulatory gesture and their combinations to produce functional speech. We expect generalization. Without it, prognosis is bleak. So, in our prognostic treatment, we set the contingencies to see if generalization occurs. Again, the multiple-baseline design is the tool we use. Production of two or more responses are baselined, one is treated, and the other or others continue in the baseline condition. Generalization is indicated by improvement or the lack of it on the untreated productions.

A.K. is shown in Figure 4. He suffered a left-hemisphere CVA and was

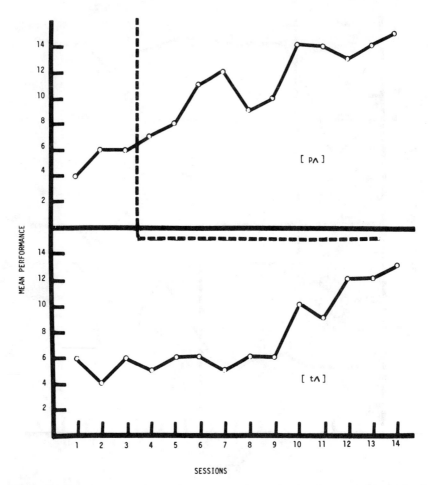

Figure 4. Response to prognostic treatment by A.K. showing generalization of treatment for /pʌ/ to production of /tʌ/. Performance is shown as the mean of 20 productions scored with the PICA multidimensional scoring system.

severely aphasic and apraxic at two weeks postonset. We gathered our multiple baseline materials to determine his ability to learn and to generalize, but we had to shelve them for two months. Pneumonia sent A.K. to the Intensive Care Unit for a month and to the pulmonary ward for another month. At two and one-half months postonset, we gathered again. We baselined /pʌ/ and /tʌ/, and we treated /pʌ/ while continuing to baseline /tʌ/. Production of /pʌ/ took off in sessions six and seven, was a bit fragile in sessions eight and nine, and convinced us of its stability after session ten. The /tʌ/ wandered alone until session ten. Generalization of treatment for /pʌ/ appeared to influence production of /tʌ/ thereafter. Or, perhaps /tʌ/

was influenced by spontaneous recovery at approximately three months postonset. Nevertheless, what we were looking for—generalization—occurred, and we predicted that A.K. was on his way to achieving return of speech.

Retention

When they get fixed, be it from treatment or from spontaneous recovery, we want them to stay fixed. Staying fixed we call retention. Pure single-subject research predicts a sag in performance after treatment is withdrawn. Typically, it does during the relatively short course of a withdrawal design. If treatment is protracted, however, performance rebounds, and we get retention. In the management of apraxia of speech, there is too much to mend to permit applying patches to what has been rendered acceptable by treatment. Performance may drop a bit when treatment stops or moves on to new targets, but if it drops too much or does not rebound, it is bad for the prognosis.

Figure 5 shows data for B.S. He arrived at one month postonset from a left-hemisphere CVA displaying global aphasia indicated by 10th percentile performance on the PICA. We were willing to wager that he was also severely apraxic, but his paucity of verbal production did not provide the evidence for us to collect the bet. One month of Visual Action Therapy (Helm-Estabrooks et al., 1982) riding on the flow of spontaneous recovery improved this man's language to the 27th percentile on the PICA and unlocked his sparse speech to confirm our early suspicion about his being apraxic. A series of sessions similar to those shown in Figures 3 and 4 brought him to the point where he was ready to tackle monosyllabic words. His performance is shown in Figures 5. We baselined two sets of CVCs, one beginning with /s/ and one beginning with /f/. We treated /s/, and it responded. We followed with treatment of /f/, and, though shaky at first, it too took hold. To test retention, we withdrew treatment of /s/ after the 11th session but continued to baseline it. B.S. maintained his gains on /s/ productions. He retained, and prognosis smiled.

Willingness to Practice

One of the reasons treatment helps patients suffering apraxia of speech, we believe, is because it structures the patient's practice. Unlike the more general stimulation techniques that may unlock aphasia, practice is the pivot that produces improvement in the apraxic patient's speech. We drill, and we drill some more. The patient must be able to participate, and must be willing to participate.

So, we want our patients active, and we want them to want to be

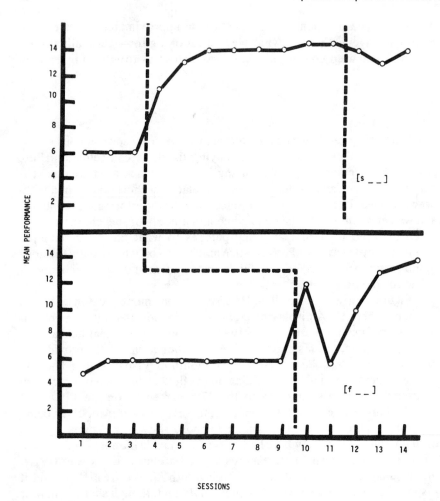

Figure 5. Response to prognostic treatment by B.S. showing retention of /s/ CVC words after the treatment of them was withdrawn but continued on /f/ CVC words.

active. Speech therapy for apraxia of speech bears no resemblance to intravenous feeding. If patients take an active part in treatment, they will conquer all but the most stubborn apraxia. If they do not, no clinician can make them talk better. A torpid patient can only hope that physiologic recovery smiles warmly upon him or her.

Typical of what the dedicated do is represented by the data shown in Figure 6 for J.N. He saw us three days a week as an outpatient. We had moved through a series of single subject designs with a variety of stimuli. J.N. learned these, and he learned the game. Following the first baseline on words with /pl/ in the initial position, he informed his wife what was coming

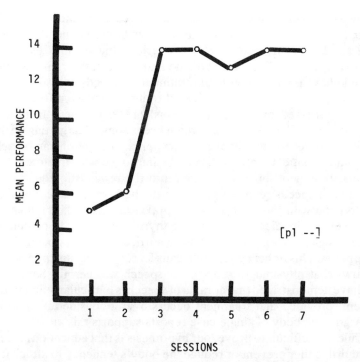

Figure 6.   Influence of J.N.'s home practice without our knowledge after the first baseline session. Baseline continued for seven sessions with no treatment intervention. Performance is shown as the mean of 20 productions scored with the PICA multidimensional scoring system.

next. He convinced her to assist him in practicing /pl/ at home, without our knowledge. What we thought was the third baseline revealed the results of his efforts. We were bemused; he was amused. Such efforts are bad for the design, but they are wonderful for the prognosis.

SUMMARY

We build our prognostic equation with biographical, medical, and behavioral variables that may predict improvement or the lack of it; with behavioral profiles that can be compared with those of previous patients who improved and those that did not; and with what the patients tell us about their prognoses when we submit them to prognostic therapy designed to measure learning, generalization, retention, and willingness to practice. We solve the equation to find a descriptive adjective to forecast the future and a statement about prognosis.

The patients presented as examples improved, some more than others. All were treated. Would they have improved without treatment? One might as well ask how many undiscovered American Indian ruins exist in the Four Corners area of Colorado. No one knows the answer. Some, probably, would have improved without treatment. The body is resilient. It can recover from all but the most horrible of traumas, and even from some of those, as witnessed by Norman Cousins' (1979) recovery from a rare collagen disease. The assumption, which keeps some of us getting up in the morning, however, is that recovery from apraxia of speech can be helped along, that the patient's prognosis can be improved with treatment.

Thus, treatment must be entered into the prognostic equation. We believe that it speeds recovery, because the body may make mistakes in trying to cope with the frustration of apraxia just as a child's body may produce auto-antibodies against its own thyroid hormone. For a child, the antibodies mean lethargy and fever and a hurried trip to the doctor. For the apraxic patient, his or her condition means fear, struggle, and performance far below what physiologic support for speech will permit. Sands et al. (1978) have demonstrated that apraxia of speech is particularly amenable to treatment, provided that treatment occurs over a considerable period of time. A growing body of single-case reports supports this view.

While it is difficult to prove, our hypothesis is that education, counseling, and drill either prevent or reduce the body's tendency to attack itself. The counseling is a crucial component. Heaton et al. (1978) point out that some brain-injured patients deny or are unaware of their deficits and set themselves for failure by attempting that which is beyond the limits of their current skills. Others underestimate and put a ceiling on their functioning that is below their current capacity. Counseling assists the patient in finding the just right. The combination of the three—education, counseling, and drill—improves the prognosis for improved speech. Placebo effect? Maybe. Influences on the psyche? No doubt. Also, there is no need to apologize. Helping a person reach a goal that may have been attained anyway is legitimate, especially if the trip made alone is halting and frightening.

We suspect, even though we cannot currently prove it, that many untreated apraxic patients do not reach the same competence that their treated brethren do. Neither their neuromotor systems nor their psyches allow it. Thus, the prognosis for functional recovery is poor without treatment, fair with treatment for the severe patient, and good with treatment in the moderate-to-mild patient.

All is not guesswork. What patients bring with them, what they can tell us about their disorder, and what our measures show can support specific prognostic statements for those patients. The statement should include the cost in time, money, and emotion necessary to reach what is predicted. It should not include a return to normal speech. We asked a patient, as we do most patients, "How long do you think you will have to work on your speech?" "Every day," he replied. It is not easy when you are a young clinician—or any age—to say a man you have thought of as old and a bit foolish is not only not foolish but almost a poet and a prophet. Every day, Joan Didion wrote, is all there is.

7

Introducing Treatment of Apraxia of Speech

Writing about treatment is like dissecting an earthworm. The worm lying against the cardboard with freshly sliced skin pinned back to expose hearts and reproductive organs, or as it appears in even the most graphic of lab drawings, bears only a slight resemblance to the one confidently protruding from its home in search of a meal or a mate. The best the biology teacher or student can hope for is that the skewered specimen or the exacting drawing will increase someone's knowledge and curiosity about earthworms and (even better) inspire respect for that sly fellow who disappears at the hint of footsteps. So it is with treatment. The lively interaction of clinician and patient cannot be described fully. The best a writer can hope for is an accurate, detailed description so that readers (practitioners) will learn a little and will want to dig into other literature and their own clinical practices for additional answers. Our lab specimen—in five pieces—follows.

A PHILOSOPHY OF TREATMENT

Judson (1980) in *The Search for Solutions* quotes from Eddington: "Observation and theory get on best when they are mixed together, both helping one another in the pursuit" (p. 162). Eddington was talking about science. He could as well have been talking about treatment. Methods and philosophies of management are intimates. Separated, they languish. United, they aid one another and patients.

Our philosophy about managing apraxia of speech is not elaborate. We believe that apraxia of speech treatment is *speech –language* treatment. It is not merely articulation training. The movements of that lovely pink fellow, the tongue, are not the sole target or emphasis. Meaning as well as movement are emphasized as soon as and whenever possible. Apraxia of speech treatment also requires drill or the orderly, intensive repetition of carefully selected responses. It requires knowledge of results and that speakers be successful more often than they are unsuccessful and that both successes and failures be used to their benefit. It requires an organization for each session that allows speakers all possible freedom or independence and one that moves them systematically toward as much control over movements and meanings as their motor speech and linguistic systems can accommodate.

Apraxia of speech treatment cannot be planned or completed by just anyone, not even one whose greatest need is to help those with speech defects. Certainly the need to help may make a clinician energetic enough to keep up with rapidly improving apraxic speakers and those who are willing to work for hours each day. It may make a clinician strong enough to endure the months of grueling drill required by those whose apraxia of speech is slow to respond. It may even allow a clinician to tolerate the patient who is easily bored or cynical about treatment's value. But even a quenchless yen to help is feckless as a guide to the selection and ordering of stimuli; to the application and evaluation of methods; and to the counseling which are the flesh, blood, and soul of apraxia of speech treatment. These require that clinicians know the influences that guide each decision they make about how to treat. This knowledge converts professional speech pathologists from caretakers to clinicians.

We have identified six major influences:

1. The nature of apraxia of speech;
2. the relationship of physiologic and linguistic processes;
3. the influence of nonspeech residuals of brain damage on responses to treatment;
4. the data and heuristic notions about how people learn skills;
5. the clinician's education and experience; and
6. the patient's abilities, attitudes, and expectations.

These six are not separate influences; a clinician and patient's moment-by-moment interactions are simultaneously governed by all of them, but we will discuss the first four separately, nonetheless. We will not discuss sources five and six because of their idiosyncrasies, except to say that treatment outcomes are profoundly influenced by them. Methods work in part because clinicians are comfortable with them and want them to. Patients learn in part because they will not have it otherwise. But neither clinicians nor patients would prosper if their clinical interactions were random or capricious. Order comes from the other four.

The Nature of Apraxia of Speech

Clinicians are helped by envisioning acquired apraxia of speech as a nondysarthric, nonaphasic, movement disorder or loss of skill whose main perceptual symptoms are articulation errors (primarily substitutions and distortions) and prosodic disturbances. Furthermore, it responds predictably to a variety of stimulus conditions. This view separates apraxia of speech from the dysarthrias and aphasias, highlights the therapeutic targets (articulation and prosody) and justifies both the search for patterns in the disturbed speech signal during evaluation and their systematic manipulation during treatment. It also reminds clinicians that treatment is the structured relearning of skilled speech movements. Other of apraxia of speech's accouterments, however, are less helpful.

Automatic –Reactive and Volitional –Purposive

The traditional automatic –reactive and volitonal –purposive dichotomy contained in many definitions of apraxia, including apraxia of speech (see Chapter 4), is of little use therapeutically. First, it fails to distinguish apraxia from dysarthria, as anyone knows who has seen a paralyzed tongue and arm move during a yawn. Second, "automatic" and "volitional" lack accepted operational definitions. Most experts would probably agree that a yawn is automatic or more automatic than a spoken word, but finer distinctions are more controversial. Is counting automatic or volitional? What is a social greeting or a 2-minute lecture after one has given it several times? Third, it may be that for some apraxic talkers what have been called volitional –purposive utterances are better preserved than what have been called automatic –reactive ones despite the traditional, nonexperimental view that automatic responses are always superior. We have seen several patients whose best speech was nearly always produced in imitation of the clinician. Imitation, it seems to us, is the epitome of volitonal –purposive speech, although we realize that this is an arguable view. Because of our disenchantment with the traditional dichotomy between the automatic –reactive and volitonal –purposive, we choose to disregard it and consider apraxia of speech simply as a movement disorder which is distinct from the dysarthrias and which is present in varying degrees on all tasks.

Types of Apraxia

Types of apraxia—kinetic, ideomotor, ideational; center, disconnection; planning, executive, unit—are only of heuristic value in treatment planning, given present knowledge. It can be posited, for example, that apraxic talkers with more distortions than substitutions have a kinetic, center, unit, or executive apraxia, and that those with more substitutions than distortions have an ideomotor, disconnection, or planning apraxia. One might also hypothesize that the prognosis for the two types is different and that responses to different modes of stimulation will differ. At present we do not even know if subtypes of apraxic talkers exist, although it has been suggested that they do (Canter, 1969; Deutsch, 1979). If apraxic patients who sound different, who recover at different rates, and who respond in distinct ways to a variety of therapeutic conditions are eventually discovered, the nineteenth century models (see Chapter 1) that generated the original types of apraxia may be supported. The clinician's best chance of contributing such support, however, is to collect diagnostic and therapeutic data with an eye only on what is happening with each patient. An analysis of what the data may mean for models or types of apraxia should be conducted by unimpassioned others. This is not to say that therapists should only be pragmatists. It does reflect our feeling that therapists have a problem when they set out to prove something: they prove it, no matter how far-fetched. The reason is simple: patients usually respond the way clinicians want them to. A clinician interested in treatment beyond what it may accomplish for each patient needs colleagues to monitor the treatment activities and analyze the data.

Relationship of Physiologic and Linguistic Processes

Physiologic and linguistic processes interact in normal speakers (Lenneberg, 1967) and in most apraxic talkers. It may even be that language contributes to the programming or planning mechanisms mentioned in classical definitions of apraxia of speech. This interaction in apraxic patients makes their errors predictable from linguistic constructs—frequency of occurrence, phrase type, and so on. That apraxia of speech can be analyzed linguistically does not mean that apraxia is a linguistic disorder, however. Kent and Rosenbek (1983) have warned against confusing the assumed neuropathology of a disorder with the method of analysis of that disorder.

The traditional, and perhaps reflexive, clinical use of the physiologic–linguistic interaction has been to justify using meaningful rather than meaningless stimuli to treat apraxic speakers. We subscribe to the traditional view. Because meaningful responses are both facilitating of adequate movements and motivating for the patients, we rely heavily on words and phrases as treatment stimuli. Others, such as Dabul and Bollier (1976), however, do not. They suggest using nonsense syllables during treatment's early stages. They say that nonsense syllable drill leaves the speaker freer to concentrate on movement adequacy, and they imply that relearning is faster than if meaningful stimuli are used from the beginning. They are not alone. Patients sometimes challenge the perfunctory use of meaningful stimuli. Some severe patients simply cannot say words. It is as if they have a dissociation of movement and meaning so that meaning has no influence on their articulatory movements. A group of chronic, moderately, and mildly involved speakers presents an even more interesting challenge. Members of this group are identified by their successful speech in the clinic and their difficulty self-correcting errors outside of the clinic. Clinicians can help such patients by separating the linguistic and physiologic, by lifting movement out of the linguistic stream and having them practice nonverbal movements, speech movements without voice, and sounds in isolation. These patients must learn careful planning, execution, evaluation, and self-correction. A motor system swept along by linguistic currents often moves too rapidly for these activities. The portage forced on the speaker by separating the physiologic and linguistic may make the trip through therapy more successful. Nor need the journey be slowed. Considerable time can be lost by getting hung up on unsuccessful attempts to self-correct when the linguistic flow has swept the speaker on but not over troublesome sounds and sound combinations.

Enlightened rather than ineluctable use of meaning, then, is the rule in apraxia of speech therapeutics. Perhaps the most thoughtful use of the linguistic–physiologic interaction is to consider it but one of a host of variables influencing stimulus selection and ordering. Others are the success rate a clinician wants to achieve in a particular session, the speaker's severity, and the clinician's long- and short-range goals.

Apraxia and Brain Damage

The brain damage that makes patients apraxic also alters them emotionally and behaviorally. The lability, irritability, depression, hyperactivity, distractability, easy fatiguability, perseveration, rigidity, and a potential ruck of other symptoms interact with the apraxia to make it worse and are themselves influenced by the speech disorder. These interactions need to be discovered during diagnosis and either accommodated or modified during threatment. Apraxia therapy cannot merely be speech therapy. Indeed, if one analyzes everything—stimuli, methods, timing, reenforcements, explanations—about a treatment session, one usually finds that only the stimuli are governed by the apraxia. The rest are introduced to accommodate and manipulate the other sequelae of brain damage. High success rates and reenforcements reduce emotionality; frequent changes in activity reduce perseveration; frequent rests reduce fatigue; frequent explanations reduce anxiety; demonstrated progress is an all-purpose balm.

The Learning of Skills

The emphasis in motor control and motor learning has moved from what Kelso and Stelmach (1976) call a "global product-performance orientation'' to an orientation ''predominately involved in understanding the processes underlying movement'' (p. 2). Discussion of these orientations is outside this book's scope; the interested reader can begin with Fitts and Posner (1967) and Stelmach (1976). In this short section, we want only to discuss a few observations primarily from the ''product-performance'' orientation for the illumination they provide on apraxia of speech and its treatment.

Characteristics of the Learner

Normal subjects trying to learn a new task resemble apraxic speakers struggling to relearn how to talk. Depending upon the instructor's acumen, normal learners are at first erratic and slow, and a few errors may create a flurry of errors. Apraxic speakers, especially during early sessions, are also variable, slow, and their errors snowball. The highly touted variability of apraxic speakers, especially during treatment, may, in part, be symptomatic of their learning rather than of their apraxia. If such is the case, variability, especialy if a speaker is aware of being observed, may be of limited diagnostic importance. Reductions in variability with treatment, on the other hand, may be a sensitive measure of progress.

Influences on Skill Learning

Influences on the way normal people learn skills may also be influences on learning by apraxic talkers. Understanding some of these influences affects our treatment and our general understanding of apraxia. If we realize, for example, that in the early stage of learning, the normal subject relies heavily on visual and tactile–kinesthetic feedback, we are less likely to marvel at the apraxic talker's ability to say visible sounds better than ones that are hard to see, and we are more likely to measure the treatment potency of visual, tactile–kinesthetic, and auditory inputs alone and in controlled combinations during diagnostic testing. When we remember that length of response influences normal learning, we are less amazed that it affects apraxic learners. We are also less infatuated with the influence of length on speech adequacy as a differential diagnostic characteristic of apraxia of speech. Finally, when we realize that normal skill learning is influenced by what Fitts and Posner (1967) call coherence and what others call meaningfulness, we are less likely to use the apraxic speaker's greater success with meaningfulness as evidence that apraxia is aphasia. We are also more likely to manipulate meaningfulness in our treatment paradigms.

Other observations about normal skill learning influence our treatment even if they do not influence our specific attitudes about apraxia of speech. Skill learning, including relearning how to talk, requires conscious, active participation on the learner's part. For speech retraining, this means increasing the patient's attention and conscious, closed-loop control of all articulatory movements. We call this state of attention and conscious control the "treatment mode," and prior to each treatment activity we tell each patient to "get into the treatment mode" (although we change the terminology to fit each speaker's background).

Three other observations from normal skill learning are also helpful in treatment planning. The interaction of success rate and normal learning rate is complex and variable, but the data are consistent enough to convince us that apraxic patients should be extremely successful, especially in the beginning of treatment, and that they can be allowed to taper off to a success rate of about 70 or 80% as treatment progresses. Also, because most skills seem to be most efficiently learned if presented in chunks or units, we first introduce patterns of spech movement and break these patterns down only if the patient cannot learn the chunks. If they cannot say, "sny" or any other S-words, for example, we see if they can say /s/ in isolation. If they cannot, we see first if they can close their mouths, then bare their teeth, and then direct an airstream through the valve that they have created. Once a serviceable /s/ arrives, we try immediately to combine it with other sounds. This is to say, we work with integrated movements if the patient can, break these integrated movements into subroutines as the patient needs to, and then recombine these subroutines as quickly as possible. Finally, we provide intensive, spaced drill and immediate, unequivocal knowledge of results from the first treatment session until the last.

GOALS OF TREATMENT

Apraxia of speech therapy's first goal is systematic, painless, and efficient reinstatement of as much speech as each patient's battered system allows. The second goal is to help the patient adjust to treatment and then to whatever disability remains when treatment is done. The third goal—but one that is unnecessary for some patients—is to teach the patient to augment speech with communication in other modes. These goals require that systematic drill be combined with counseling. Drill alone, even of the most carefully selected and ordered stimuli, must be blessed if it is to succeed. Since so much in medicine and the other helping professions must be left to the fates under even the best conditions, it seems reasonable that clinicians should want to exert more earthbound control whenever they can. Counseling can provide that control. If patients and families know what is happening, why it is happening, and what the possible outcomes will be, they are better able to accept therapy's sweaty labor and the reality that recovery almost surely will be incomplete—but worth it nonetheless. Taken together, drill and counseling can help a patient talk better, can improve communication within a family (assuming family members communicated before), and can prepare patient and family to make the best of their remaining time and abilities (assuming they were doing their best before). Patients who are both drilled and counseled are likely to begin communicating even when they cannot talk very well and to continue communicating regardless of how much speech they regain.

APRAXIA OF SPEECH TREATMENT COMPARED TO OTHER TREATMENTS

Apraxia of speech is not dysarthria, a simple phonological disorder, or aphasia. Its treatment, too, is unique. Unfortunately, these two opinions are not universally accepted and debate (Martin, 1975; Aten, Darley, Deal, & Johns, 1975), some of it acrimonious, continues, especially about the nosology and differential treatment of apraxia of speech and aphasia. Aten, Darley, Deal, and Johns (1975) and Johns and Darley (1970) led the group who argued that aphasia therapy would not help apraxic speakers, or at least would not help them as efficiently as would treatments specific to their symptoms and underlying neuropathology. Rosenbek (1978) said much the same thing about the differences among apraxia of speech therapy and that for the dysarthrias and for phonologic disorders. Probably the treatment issues are not so simple, however. By comparing and contrasting apraxia of speech treatment with treatment for the dysarthrias, for phonologic disorders in children, and for the aphasias, we hope to make the complexities more trenchant, while simultaneously adding further to our definition of what apraxia of speech treatment is.

Apraxia and Dysarthria Treatment

Comparing and contrasting apraxia of speech and dysarthria therapy is difficult. The variability within both populations to which treatments must respond and the lack of agreement about what apraxia and dysarthria treatment are make it hard to grasp similarities and differences. Nonetheless, let us try, beginning with the differences.

Differences Between the Two

Differences in apraxia and dysarthria treatment arise in part because some of the reasons for apraxic and dysarthric errors are dissimilar. The primary reason for apraxic symptomatology is a disruption in the planning and execution of gestures or movements. Apraxia then results from a breakdown at one of the highest levels of motor control. Dysarthric symptoms, according to Netsell and Daniel (1979), result from a variety of conditions including weakness, abnormal tone, impaired timing, and dys-coordination. The weak dysarthric speaker therefore may need muscle strengthening exercises; the apraxic speaker will not. The hypotonic dys-arthric speaker may profit from increased tone; the apraxic speaker will not. Further contrasts based on the disturbed neurophysiology underlying apraxia of speech and the dysarthrias are impossible to draw. Indeed, suspected similarities in some neurophysiologic features generate further commonalities in the treatments. Hypertonicity may contribute to both conditions and when it does, treatment can either accomodate it, reduce it, or prevent its getting worse. The abnormalities in timing and coordination that seem to plague some apraxic and dysarthric speakers seem to be similar enough, at least clinically, so that treatments for both kinds of patients may attend in similar ways to these abnormalities.

Some treatment differences result because apraxia and dysarthria may invade different functional components (Netsell, 1976) of the speaking mechanism. Respiratory structures are unaffected in apraxia, but often are affected in the dysarthrias, making improved respiratory support for speech a frequent goal of dysarthria but not of apraxia programs. Only the articulatory function of the larnyx will be disturbed in apraxia of speech, whereas the dysarthric speaker may not only make voicing errors but may have abnormalities in fundamental frequency, intonation, and quality as well. The dysarthric larynx, unlike the apraxic larynx, therefore, cannot be managed solely with articulation drills. For example, dysarthric speakers may need their fundamental frequency altered or quality improved. The articulatory function of the velopharynx may be impaired in both apraxic and dysarthric speakers and be a target of treatment of both. On the other hand, hypernasality is infrequent in apraxia but frequent in dysarthria, and therefore a target for modification only in dysarthria. Apraxia of speech treatments are directed primarily at the upper airway and are concerned with the other functional components of the speaking mechanism only as these contribute to speech sound and prosodic production. In contrast, dysarthria therapy may ignore the upper airway altogether or delay work on it until other functional components are performing better. Finally, apraxia of speech therapy seems to rely much more heavily than dysarthria therapy on linguistic or language variables. Frequency of usage, for exam-ple, influences both kinds of talkers but influences the apraxic more.

Similarities of the Two

Because both apraxic and dysarthric speakers may have disturbed articulation and prosody, some of the treatment targets—specifically artic-ulatory movements and the movements of the entire speaking mechanism that produce the intonational, stress, and rhythm profiles of speech—will be the same. Second, it appears that both apraxic and dysarthric functions of the jaw, lips, tongue, palate, and larynx can be influenced by the enlightened manipulation of articulation time and pause time. Specifically, if apraxic and dysarthric speakers can be slowed down, they sound better unless they are horribly severe, or profoundly aphasic, or already talking as slowly as they can. A third similarity is that drill is good therapy for both conditions and general facilitation or stimulation is feckless. Lectures, explanation, encouragement, and warm support are as helpful to them in regaining speech as similar activities would be in teaching skiing to a one-legged man. Such activities may motivate and sustain, but if the one-legged man is to negotiate a slope, he will need to don a ski and begin moving downhill under the constant guidance of a professional. So it is with both apraxic and dysarthric speakers. They relearn by doing.

Apraxia and Articulation Treatment

Therapy is not for the misoneist, because new knowledge constantly alters the features of all treatment. One has the feeling, however, that the specific methods for managing children's phonologic disorders have not changed as much as have the systems for analyzing performances and for selecting and ordering therapeutic targets (Ingram, 1976). Apraxia of speech clinicians have borrowed extensively from articulation therapy's traditional methodology. Despite the borrowing, however, apraxia of speech therapy is no more only articulation therapy than a person with a library card is a library. The therapies differ because (1) the apraxic adult usually has had a history of normal speech–language which the child for whom most articulation therapies were devised has not, and (2) the apraxic adult is brain damaged and is usually plagued by myriad coexisting speech–language and sensory-motor deficits while the child usually is not.[1]

Differences Between the Two

The apraxic adult's history of normal speech makes auditory training less important for him than for a child with a developmental phonologic deficit. According to Winitz (1969), a child's speech and sound learning is helped if discrimination training precedes production. Ingram (1976) is not so sure. Fortunately, we can leave those experts and their followers to

---

[1]We are excluding apraxic children from this comparison. When traditional therapies for children were being created, developmental apraxia of speech was seldom, if ever, diagnosed and its influence on those methods was probably small.

battle that one out in the research trenches. The adults about whom this book is written know how their speech should sound, and they may have even more rigid standards of adequacy than their clinicians. What they sometimes lack is either the willingness to listen to their disordered speech or a clear idea of what they are to be listening for. We are always amazed how discrimination is improved once listeners accept that they must listen and learn what to listen for. We do not precede production drills with discrimination drills, but we do precede production with counseling and education. We then combine production and discrimination training. We tell patients what we want them to say, help them say it, and then help them evaluate how well they have done.

Apraxia of speech treatment is also broader in its scope than articulation therapy, because most apraxic adults,[2] unlike most children with simple phonologic problems, have some degree of prosodic disturbance and coexisting behavioral differences such as fatiguability, perseveration, and distractibility—all of which need treatment. Admittedly, some (cf. Darley, 1968) claim that the prosodic differences in apraxia of speech are secondary, perhaps in compensation for the articulatory problem or even the result of treatment. It seems to us, however, that dysprosody is a primary symptom of apraxia, although we cannot be sanguine because the data are limited. Regardless of whether prosodic disturbances are primary or secondary symptoms, they are, at least for us, primary therapeutic targets. Improved prosody makes apraxic speech less abnormal sounding and increases its intelligibility. We also manipulate prosody to improve a patient's ability to articulate sounds and sound combinations and to provide for variety in treatment. In contrast, traditional articulation therapy seldom is concentrated to the same degree on prosodic features, at least so far as we have been able to determine. Fatigue, perseveration, and distractibility plague us all, and we do not deny that the child with a phonologic problem is sometimes perseverative, or distractible, or sad. We want to emphasize only that these conditions are daily parts of the apraxic adult's life so they must be a clinician's daily concern as well.

Other differences between the child and the apraxic adult also create treatment differences. Children and their clinicians can rely on the future and on maturation to augment therapeutic effort. Not so brain-damaged adults. For them, the past is a powerful beacon and the future, a frightening time of unpredictability and altered role. They and their clinicians must rely on physiologic improvement to supplement treatment. Unfortunately, physiologic improvement seldom sweeps as clean as maturation. Also, most children with a phonologic disorder have normal movements of their

---

[2]Apraxic children may or may not have disturbed prosody. The data are not yet in.

extremities, normal hearing and touch, and an intact—if rudimentary—concept of self. The stroke or other trauma that alters the adult's speech, on the other hand, may well create a hemiplegia, a visual field deficit, or a seizure disorder that nearly always slows progress in treatment, limits one's future, and alters one's sense of self. Such sobering realities require that an apraxic adult's clinician prepare a general rather than a specific treatment program.

One other difference between the therapies is equally as subtle but (we think) equally as real. It is the place of language in the two treatments. Phonologically impaired children and apraxic adults may have impaired language, but such impairment is more likely in the apraxic group. Both treatments recognize and control linguistic variables such as meaningfulness; but we suspect that the interaction of movement and meaning is more therapeutic for the apraxic group. Meaning is likely to summon correct movements from apraxic adults because they usually have a long history of normal speech and language. On the other hand, meaningful stimuli may be inappropriate in the early days of treatment for a childhood phonologic disorder. A real word may merely summon the phonologic error. At times, then, the child's clinician may assiduously avoid meaningful stimuli altogether.

Similarities of the Two

What are the similarities of the two treatments? Some methods are similar because apraxia of speech clinicians borrowed methods developed for children with phonologic disorders. Also, treatments for both are increasingly based on similar methods of linguistic analysis such as process analysis. Ingram (1976), for example, describes the processes that explain the most frequent childhood phonologic errors—omission, occlusion, and fronting. He could have done the same for many apraxic errors, and other researchers (Klich, Ireland, & Weidner, 1979; Kearns, 1980; Crary & Fokes, 1979) are beginning to. While the processes described by Ingram and others do not predict all of the adult apraxic's errors (distortions resulting from abnormal timing and coordination, for example, are not predicted), they do predict some of them. If processes predict a portion of the apraxic patient's pattern, then those same processes may also be used to guide the selection and ordering of treatment targets, as is apparently now happening in the treatment of childhood phonologic disorders (Singh & Polen, 1972).

Some specifics of stimulus selection and ordering are already similar for the two groups. Consider these examples. McReynolds and Bennett (1972) successfully taught a group of children selected sounds in the initial and then the final position of simple, nonsense syllables. The majority of apraxic clinicians also treat the initial position first, especially if a speaker is severely involved. Ingram (1976) advocates working on processes that occur infrequently because they are probably going to be easier to change. In addition, he defends trying to change processes most damaging to intelligibility. Apraxia clinicians make similar decisions (although their terminology for what is being treated may differ) because they want quick changes that make big differences. Also, clinicians working with children rely, in part, on normal developmental patterns to help them decide what to work on. In a child's speech development, velars emerge later on the average than sounds made in other places, so, velars are not ideal treatment targets for the phonologically impaired. Apraxia clinicians also use developmental criteria, along with several other criteria, for deciding what to work on. Finally, as more clinicians begin measuring their effectiveness, treatments for a variety of communicative disorders including apraxia of speech and developmental phonologic disorders will have similar structures. For example, the structure of single-case design research (see Chapter 8) is largely indifferent to the kind of person being treated.

Apraxia and Aphasia Treatment

Identifying the differences between apraxia and aphasia therapy requires a keen eye, a large sample of both treatments for comparison, and perhaps even a limber imagination. This is not to suggest that the differences are inconsequential or that they exist only in the minds of clinicians devoted to preserving the apraxia–aphasia distinction. It is to suggest that the differences are more like those between dusk and dawn than between night and day. The similarities, on the other hand, are a bit more obvious. First the differences.

Differences Between the Two

We agree with Alajouanine and Lhermitte (1964) that the apraxic speaker is more likely than the aphasic speaker to profit from drill, especially (and this is our qualification) during the acute stage. According to Alajouanine and Lhermitte (1964), "procedures of didactic learning have maximal efficiency in motor and perceptive disorders . . . Such procedures, however, are no longer efficient when the central problem is one of a disorder of symbolic formulation" (p. 215). Related to the appropriateness of drill is the appropriateness of explanations. The apraxic speaker may profit from knowing how and why; the aphasic speaker, unless mild, seldom does. Disordered language is improved by restimulation, not explanation. Indeed, one might posit that an apraxic speaker's ability to profit from explanation is an index to his or her coexisting aphasia.

Another difference between the treatments is that imitation is more therapeutic for the apraxic speaker than for all aphasic speakers except possibly those with transcortical motor or transcortical sensory aphasia. Even the anomic aphasic speaker, whose repetition initially may be superior to the apraxic patient's, does not transfer to propositional speech the competence gained from imitation the way the apraxic does. The reason for imitation's impotence in apha . treatment may be that imitation is more often dissociated from other kinds of performance in aphasia than in apraxia, although admittedly it can be dissociated in apraxia of speech as well.

The most trenchant difference between the two therapies involves the *principal* targets. Depending on severity and coexisting symptoms, the targets of apraxia of speech treatment are vocal tract shapes and their ordering. The emphasis, to borrow from Lenneberg (1967), is on *physiologic processes*. In aphasia treatment, the emphasis is on *linguistic processes*—on morphosyntax and semantics. We emphasize "principal" because, at any moment in apraxia treatment, the emphasis may be equally on physiologic and linguistic processes as when meaningfulness is invoked to stabilize shapes and movements, or when the clinician drills a set of words in several modalities, or tries to strengthen an apraxic talker's associational network for an utterance by using question-and-answer drill and other techniques that might be called pragmatic. This simultaneous emphasis on physiologic and linguistic processes is nowhere clearer than in the treatment of the severely apraxic. Treatment of this patient *must* emphasize the linguistic if the patient is to improve. On the other hand, no aphasic speaker in our experience has profited from practicing movements. The jargon aphasic speaker does not say "goofy newson" for "speech pathologist" because his motor system substitutes /g/ for /sp/ or /n/ for /p/. Nor will "speech" emerge from "goofy" if the clinician reminds the aphasic talker that /s/ is a fricative and /g/, a plosive.

Similarities of the Two

The similarities of apraxia and aphasia treatment, however, outnumber the differences. Linguistic variables such as phrase type, frequency of occurrence, and length are controlled in both. Both apraxic and aphasic patients have deficits resulting from their brain damage that influence their communication and which treatment must modify or accommodate. They perseverate, are distractible, are slow to rouse, and quick to tire. These and other general conditions threaten their performance, causing them to look more apraxic or aphasic than they otherwise would. Treatment then must be broader than drill or facilitation of motor and linguistic processes. It must be organized, paced, and spaced so that these general influences have minimal effect. To reduce perseveration, for example, the clinician changes stimuli and tasks frequently, tries to keep the patient successful, and takes periodic breaks. To minimize emotionality, the clinician explains, supports, and helps the patient do things that are otherwise impossible. Finally, in both kinds of treatment clinicians are likely to restimulate rather than correct, especially if a speaker is frustrated by failure; and in both kinds clinicians encourage self-monitoring, self-correction, and other forms of independence.

How then is the relationship between the treatments to be summarized? In our view, the difference is what receives top billing on the marquee. In apraxia of speech is is movement. In aphasia, it is meaning.

SENSORY MODALITIES IN TREATING APRAXIA OF SPEECH

We have two reasons for believing that the antecedent event is of greater concern than the consequent event in apraxia of speech treatment. Good speech (or improved speech) is its own reward. Apraxic speakers generally are keen judges of how well they have done each time they talk. In general, then, if apraxic speakers are helped to say something, they will take care of the rest. Methods and stimuli, the guts of the antecedent event, are discussed in subsequent chapters. In this section we will devote brief attention to the modalities, the other major component of the antecedent event. In addition to being critical components of the antecedent event, modalities are of importance for what they may indicate—in interaction with response adequacy—about the underlying neuropathology of apraxia of speech. For example, it might be hypothesized that apraxic patients with what Buckingham (1979) called a center apraxia will be insensitive to modality effects, while those with disconnection apraxia will show a striking perference for one modality over others.[3] This section therefore is included for both its clinical and theoretical significance.

Auditory Modality

Most clinicians present their stimuli through the auditory modality, because apraxic talkers, unless they have severe coexisting aphasia, understand what they hear. They understand directions, recognize stimuli, and in general react like normal speakers, except perhaps for being a bit delayed and requiring a slightly slower or simpler presentation of the material. This relative intactness in the auditory modality no doubt helps explain LaPointe and Horner's (1976) finding that listening to a model helps

---

[3]Lemme, Wertz, and Rosenbek (1974) examined the disconnection hypothesis and failed to find any data in support of it; however, more research is justified.

apraxic patients talk better than reading alone, or listening to and watching the clinician, or listening to the clinician while simultaneously reading the stimulus. Despite findings such as those by LaPointe and Horner, however, the clinical platitude persists that stimulation should be multimodality, and those authors themselves were quick to point out that clinicians should evaluate each patient's individual pattern and adjust treatment to it. We will return to this issue when we discuss the other modalities and our own clinical practice.

Auditory Discrimination Training

More controversial yet is how much auditory discrimination training an apraxic patient requires. To mention auditory discrimination training in a discussion about apraxia of speech rehabilitation (for the second time in this chapter) is to elicit the same quizzical looks given a bowling shirt in a fine lingerie shop. Johns (1970) and many others have ruled that discrimination training is unnecessary because apraxia of speech is a motor speech disorder. This may be too simple. If we hypothesize that movement planning requires sensory motor integrations (cf. Roy, 1978), we might hypothesize in turn that improving auditory processing abilities will improve planning and execution. This hypothesis deserves testing. We do not mean to divert this discussion into a darkened room where nothing can be made out. We do however, want to warn against rejecting discrimination training perfunctorily. In our view, we know too little about the mechanisms underlying apraxia of speech to make such an exclusion advisable. We also have seen too many apraxic speakers with only minimal amounts of aphasia who were nonetheless poor listeners during treatment's early days. However, because we are unwilling to risk preceding production with even short periods of traditional auditory discrimination training, our solution is to pair production and discrimination by having patients first listen and watch as we provide the model and then listen to and evaluate their own attempts.

Learning How to Listen

Our methods for improving listening are prosaic. We usually begin by having patients produce slow, careful speech which we ask them to evaluate, preceded in most instances by instructions about what to listen for. Some patients reject weak but otherwise adequate utterances. They need to understand that stroke or other trauma always steals the strength, and that they are to evaluate clarity rather than loudness. Some patients reject slow responses. Such patients need assurance that speed is unimportant and may even retard progress; an apraxic tongue needs time to get where it is going. Still others reject hoarse or strained but otherwise adequate responses. They need help in separating quality from adequacy. Some reject all responses because they are not the way they used to be. We remind these speakers that normal may never again be possible, that longing for it is enervating, but that improvement is likely (if it is), and that criteria for adequacy can change as performance does. During early drills, we help patients set criteria by comparing their judgments with ours and any time criteria can be changed we again resort to such comparisons so that the new criteria are learned. Throughout treatment, we reward any sign that a patient is listening. The usual first signs are attempted self-correction or a disgruntled look after an error.

Our most industrious and successful patients share a common talent: they listen and judge accurately. Some arrive at treatment with this ability. Most of even the best ones, however, develop good ears after being erratic judges during the severe, acute period. Patients who fail to develop as listeners have the devil's own time carrying over therapy's gains to everyday speech. They may not even improve within clinical sessions. So all efforts to improve a patient's listening are justified.

Relation of Speech to Listening

Before ending this short section on the auditory modality, it is perhaps worth noting that apraxic speech errors may have disastrous effects on listening. It seems to us that the ears can be blocked by the tongue, and a rash of apraxic errors or even the struggle to make an apraxic tongue perform can create so much "neural interference" that the patient is unsure about what has been heard. The other senses may be disturbed similarly. The point of all this is that improved comprehension may arrive on the heels of more predictable movements.[4] In therapy, this means for us that the patient should be encouraged to listen from day one but that the clinician should emphasize production first and assume much of the burden for knowledge of results until the patient is producing more predictable noises and has learned how to listen.

Tactile – Kinesthetic Modality

Tactile –kinesthetic cues associated with position and movement may be as important for some speakers as auiditory ones, especially during treatment's early sessions. Patients whose inability to plan because of an impairment in the tactile –kinesthetic network assumed to be important for motor planning may be improved by enhanced processing of tactile –kinesthetic information. Tactile –kinesthetic awareness can also improve ongoing articulatory accuracy, especially at slow rates. In addition, it may help a patient self-correct before making an audible mistake. In

---

[4]For a recent review of auditory discrimination, read Locke (1980a, 1980b).

fact, groping in apraxia of speech may result partly because some patients sample the adequacy of a placement before adding noise. Teaching patients to process tactile –kinesthetic cues may make them more efficient gropers and, therefore, more efficient speakers.

A potential complication is that oral sensory –perceptual integrity may be compromised in apraxia of speech (Rosenbek,Wertz, & Darley, 1973), although some researchers (Deutsch, 1981) have not confirmed such deficits. Even when such deficits are discovered, however, they appear to be more frequently unilateral than bilateral, resulting in tactile –kinesthetic cues to movement that are muted or distorted but not absent. Regardless of whether patients have normal or abnormal sensation and perception, clinicians will likely have to work assiduously at helping them learn how to use such sensory information because most of us are ignorant of our mouth's interior. Slow productions which the patient is instructed to both hear and feel, and silent posturing during which the patient makes a correct shape without producing the sound, are demanding but effective ways of enhancing a speaker's awareness of tactile –kinesthetic cues.We do not precede production with oral sensory –perceptual training although it has been advocated (Macaluso-Haynes, 1978). We combine the two.

Visual Modality

"Make the patient visually minded" resounds in nearly every piece of apraxia of speech treatment literature. Unfortunately, it is easier by far to watch one's feet and hands than one's tongue, and the only way patients can watch themselves is to use a mirror or a videotape monitor. We do not use mirrors or monitors. In the acute stage, we worry that patients will be distressed by their appearance, altered as it often is by weakness; and at all stages of treatment we are likely to eschew the mirror for another reason. We never had much training in its use and so feel more comfortable with other techniques. This is not meant as condemnation. The mirror may speed learning; many experts seem to think so. We will leave the proof to them.

We do use the visual modality, however. We have patients watch us, and we repeatedly explain what they are to watch for. We try to pair what patients see and hear us doing with what they hear and feel themselves doing. We also have some patients read aloud. Our specific uses of the visual modality will be described in detail in subsequent chapters.

Combining Modalities

It may be that like the cross-country skier who dons four layers of clothing and then roasts after ten minutes on the trail, our treatment has too much outerwear. Perhaps auditory, tactile –kinesthetic, and visual cues are unnecessary and even retarding. For some patients listening may be enough, and if the ears fail to guide the tongue toward independence, feeling and seeing will not help either. We continue our multimodality training anyhow. Roasting is what comes of wanting to be absolutely warm, and like a skier we can always strip a few items away when we get too hot. We can strip away certain inputs, for example, if a patient shows a preference for one set of sensory associations over others. Until the research of the type done by LaPointe and Horner (1976) is complete, we will continue to overdress.

OUR LEGACY

The methods described in this book are not unique. We have inherited a rich lode of methods from past and contemporary clinicians. Our wealth we owe to Halpern (1981); Shewan (1980); Broida (1979); Deal and Florance (1978); Lebrun and Hoops (1978); Holtzapple and Marshall (1977); Wilson (1977); Love and Webb (1977); Warren (1977); Keenan (1975); Darley, Aronson, and Brown (1975); Stryker (1975); Eisenson (1973); Keith (1972); Kreindler and Fradis (1968); Johns (1970); Luria (1970); Buck (1968); Agronowitz and McKeown (1964); Schuell, Jenkins, and Jiménez-Pabón (1964); Wepman (1951); Goldstein (1948); Granich and Prangle (1947); and Weisenberg and McBride (1935), to name only a few. What specifically is this inheritance? Almost everything that is to be discussed in subsequent chapters. Other clinicians have told us about the importance of the visual modality, about the proper ordering of stimuli, about reorganization, about facilitation, about imitation, about minimal contrasts, about reading, about rules for combining sounds with prosodic features and with gestures, about counseling, and about treating the whole patient. So why does this book contain four more chapters? Because we try to combine in them the best that we have extracted from the literature with the best in our clinical practice to produce a durable alloy capable of withstanding the buffeting that all clinical interactions impose on all methods and practitioners.

THE NEXT FOUR CHAPTERS

In the four chapters to follow, we will provide a set of guidelines on stimulus selection and ordering and chapters on counseling and specific treatments for severe, moderate, and mild apraxic speakers. All clinicians know that to divide a book into treatment chapters is to risk autopsy rather than surgery, because methods and the thing to be learned—speech in this instance—interact. We hope our intended cuts (chapters) will be kind to treatment and therefore to the apraxic patients for whom this book is intended. It seemed to us that a separate section on stimulus selection and ordering (Netsell, 1978) would prevent the redundancy that might crop up if we tried to discuss stimuli in each of the three specific treatment chapters. Separating stimuli from methods seemed also to reenforce our view that stimulus selection is determined by many variables, severity being only one. Three treatment chapters with methods grouped according to their appropriateness for patients of different severities seemed appropriate because patients divided by severity appear to distribute themselves according to a series of three overlapping, bell-shaped curves. Certain patients will be from the middle of one of the distributions. They will be easily identified, and the therapy to be described will fit them best. Other patients will be at the overlap of two distributions. The clinician will not want to force them into one distribution or the other, and should not. Treatment for these patients can be created out of the materials from more than one chapter. Still other patients will not fit any of our distributions because of coexisting sensory-motor, psychiatric, educational, and developmental differences. Their management will have to be inferred and the inferences checked against their response to treatment.

Each treatment chapter ends with data on selected methods. These data are drawn from single-case designs (Hersen & Barlow, 1976), conducted according to traditional restraints. In our view, it is unconscionable for speech pathologists to spurn data collection and to seek refuge in that tired old disclaimer, ''At least it doesn't hurt.'' Wrong speech treatments do hurt, although the wounds do not weep nor does the patient expire. Failure to improve, when improvement is possible, is frightening. Being shuffled from one method to another for short, ineffective blasts of therapy is debilitating. Being greeted by a benign smile, a cup of coffee, and a few minutes of meandering, vapid conversation when drill is required is confusing and disheartening. We have also included data because so few have been published. The pitiful state of affairs in aphasiology (including the study of apraxia), even after all our years of practice, is that we do not know for sure what works, how rapidly, and with whom. Someone's word is not proof of a method's efficacy. Our data do not prove that the methods work, only that they can work for some patients in the hands of some clinicians. Throughout, we will label untested methods with a skull and crossbones.

A CAVEAT

What follows is only the way it seems to us. We hope that our methods will form a useful clinical guide and that they will become a pleasant history. To make them history quickly was our major aim in writing this book.

8

Selecting and Ordering the Stimuli

Methods and stimuli interact, but they are separated in this book. Prescribing methods is confining enough. To prescribe stimuli as well is to create a manacle from which only the most adroit clinician can escape and which only the most experienced clinicians can avoid altogether. Perhaps our compromise—assigning a separate chapter to stimuli—is like providing one cuff at a time. Regardless, it did seem less cumbersome and fairer.

Three issues are raised in this chapter: (1) what stimuli can treatment begin with, (2) how many stimuli can be worked with simultaneously, and (3) how can stimuli be ordered once treatment has begun? Differences among patient histories, futures, symptoms, and responses to treatment, as well as differences among clinicians make fiat impossible. Instead, we have summarized our criteria for resolving each issue for individual patients.

SINGLE-CASE DESIGNS

Featuring a research criterion to guide the selection and ordering of treatment stimuli may seem queer to some. We have chosen to do so because we think clinical research is as intimately related to clinical practice as smell is to taste. Experimentation gives form to treatment. It helps clinicians evaluate the opinions and actions of colleagues. It gives them answers about which of their methods works and with whom. For a long time speech pathology has had treatment techniques, dedicated clinicians, and patients needing treatment. The research methodology that can provide a data base for the interactions of methods, clinicians, and patients has been slower to arrive, but arrive it has in the form of *single-case design research.*

To understand the influence of single-case design or the systematic study of single patients on stimulus selection and ordering, one first needs to understand something about the types and requirements of such designs. We most frequently use (1) the withdrawal or ABA design, (2) the multiple baseline design, and (3) the alternating treatments design. Hersen and Barlow (1976) and Kratochwill (1978) have written extensively about these, and their specific uses in speech pathology are described by Silverman (1977) and McReynolds and Kearns (1982). Our discussion owes almost everything to Hersen and Barlow (1976) and McReynolds and Kearns (1982).

The Withdrawal or ABA Design

The *withdrawal design's* essential components are (1) a period of baseline testing of the target response(s), called the A period; (2) a period of treatment during which the target response(s) are treated and periodically tested, called the B period; and (3) a period of withdrawal when treatment is withheld and retention of the response(s) is periodically tested, called the A period. Baseline, treatment, and withdrawal periods should be about the same length; the treated response(s) should be tested about the same number of times; and treatment should be reinstated after the withdrawal period whenever possible, making the design an ABAB. Evidence for a treatment effect potentially comes from two sources: (1) the superiority of treated performance over baseline performance, and (2) disintegration or leveling off in performance once treatment is withdrawn. An idealized withdrawal design appears in Figure 1. We took the liberty of portraying a stable baseline, an immediate and clinically significant jump in performance with treatment, a convincing but less than total collapse after withdrawal, and a return to excellent performance once treatment was reinstated.

Clinicians worry about the ethicality of withdrawing treatment. We do too, so we keep withdrawal periods short and follow them with additional (but not necessarily the same) treatment. We worry more, however, about the ethics of using untested treatments. The withdrawal design, properly handled, allows one to test methods without sacrificing patients. Our procedure is to reintroduce a method after the withdrawal period, if the data show that it is working. If the data show that it is not, we change treatments. In the first case, patients get more of what helps. In the second, they are spared what does not help. Either of these possibilities seems fairer than unstructured treatment that goes until time, money, or patience runs out or until a clinician "gets a feeling" that a method is good or bad.

Clinicians are also puzzled by the experimental convention of using the deterioration in a response's adequacy after withdrawal of treatment as evidence for a method's efficacy. The leveling off of a response is less

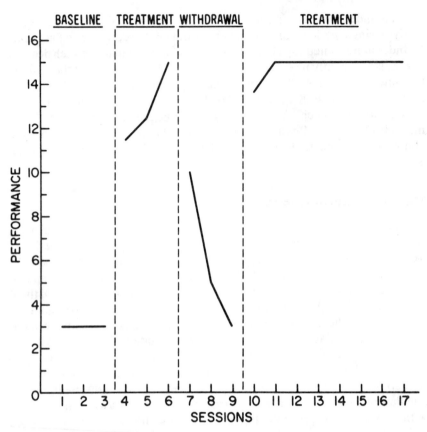

Figure 1. An idealized withdrawal design, showing a flat baseline, improvement with treatment, a sag in performance during withdrawal, and a return to good performance when treatment is resumed.

puzzling. We think that the convention is especially appropriate with brain-damaged adults. In our view, the only responses that reappear after brain damage are those that physiologic recovery and treatment bring. So if a treated response improves during the *acute* state of recovery but does not deteriorate or plateau when treatment is withdrawn, the clinician seldom has any choice but to conclude that improvement was caused by physiologic recovery. Failure of a treated response to deteriorate or plateau after withdrawal of treatment during the chronic stage is a bit more difficult to interpret. But even during the chronic stage, unless a response has been treated for several months (an unlikely condition in most withdrawal designs where baseline, treatment, and withdrawal stages are approximately the same length) failure to deteriorate or to plateau compromises

.the design and the clinician should not be sanguine about specific treatment effects. Clinicians who can remember their own undergraduate and graduate educations should not be surprised by our position. Material learned in school—the cranial nerves, the International Phonetic Alphabet, the number of subtests on the Porch Index of Communicative Ability—are not retained completely once school is over.

Responses that have been treated for a long time are a special case. They may not sag even though their integrity results solely from treatment. Protracted treatment usually is characteristic of the second treatment phase of an ABAB design. In this sense also treatment is like graduate school. Nothing keeps phonetics fresher than daily transcription for a period of months or years.

The Multiple Baseline Design

The *multiple baseline design* requires that a number of targets be ordered according to sound clinical or experimental criteria, that all receive baseline testing, and then that the same treatment be directed systematically toward each of the targets in turn. Each treated target continues to receive progress testing, and the untreated targets continue to receive baseline testing. This pattern can continue until targets have been brought systematically under therapeutic control, or some targets can go untreated and serve as measures of generalization. For example, the clinician might choose to place initial /p/, /b/, /t/, and /d/ words in such a design. Treatment would begin with the /p/ words, then move to /b/, then to /t/, and finally to /d/. An idealized multiple baseline design appears in Figure 2. Proof of therapeutic effectiveness is in the response of each target as therapy is introduced. This design is less offensive to some clinicians than the ABA design because treatment need not be withdrawn. A significant drawback is that generalization across targets may cause them all to move even though only one or two are being treated, an effect that may be hard to separate from physiologic recovery. Generalization can be reduced by selecting dissimilar targets and by selecting some targets that are very difficult.

The Alternating Treatments Design

In the *alternating treatments design* (Barlow & Hayes, 1979) a target is treated with two different methods. For example, a set of words or phrases could be treated with an imitative program and with a reading program. Performance is measured in both and the results compared as in the idealized example shown in Figure 3. This design has been infrequently used in published speech pathology work, and is less popular generally than the withdrawal and multiple baseline designs. It has the values of

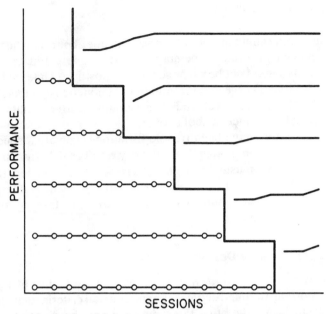

Figure 2. An idealized multiple baseline design. Baseline performance is represented by the circles to the left of the dividing line and response to treatment is represented by the solid lines to the right of the dividing line.

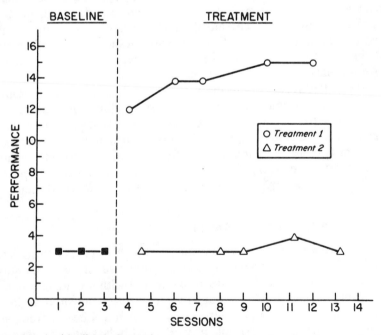

Figure 3. An idealized alternating treatment design, showing the superiority of treatment one over treatment two.

allowing for comparison of methods and obviating treatment withdrawal. A clinical drawback is that generalization from one treatment to the other may make interpreting results difficult. Despite this complication, Rubow, Rosenbek, Collins, and Longstreth (1982) successfully used a slightly modified alternating treatments design to compare simple imitation and imitation with vibrotactile stimulation with one moderately apraxic speaker.

General Guidelines for Constructing Single-Case Research

Despite differences in structure, the three previously described designs all require that the clinician cleave to certain common guidelines. Hersen and Barlow (1976) have described these at length; we will only summarize them here.

Limit and Specify Treatment

Single-case designs do not allow for the testing of a treatment package—for this one needs group designs—but they offer the best possible mechanism for testing the specific techniques that might ultimately be part of such a package. For this reason, and because clinicians want both to enhance their chances of identifying what it was that helped individual patients and to produce studies that other clinicians can replicate, they must limit and specify the treatment. This guideline can frustrate early attempts to complete a single-case design because clinicians—at least the ones writing this book—use an extensive and protean approach during each session much like a person destroying crabgrass by bulldozing the yard. With practice, however, treatments can be conducted with greater finesse and focus.

Use Specific, Complete, and Replicable Measures

The clinician needs to select or create measures of baseline performance, progress, and retention that are specific, complete, and replicable. Once the clinician has decided what is to be asked with each single-case design, test selection is relatively easy. For example, if the clinician is interested in finding out if a particular method such as phonetic placement helps a patient learn sounds in isolation, testing will be of sounds in isolation. If the question is whether such training makes it possible for the patient to say the sounds in words, words will have to be tested as well. Measurement of carryover to spontaneous speech will require adding a spontaneous speech measure. As a general rule, tests clinicians create are as useful as standardized tests if they are constructed according to phonetic and linguistic principles and are carefully specified.

Control When Testing is Done

The timing of testing should be controlled. Questions to be answered usually determine schedules for testing. Testing at the beginning of a session will answer questions about retention from session to session; testing at the beginning and end of a session will document learning within a session. Rapidly improving patients and questions about rate of learning require frequent testing. Chronic, slowly changing patients whose clinicians are interested in the final amount of learning rather than in the rate can be accommodated with less frequent testing, and so on. Once a measurement schedule is specified, the clinician is less likely to forget to test or to be lured into opportunistic testing timed to show maximum and perhaps misleading effects. Altering any schedule is always legitimate as long as the reader of any subsequent report is informed of the change and why it was done.

Establish a Predictable or Stable Baseline

Prior to intervention, the clinician will want to establish a predictable or stable baseline, because it is only from predictability, including stability, that convincing treatment effects can be seen. If nontreated performance is improving as in Figure 4, any change with treatment would need to be big

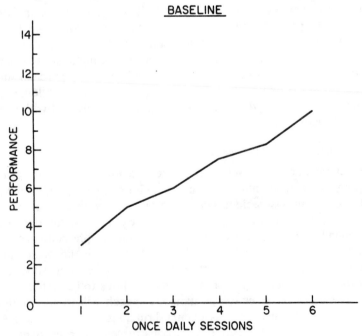

Figure 4. A baseline showing improvement without treatment.

and immediate to be credible. Preferable to such an improving baseline are flat, deteriorating, or minimally variable ones as shown in Figure 5. A minimum of three measures is usually necessary to determine a baseline's shape. In scheduling these baseline measurements, the clinician needs to consider the influence of spontaneous recovery (if it is operating), incidental learning as a result of repeated testing, and clinical realities such as the patient's physical therapy schedule.

Make Testing Unobtrusive

Testing should be as nearly unobtrusive as possible. Patients want to please; the clincian's well-being seems important to them. Therefore, when they have the idea that it matters more than usual they will behave better than usual. The result may be inflated scores and spurious conclusions about a procedure's vigor. In our bid for unobtrusiveness, we are not above a bit of deception. We try to introduce a number of activities that resemble testing and not allow the patient to know which are tests and which are not.

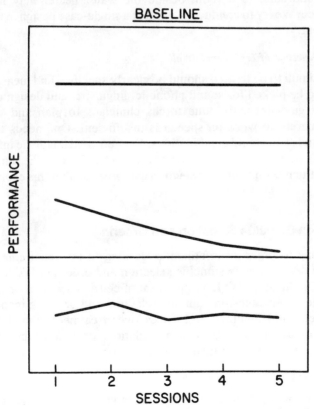

Figure 5.   Flat, deteriorating, and minimally variable baselines.

We also use other clincians to score responses—preferably out of the patient's sight—while we administer the stimuli. Probably they are not fooled, but we do the best we can.

Specify Personnel and Conditions

Treatment, test personnel, and conditions should be specified beforehand. A common fear, especially among experienced clinicians, is that what works for them does so because of something in themselves as well as something in the methodology. The fear may be justified, and one way to find out is for a variety of clinicians to attempt replication of their colleague's designs. Another way of helping to guarantee that treatment effects are the results of methods rather than specific clinicians is for disinterested clinicians to score the baseline and progress data. Treatment clinicians should not even collect data during a treatment experiment except that changing clinicians obviously threatens unobtrusiveness. Finally, testing and treatment conditions should be controlled. Moving from a sound suite to a room beside the water heater may influence performance. We try to conduct all parts of a single-case design in the same environment.

Control the Selection of Treatment Stimuli

The stimuli to be treated should be clearly specified and measureable; they should be picked for sound phonetic, linguistic, and design reasons. Like other guidelines, this one forces clinicians to plan and winnow. Deciding merely to work on speech is insufficient. One needs to select certain sounds and sound combinations. Phonetic and linguistic influences on stimulus selection will be discussed later on. It is to the single-case design's influence on stimulus selection and ordering that this chapter now turns.

Influence on Stimulus Selection and Ordering

Deciding to organize treatment according to the requirements of a single-case design affects stimulus selection and ordering. We think that the effects are healthy. We have never sacrificed a patient to a design. Nor are a design's influences on stimulus selection and ordering inconsistent with phonetic and linguistic influences over treatment stimuli such as frequency of occurrence, ease of articulation, or manner and place of articulation. All of these influences merely interact.

Influence of the Withdrawal Design

A withdrawal design requires a single target. A single target does not mean a single syllable, word, or phrase. In apraxia of speech treatment, it means a single sound or sound combination in some manageable number of syllables, words, or phrases. For example, a clinician interested in measuring an imitative paradigm's potency can select a high frequency of occurrence sound such as an /s/, and drill it in appropriate stimuli such as words. To test the treatment's effect, the /s/ can be tested in both treated and untreated words, in sentences, and even in connected speech.

Influences of the Multiple Baseline Design

If the clinician chooses, for whatever reason, to treat several targets, the multiple baseline design is the design of choice although it may sometimes be appropriate to complete a series of individual withdrawal designs. Multiple baseline designs encourage creative stimulus selection and ordering by allowing the clinician to answer reasonably sophisticated treatment questions. Techniques can, of course, be evaluated. In addition, clinicians interested in generalization can select sounds of known relationship and, by systematically testing and treating, find out if generalization occurs. For example, a clinician might select /p, b, t, d, s, z/ in word-initial position and begin treatment of the /p/. Improvement in /p/ is evidence that treatment has helped. If spontaneous recovery can be accounted for—if the speaker is a chronic apraxic speaker, for example—simultaneous improvement in other sounds suggests generalization. Indeed, generalization itself may help a clinician separate treatment effects from those of physiologic recovery. For example, treatment of /p/ might reasonably be expected to influence the cognate /b/ and even /t/ and /d/, which are similar in manner. It would be less likely to influence /z/, which differs from /p/ in place, manner, and voicing. Simultaneous changes in /p/, /s/, and /z/ would suggest physiologic recovery or that the speaker has learned some general strategies, such as slowing down, that influence all sounds. A general strategy might be inferred from how the patient approaches each task, but simultaneous changes in a variety of unlike targets forces clinicians to be conservative in discussing their findings.

Learning one treatment target may generalize to others, but it may also interfere with the learning of others. Patterns of interference can also be inferred from patient responses within a multiple baseline context. Consider the same example of /p, b, t, d, s z/. It may be that learning /p/ makes it harder to learn a /b/. If so, as /p/ performance improves, the integrity of /b/ might deteriorate from the pretreatment baseline. Or /b/ might be slower to respond if training of it follows rather than precedes training on /p/. Examples of such interference are common in clinical practice. One of our trainees once worked so hard on final /ks/ that final /s/, which had previously been intact, deteriorated. Each time the speaker attempted an /s/, a /ks/ emerged. Work on /ks/ was abandoned, drill of /s/ was intensified, and the two targets were contrasted in paired stimuli with each getting equal attention. Serendipitously, final /s/ had been in a withdrawal design and we continued to test it after /ks/ in the final position began to be treated. Figure 6 shows how /s/ deteriorated after /ks/ was introduced during session 15.

In apraxia of speech's acute stage, when physiologic recovery threatens any measure of treatment, a multiple baseline can include difficult targets such as the affricates, the diphthongs, and consonant clusters. Such difficult targets may be immune to spontaneous recovery, and may wait patiently for the clinician's attention. If hard targets are included with frequently occurring sounds which improve intelligibility, and if those hard targets improve with treatment, the patient is well served and clinician and profession benefit from evidence showing that some techiques help even during physiologic recovery. An enduring clinical shibboleth is that treatment speeds change, even during the acute stage of improvement. The multiple baseline design and sophisticated stimulus selection and ordering will help us test this notion.

Influences of the Alternating Treatment Design

The alternating treatments design, like the withdrawal design, limits the number of treatment targets to one, depending upon how its require-

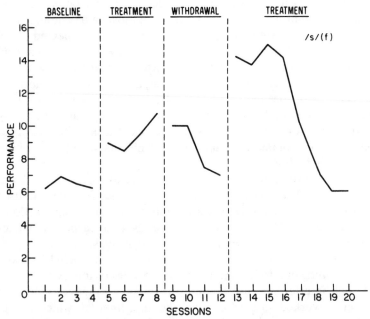

Figure 6.   Withdrawal design showing deterioration in word-final /s/ once word-final /ks/ was introduced during session 15.

ments are interpreted, but it allows the clinician to compare two methods. Clinicians are not free to select any single target or any two methods, however. The alternating treatment design imposes some restrictions (Barlow & Hayes, 1979). Foremost among the influences on stimuli is the design's requirement that the treated behavior admit to rapid change. In general, therefore, clinicians should use relatively short, simple stimuli rather than sentence length or longer ones unless the patient is only moderately or mildly imvolved. Shorter stimuli are more likely than longer ones to show quick improvement. Clinicians would do well to consider other stimulus variables that can reasonably be expected to change quickly. For example, familiar words are liable to change more rapidly than rare ones. Experience with each patient allows clincians to predict other relevant linguistic and phonetic dimensions and choose their stimuli accordingly.

Speech stimuli are not the only or inevitable targets of apraxia therapeutics. Attitudes, attention, and muscle tone are among the possible nonspeech targets. It is unlikely that changes in these could be measured in an alternating treatment design, because they cannot be altered quickly (tone may occasionally be an exception).

Coping With the Interaction of Stimuli and Methods

Stimuli and methods may interact. Clinicians can try to anticipate such interactions and avoid them in designing their research, or they can try to anticipate them and select their stimuli accordingly, or they can recognize them when interpreting their data. A study by Love and Webb (1977) helps bring at least a portion of this issue into focus. They demonstrated that imitation improved apraxic speakers' production of single words more than did providing them with each word's initial syllable, sentence completion, and reading. Providing the initial syllable was next most potent. Sentence completion and reading were not appreciably different and were in third place. This study was not a treatment study, but it might be used uncritically by some clinicians to defend the ubiquitous use of repetition in apraxia of speech treatment. The data, however, do not support the exclusive use of imitation. It is possible that other stimuli, because of their difficulty or for some other reason, might have yielded no significant differences among any of the stimulus conditions or might have yielded a different hierarchy of potency. Love and Webb probably could not have anticipated the hierarchy that emerged, although their discussion suggests that they recognized the hierarchy as logical given the nature of apraixa of speech as they understand it.

Other interactions of methods and stimuli are somewhat easier to anticipate. A method that requires the patient to watch sounds being made will have a less profound influence on sounds that are difficult to see such as /k/ and /g/ than on highly visible ones such as /p/ and /b/. Delayed auditory feedback does not appear to influence the single-word productions of apraxic speakers (Lozano & Dreyer, 1978) but it may improve their sentence productions. Interactions that can be anticipated can be controlled lest their effects cause clinicians to misinterpret the efficacy of certain of their techniques.

Sometimes clinicians choose not to worry about an interaction and opt instead to design their study and interpret their data with it in mind. In a study of imitation plus vibrotactile stimulation and imitation alone, Rubow, Rosenbek, Collins, and Longstreth (1982) randomly assigned what they called "predominately plosive words" to simple imitation and "predominantly fricative words" to the vibrotactile plus imitation condition. They did not use the same words for both, although strictly speaking the design required it, because they wanted to minimize generalization across treatments that would have obscured the potentially different effects. To control for familiarity and relative difficulty of the two lists, they selected words of equal difficulty as determined by the patient's inability to produce them correctly on any of three baseline tests. The weakness of the study was that they had no answer for the charge that the vibrotactile stimulation might have been therapeutic only for fricative words. All they could say was that the fricative words treated with imitation plus vibrotactile stimulation were significantly improved over the plosive words treated with imitation alone. Because so few studies of techniques have appeared, they felt it more important to control for a confounding generalization than for the possibility that vibrotactile stimulation was specific in its effects.

With careful planning, clinicians might even use alternating treatment designs to confirm expected interactions of methods and stimuli and to discover unexpected ones. Clinicians with a sufficient number of patients can measure the relative influence of a number of methods and monosyllabic word, polysyllabic word, and sentence stimuli, for example, or on rare and frequent words, or on clusters in word-initial and word-final positions. Such findings are not nit-picking. Too often in speech pathology methods are described as being successful without being described as successful for what.

Patients should not be sacrificed to designs. Designs, however, are not the only potential Molochs in clinical practice. Patients are as quickly sacrificed by inefficient treatment—treatment that improves them more slowly than need be. It is only a slight exaggeration to say that most things clinicians do help apraxic speakers. Efficient help is what superior clinicians provide. Pursuing efficiency will also influence a clinician's stimulus selection and ordering.

EFFICIENCY

Unless the patient is receiving team treatment with spontaneous recovery as one of the clinicians, apraxia of speech treatment can be protracted. For this reason, and because clinicians want to work quickly and well even if a patient is to be seen only for a week, treatment must be efficient. A number of plausible but mostly untested bases for efficiency in treatment can join single-case design requirements as guides to stimulus selection and ordering.

Frequency of Occurrence

Frequently occurring sound are usually good stimuli, especially during treatment's early days. If improved by treatment, their frequency has a substantial effect on intelligibility. While the exact ranking is controversial, among the most frequently occurring sounds in American English are /s/, /t/, /d/, /p/, and /l/. Among the most frequently occurring vowels are /i/, /ʌ/, and /ɑ/. Early in treatment, we test all speech sounds in a variety of contexts to see which sounds patients have, how well they have them, and what appears to be necessary to improve them. If we have a choice because of a patient's responses, we begin by stabilizing the common sounds. If a speaker is speechless or nearly so and it appears that most sounds are going to have to be taught, we first teach the common ones. Only if for some idiosyncratic reason a speaker can produce one or more rare sounds and no common ones would we be tempted to abandon our emphasis on frequency. Even then we might not and would choose instead to work harder at eliciting the common ones.

Stimulability

How easily a sound or combination can be elicited is another powerful influence on stimulus selection and ordering. Some sounds may be absent from a patient's connected speech but be rousable after only seconds or minutes of simple imitation, phonetic placement, or phonetic derivation. The most stimulable and the most common become the first treatment targets. Less stimulable sounds are reserved for later in the hope that they will become more tractable with time.

Position

Position in the word is also an influence on stimulus selection and ordering. A good start is more important than a good finish; listeners can predict many word-final position occupants. Given a choice between teaching a sound or combination in initial, medial, or final position, we would nearly always opt for beginning with the initial. Indeed, we often ignore word-final position altogether unless a patient has entered the moderate or mild part of the apraxic distribution without most final sounds in tow—an unlikely circumstance.

Occurrence in Connected Speech

Sounds heard in connected speech deserve special consideration. It is important to distinguish between sounds that occur inconsistently but in varying environments and those that may appear consistently but only in one or a few phrases. Sounds that exist only as part of a few cast-iron phrases are generally difficult to transfer to other environments. More readily transferred are those that inconsistently appear when they are supposed to and even those that appear as substitutions for other sounds. Such sounds are probably more or less independent of meaning, an independence that makes them easier to treat and good choices as stimuli with which to begin treatment.

Distinctive Features

Some subtleties of distinctive feature analysis in apraxia of speech have been described in Chapter 2. Its therapeutic exploitation is only now beginning, and that beginning is with phonologically impaired children. The literature on treating such children seems to suggest that to treat features rather than sounds is efficient (McReynolds & Bennett, 1972; Costello & Onstine, 1976). We do not know if the same is true for apraxic adults. The studies have not yet been done.

Heuristically, to treat features such as voicing or plosion is logical and efficient, and we try to do it, especially with the severe patient. For example, we sometimes encourage the speechless patient to make a predictable air stream, whether voiced or voiceless, and then to valve it in different ways. If the air stream is unvoiced, the lower lip against the upper teeth produces an /f/ or its approximation; with the tongue protruded and gently contacted by the upper teeth the stream makes a /Θ/. The voiced air stream produces the cognates, /v/ and /ð/. Because severe patients perseverate, we usually introduce the idea of plosion simultaneously with that of frication; otherwise plosion becomes too hard to teach. Once the ideas of a disturbed air stream for the fricatives and that of a stopped and quickly released air stream for plosives have been established, we begin teaching the appropriate valves—bilabial; labiodental; apricoalveolar; postdorsal, postvelar. To prevent the patient's perseverating on voicelessness or voicing, we try early on to teach the voiced–voiceless distinction.

Generalization

Generalization of training also increases efficiency. Ideally, clinicians consider generalization across sounds and environments when selecting and ordering stimuli. Unfortunately, few data on generalization in apraxia of speech are available. We have not studied generalization in apraxia from one sound to another. We have collected some data on generalization from word-initial to word-final position. For example, the influence of treating /st/ in the initial position on /st/ in word-final position for one apraxic adult is shown in the top half of Figure 7. Because he had almost no aphasia and was an eager practitioner, he could recognize the /st/ when it occurred outside word-initial position, and he was careful to begin producing it in these other environments. He was successful. His /tʃ/, however, did not want to generalize as is evident in the bottom half of Figure 7. He knew what we were doing despite our secrecy, because he laughed each time we tested /tʃ/ in word-initial and word-final positions. We have similar findings for /st/ and /tʃ/ for two other patients: the /st/ generalized, the /tʃ/ did not. The profession needs similar data on other sounds and sound combinations; on the generalization from short to long stimuli; on the effects of beginning with harder rather than easier stimuli and vice versa; on transfer across manner, place, and voicing; and on a host of other variables. Until such data are forthcoming, clinicians will have to rely primarily on other bases for making decisions about stimulus selection and ordering.

Stimulus Pairs

Efficiency also dictates that even severely apraxic speakers practice at least one pair of stimuli as soon as possible. Practicing one sound or word may well leave a speaker saying that sound or word and no others. Even in the most laconic family, one word is inadequate. What of the speechless patient who can make only one noise, and that only with considerable help from the clinician? We work to establish that noise, but only as a contrast with some other noise. If the patient is unable to make even one contrast after a few sessions, we change our treatment. Such patients are probably not apraxic and even if they are, an alternative to speech communication is indicated. Patients capable of learning contrasts begin drilling pairs of vowels, pairs of consonants, and vowel–consonant pairs. Learning just one sound is inefficient, but practicing just any two may be little better. What are the indications that particular stimulus pairs will be more efficient

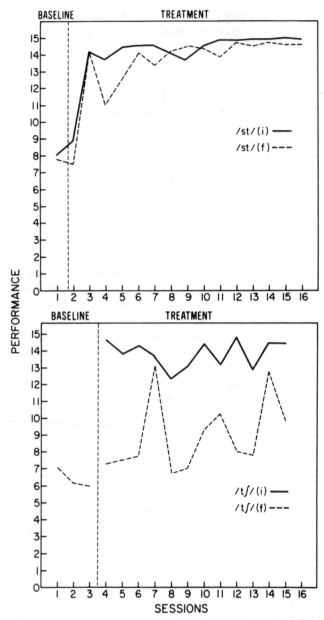

Figure 7. Generalization of word-initial /st/ to word-final position and failure of word-initial /tʃ/ to generalize to word-final position.

than others? Variables such as frequency of occurrence, what the speaker can say even without treatment, distinctive feature differences among members of a pair, and predicted generalization (and interference) can all be used to plan pair selection.

Strategies to Hasten Learning and Carryover

Efficiency dictates that apraxic talkers not only be presented with particular arrays of stimuli but that they learn general strategies to hasten learning and generalization. Our nominees for strategies are four. The first is taking time to plan. The second is attending to all possible cues from the clinician and from one's own production. The third is exhalting in success and repairing failure efficiently. The fourth is recognizing when failure can be converted to success by going on to some other response or by resting. What have these strategies to do with stimulus selection and ordering? For us, they primarily mean discussion so that the speaker understands what they are and how they may help, especially early in treatment; drill with a number of relatively easy stimuli during a portion of each session so that the patient is free to concentrate on these general strategies; and immediate knowledge of results about how well the strategies are being learned. Apraxia of speech cannot be overpowered; it must be finessed.

SUCCESS

Success is crucial to learning. If patients fail continuously even in the clinic, they are likely to leave therapy. On the other hand, a 100% success rate is unlikely to keep them coming back. Patients want challenge, Materials with which they have no difficulty will be perceived as "childish" or "too easy." Also, relearning of a motor skill seems to require some failures which can then be evaluated. A patient can be nearly 100% successful with treatment tasks and learn more slowly than a patient allowed to make and analyze mistakes. Stimulus selection and ordering are influenced by the ratio of successes and failures that a clinician tries to establish at any given time.

Ratio of Success to Failure

A problem is that the proper ratio of successes to failures has yet to be determined. The optimum ratio probably depends upon the patient and the stage of treatment. Individual differences are not easily accommodated in a written discussion; however, the interaction of ratio and stage in treatment is a bit easier to manage. During the first few sessions with new patients as clinicians try to find the right methods and stimuli, the patients are likely to have many failures. Counseling and humor can usually shield them from any disastrous effects. Later on, as they improve, the success rate can be increased. The rate can drop again as they begin work with difficult movements or as they move into the moderate or mild ranges and begin more independent practice. Even within a session, the ratio of successes to failures may vary, being high at the beginning and end and low in the middle.

Different ratios of success and failure can be achieved in several ways. The clinician can work harder so that, for example, a sound or syllable which does not respond to imitation is elicited with phonetic derivation. The clinician can go slower and do more counseling and cheerleading. The criteria for success can be changed; progressively greater articulatory precision can be required for a given response to be called successful. Also, as suggested previously, stimuli can be selected and ordered in different ways depending upon the ratio a clinician is trying to achieve.

What the Literature Says About Stimuli and Success

One can select stimuli to be easier or harder. It is in planning these selections that the literature summarizing the speech of groups of apraxic talkers has been of the greatest use. It teaches that, on the average, vowels are easier than consonants; that singleton consonants are easier than clusters; that shorter stimuli are easier than longer; that plosives are easier than fricatives and affricatives; that voiceless sounds are easier than voiced; that front sounds are easier than back; that visible sounds are easier than the hard-to-see ones; that frequently occurring sounds are easier than rare ones; that sounds in the final position are easier than those in the initial position; and that nonspeech gestures are easier than speech ones.[1] These and other influences on the apraxic talker's movement adequacy have been bountifully described in Chapter 4. A question remains: What is the clinical use of such group data?

Unfortunately, these data are only weak predictors of what an individual patient will do. Individual patients are indifferent to the literature. One person does better on short stimuli, the next on longer ones, and the next shows a mixed pattern, being better on some sounds in short stimuli and on others in longer stimuli. One patient finds affricatives easier than plosives and some diphthongs easier than vowels; the next does what the literature predicts. Another has success with a sound in some meaningful stimuli but is incapable of saying it in others. A further complication is that

---

[1]This idea needs further study. Not only may nonspeech movements be harder, they may be different in neuromotor control (Netsell, 1982).

stimulus characteristics (length, voicing, position, and the rest) interact, making traditional lists of variables misleading. For example, voicing and position in the utterance interact. Voiceless sounds are more often correct in the final position, and their voiced cognates are more frequently correct in word-initial position. The clinician then is faced with the same problems as a farmer. Seed, fertilizer, water, and warmth interact; and to concentrate only on fertilizer is inadequate. The clinician cannot decide merely to teach voiceless fricatives without simultaneously considering their position in the utterance, what sounds they will be combined with, the length of utterance, and the speaking rate. Fortunately, patients, like crops, thrive year after year because those responsible for their care have learned how to balance these interactions. A final complication which makes the experimental data difficult to transfer into the clinic is that clinicians have a different influence on patient's speech than do researchers. Clinicians make patients successful. Researchers make them respond. What the researcher reports to have been difficult, the clinician can sometimes make easy.

Carefully handled, however, weak predictions based on the literature are better than none at all. They guarantee that stimulus selection is never random. The experienced clinician, by combining clinical experience with the literature, can predict easy and hard stimuli and then test each prediction in the clinic. If a prediction holds up, if shorter stimuli are easier than longer, for example, part of stimulus selection is settled. When predictions fail, they can be replaced by new ones and the failure can be stored away so that it does not intrude on a future patient's treatment.

Stimulus Variables That Influence Success

Stimuli seldom are capricious in their effect on the apraxic patient's speech. A pattern can usually be discovered in what each speaker finds easy or hard. Some dimensions of stimuli that are associated with their success, such as frequency, are the same as those that influence efficiency. Others are not. It seemed worthwhile to risk a bit of duplication.

Place of Articulation, Visibility, and Frequency of Occurrence

Considerable ink has been spread about discussing these three items and apraxia of speech. The conclusions: front is better than back, visible is better than obscured, frequent is better than rare. We also know that the three interact. The apicoalveolar sounds such as /t/ and /s/ are visible; they are also among the most frequent. Blumstein (1973) believes that frequency is the most potent of all stimulus dimensions. She has convinced us, and frequency is one of our main criteria for selecting the sounds an apraxic talker will begin with. Stimulability is the other. We first see if the /t/, /s/,

/p/, and /l/ are available to the patient. If they are, we pair these with vowels to make words, and treatment is launched. To these we add whatever other sounds are stimulable. Frequently occurring, stimulable sounds keep a patient successful. They are good for early treatment sessions and at other times when the patient needs successes. They also make good companions for more difficult sounds once the time in treatment arrives when a clinician has to work on sounds the speaker finds very difficult and wants to put these difficult sounds in a variety of otherwise easy syllables, words, and phrases.

Length

We have been taught that apraxic errors increase as stimuli increase in length. Unless the experienced clinician guards against it, this aphorism can beguile him or her into starting each patient with short stimuli. According to the rule, the severe patient starts with sounds; the moderate one begins with syllables and words; and sentences are reserved for the mildly apraxic talker. Short is not always better. In our experience, some apraxic speakers have no difficulty with words or selected phrases once they have been helped to initiate the utterance, even though they may have great difficulty with isolated sound and syllable stimuli. Drilling longer stimuli with such patients will increase their success and treatment's efficiency. Treatment of sounds may increase their failure and slow their progress.

The popular litany about length's influence on apraxic articulation can lead to other clinical mistakes (at least we regard them as mistakes) that endanger both success and efficiency. The first mistake is to proceed as if the same length is appropriate for all stimuli for a given individual. In reality, a patient may be able to complete some /s/ words but not others, or be able to produce several sounds such as /s/ and /t/ in words and phrases, but be unable to make other sounds such as the /dʒ/ in any environment. The second mistake is to forget that stimulus length and method sometimes interact. Reading, for example, may elicit certain long stimuli but be effete with others no matter how short. The final mistake is forgetting the potential interaction of progress in therapy and appropriate length of stimulus. A sound may appear to be doing well in longer stimuli but may remain difficult to self-correct outside of the clinic. A patient in this frustrating position may need drill of the sound in isolation as a way of learning additional cues to its production before returning to drill of longer stimuli and before having a reasonable expectation of being able to control the sound outside. Or, some sounds may be produced well even in long stimuli until other sounds are introduced. Competition from the new sounds disrupts the older ones. This competition may force the clinician to make changes—including changes in stimulus length—if the speaker is to remain successful.

In other words, success does not depend merely upon starting short and getting long. We try to find the interaction of stimulus type, stimulus length, method, and progress in treatment that keeps the patient successful the right amount of time.

Meaningfulness

Because we believe meaning drives the motor system and enhances its performance, we use meaningful treatment stimuli as early and as often as possible even with the severely involved. We do not find compelling Dabul and Bollier's (1976) argument that patients are freer to concentrate on movements if meaningless stimuli are used. Unlike children who may have come to associate a particular combination of wrong gestures with a particular word (such as "pour" for "four") and who need training with nonsense, apraxic adults know how words used to sound and can use that knowledge to help themselves sound that way again. The meaningfulness makes it easier for them not only to produce correct movements but to judge their adequacy, and meaningful stimuli leave adults as free to concentrate on the feel of movement as they would be with meaningless ones.

For a variety of reasons, however, the clinician may want to use a combination of meaningful and meaningless stimuli to keep a patient successful. For example, we sometimes have even moderate or mildly apraxic talkers practice some sounds in isolation or in meaningless syllables if they have difficulty correcting them in connected speech. One of our moderately apraxic speakers sometimes distorted /s/ in connected speech by investing it with a plosive quality. It was not /s/, nor /t/, nor /ts/. He profited from practicing /s/ in isolation and in nonsense syllables alternated with practice of /s/ in short, meaningful utterances. This work with short, meaningless stimuli also is often appropriate for severe patients who cannot make sounds in any word or phrase, but who can often say a few words such as "no" and "yes." It is motivating not only to talk but to say something. So we spend some time practicing sounds which we combine as quickly as possible into words, and we also have them drill the one or more words they may have as part of more or less automatic utterances.

Nonverbal Movements

Verbal movements, whether meaningful or meaningless, are not always possible. Some severe patients, for example, cannot make certain sound shapes until they have had a change to break the shapes into phonetic components. These components are nonverbal: biting the lower lip, protruding the tongue, raising the tongue trip to the alveolar ridge, exhaling air, puckering the lips, and so on. We have seen patients learn a sound in a single session once it is broken down, after having failed to learn it as a unit even after several sessions. Our rule for using nonverbal movements in therapy is to begin with speech and resort to nonverbal movements if speech is slow to come. In our view, the clinician should be quick to resort to this. To work with nonverbal movements is not to doom the patient to a snail's pace, especially if clinician and patient move back and forth between nonverbal and verbal movements as the patient needs to.

TASK CONTINUA

That stimuli should be organized into heirarchies or task contiua is the final influence on stimulus selection and ordering. "Organize stimuli into hierarchies" springs from our lips as effortlessly as "hello," and hierarchies are thought to bind treatment's fabric as tightly as good manners do society's. It is a truism that stimuli and methods should be organized. It may be untrue, however, that apraxia of speech treatment should start at the bottom or easy end of each continuum and work its way relentlessly to the top. In our view, clinicians need to know what is easy and hard, but they also need to remember that treatment is dynamic. The goal is to move up and down one or more hierarchies in response to each patient's successes. Down is as important as up. Treatment does not hunker down at step one only to wait for 27 repetitions, or 4 minutes, or until the patient has been successful ten consecutive times. Rather, the clinician urges the patient back and forth along each continuum. If someone can click off identical events as a clinician and patient are working, what must be taking place is inventory, not treatment.

PUTTING IT TOGETHER

Stimulus selection and ordering cannot be based solely on what the literature tells us. What a clinician and patient are drilling at any given time is dictated by an interaction of clinician goals; patient characteristics; the requirements of single-case design; the clinician's attitudes about efficiency, success, and task continua; and the methods selected to teach the stimuli. The rest of this book deals with those methods.

9

Treating the Severely Apraxic Patient

The methods in this chapter will not help the globally aphasic patient; they will help the severely apraxic one, even if an aphasia accompanies the apraxia (as it usually does) as long as that aphasia is less severe. Differential diagnosis is then critical. However, because diagnosis is often so difficult with any severe patient, especially during the acute period, speech—language treatment may have to begin before the clinician is sure of what the patient has. If that treatment is systematic, the patient's reaction to the methods may aid in differential diagnosis.[1] If patients fail to improve with the treatment methods to be described, clinicians can hypothesize that they either are not apraxic at all or that they have aphasia or some other condition which is more severe than their apraxia of speech. Patients who fail probably have global aphasia and perhaps bilateral brain damage. Testing an hypothesis about the severe patient's diagnosis is often easier in the chronic state than in the acute state because the chronic patient is usually feeling better, is better able and usually more willing to cooperate, and may have developed strategies for communication that are themselves clues about the diagnosis. Regardless of how long a patient has had a severe communication deficit or how much or little the clinician may know about it with certainty, patient and family deserve our best, most orderly efforts.

---

[1] A patient's response to a treatment, no matter how firmly based in concept that treatment is, may have little or nothing to do with the treatment or its underpinnings. Things are as likely to happen because clinicians want them to as because of a treatment's appropriateness or a clinician's perspicacity. Interpreting a patient's response to treatment then must be done prudently.

In this chapter, counseling and methodology for acute and chronic severe apraxic talkers will be differentiated. The acute patient is usually speechless or nearly so and generally unresponsive, and the family is usually worried and confused. Severe involvement is less shocking after people have lived with it awhile. Duration then seems to have important implications for severe patients, although some of the counseling obligations and many of the methods—at least during treatment's early sessions—will be similar. Both the differences and the similarities will be described. This attention to acute and chronic is not preserved in the chapters on moderate and mild apraxia where duration seems less important.

TREATING THE SEVERE, ACUTELY APRAXIC PATIENT

Counseling

The bulk of information on counseling the apraxic patient and family will be presented in this chapter because most patients are severely involved at first, if only for a few days. Their communication deficit is but one part of a frightening, disorienting experience that includes hospitalization, anxiety, guilt, doubts about the future, and agonizing reappraisal. In this section we will describe a number of counseling issues involving families, patients, and other health professionals. The discussion is selective rather than exhaustive.

The Medical Diagnosis and the Team

A physician usually sees patient and family during the first hours of an illness. When the speech pathologist first meets them is seldom predictable and may vary from days to weeks or months after the onset. Regardless of when speech pathologists are consulted, however, they should try to read the medical records, including the diagnosis or the hypotheses about the diagnosis, before seeing the patient or family. The medical diagnosis will help them begin settling on counseling and treatment procedures and on a prognosis. For example, it is a truism that one's activities and predictions with the stroke patient are usually significantly different from those for the patient with metastatic disease. The medical report will also list associated medical problems such as diabetes, dementia, and schizophrenia that influence rehabilitation and prognosis. When reviewing the chart is impossible or when the medical diagnosis is undetermined, our procedure is to meet the family; explain our potential role; interview them; reassure them in a general way; and then begin an evaluation adjusted to the patient's willingness and ability to cooperate. We assiduously avoid making a prognostic statement or counseling family and patients about what we will do until a treatment team consisting of physician, nurse, physical and occupational therapists, social worker, and ourselves has agreed upon a plan.[2] When the rehabilitation team has settled on its plan, counseling begins. The physician describes the patient's likely course of recovery, quotes the probability of a second episode, and helps the patient and family understand medications, diet, rest, and so on. The nurse describes the nursing care plan and often becomes the patient's leading advocate. The physical and occupational therapists explain their programs and expectations. The social worker discusses financial and discharge planning. The speech pathologist provides the speech diagnosis, prognosis, and explanation about treatment. On the ideal team, all members share the responsibility of supporting patient and family and easing them toward recovery.

Communication Disability and Ability

When the speech pathologist has determined the amount of the patient's apraxia and aphasia, patient and family—and especially the family, because patients seem to know what they can and cannot do—can be helped to understand the disability. Families are predictable. They usually overestimate, rather than underestimate, the patient's ability to understand, read, write, and even speak. We try to give them a realistic assessment of the patient's ability in each of these modalities. Our aim is not to make the patient look bad but to help the family toward a realistic assessment of the deficits. It is especially crucial that they recognize how much their loved one understands. If they think "he understands everything," and he doesn't, they can make costly decisions about insurance, guardianship, property, and a host of other potentially expensive and emotional subjects. Each clinician knows at least one clinical anecdote about a family's making a mistake because of what they assumed a patient understood.

So we tell families how much a patient seems to be understanding and show them how to confirm that a message has been understood by making a statement in two different ways. For example, if the family has a question about encouraging a brother-in-law to visit, they can ask "Shall we have Tom come to the hospital?" and "Shall we keep old Tom away from the hospital?" If the patient answers the same to both, the family will know they need to work harder to make him understand. We also tell families that we know husbands and wives are among the best communicators—usually. We let them know that we know their years of sharing make it likely that they can communicate with each other even if one or the other is

---

[2]Speech pathologists without a team, and they are numerous, need to be very cautious, especially about making prognostic statements.

reduced to glances, gestures, and a few words. But we try to help them understand that subtleties of messages about insurance benefits, college educations, and the like may require more comprehension than love and familiarity can create. When they reply that he understands the nurses and doctors "even though they are using all those big words," we try to point out that many hospital communications are stereotyped and predictable. We are quick to add, however, that they are correct to some degree. Even very severe patients understand some things such as "nursing home" in the phrase, "Howard, we are going to put you in a nursing home but only for a few weeks." What they may not understand is "but only for a few weeks," and that makes all the difference.

Because families usually have no idea about the cortical organization of speech-language activities, they have no reason to think that writing and reading suffer along with speech. Therefore, even reasonably sophisticated families are surprised at the unintelligible writing which appears on the magic slate which they have just thrust into the patient's hands.

Probably, they reason, it is because of paralysis and being forced to write with the nondominant hand. To the speech pathologist's observations that the patient is only reading single words reliably they remark that he enjoys all of his cards. Probably he does but not because of the sympathetic prose. Knowing that a sweet smelling card with roses and fruit on the front is meant to cheer requires no words. So we try to help them understand how much the patient can read and write lest they invite the family attorney out to the hospital with a new set of contracts for the patient to read and sign.

During this cataloging of the patient's disabilities we remind ourselves that families need to believe in something and that our counseling about what the patient cannot do must be exposition, not exposé. We tell them our motive. That motive is simply that an informed family is powerful medication without harmful side effects; an uninformed family can be harmful. Clinical anecdotes abound about patients being subjected to new teeth or a more exotic dental adhesive when they cannot talk; eye examinations and new glasses when they cannot read; typewriters, pens with blue rather than black ink, and magic slates with Donald Duck around the border when they cannot write; and obnoxiously loud television sets and communication boards when they cannot understand. Knowledgeable families avoid these mistakes just as they avoid talking to the patient as if he or she were deaf, or an early Hollywood version of an American Indian, or a child, or—worst of all—senile.

We also balance the discussion of what patients cannot do with a description of what they can do. They can feel your concern and appreciate your support; understand simple straightforward information about family, friends, and the world; read spouses' names and appreciate grandchildrens' homemade cards; and be socially appropriate. They have intellect. Most important they have a future.

Coping with the Future

The trip to the hospital comes while children are in school; while mother is seeking election; while Grandad is showing the first signs of forgetfulness; while husband and wife are trying to scrape together enough money to pay off the credit cards; while sister-in-law is living in the upstairs bedroom; and when life is full of promise. So families and patients naturally want to know what the future holds.

Will he talk again? One of the family's first questions of the speech pathologist is often, "Will he be able to talk again?" If the diagnoses of stroke and apraxia of speech can be confirmed in an otherwise reasonably healthy person, the family and patient can be reassured that functional recovery is likely. As part of this reassurance we let them know, but not in a cynical way, that if one has to have a speech disorder, apraxia of speech is the one to have. Families are not allowed to take this as proof that stroke and apraxia, like pneumonia, will completely disappear. They are reassured only that the patient will not stay speechless, especially if speech begins to reappear during the first four to six weeks, and that considerable return is especially likely if recovery starts within the first two weeks.

The more severe the accompanying aphasia, however, the more guarded our prognostic statements. If the patient's aphasia is more severe than the apraxia, we tell the family that recovery is possible but not guaranteed; and that we will give them weekly (or daily) progress reports and a final prognosis based on our clinical experience and the patient's pattern of change as soon as we are reasonably sure of it. In our experience apraxic patients recover more functional communication than aphasic ones, but for all patients, the amount of recovery during the first month is a more powerful prognosticator than the label. So when the family of an apraxic speaker asks, "Will he talk again?," we scrupulously avoid predicting or promising too much, but neither do we shrug our shoulders nor put on a long face. If we do not know the answer, we tell them so and get on with the business of collecting the daily progress data that will give it to us.

What to do until the future can be predicted. Most families are amazingly protean. Spouses who have shunned the check book rediscover subtraction and addition. Children learn to rouse themselves and get off to school. An aunt volunteers to shop and tend the garden. A neighbor does the chores and chauffeuring. While everyone is working and waiting, options can be evaluated. What happens if the patient never works again or if caring for home, spouse, and children is forever impossible? Most families think about such things and begin making inquiries about insurance benefits, retirement funds, and how much the business is worth. If they do not do so, we encourage them to begin. If the patient recovers, they will not have to concern themselves about such issues, at least for a while. If not, they will have at least some of the facts necessary for planning their vastly altered existences. Through all of this we try not to douse any sparks of hope. Instead, we try to fan them with realistic early planning.

Delicate Conditions

Families often talk to speech pathologists about a variety of problems, many of them unrelated to the patient's present illness and communication deficit. The wise clinician, in our view, should avoid getting sucked into a family's vortex by information about a spouse's drinking, or cruelty, or despair, or love, or strength. If family members need to talk, clinicians can listen, but only if they feel comfortable doing it. If not, they should involve someone else on the health care team. Also, if they feel comfortable, speech pathologists can point out that love, responsiveness, and balance are almost never permanently extinguished by trauma, and that the patient's anger, or volubility, or indifference will disappear with time and recovery. Sometimes it takes a year or more, but if an emotion or characteristic was there, it will return. Unfortunately, the obverse is also true. Trauma fails to improve existing problems, marriages do not get better, moods do not improve, anger is not changed to understanding. Nor can clinicians undo what the years have done. Clinicians should be good listeners but should avoid thrusting themselves into the lives of those whom history has doomed, regardless of how much families may appeal or how much they may want to help.

What Can We Do to Help Him Talk?

We make five suggestions when families ask us what they can do to help the patient talk better. We tell them first to adjust the rate and content of their speech to accommodate the patient, but in all other ways to behave as they have always behaved. We tell them to begin assuming most of the responsibility for communication. We ask them to learn methods that may help the patient respond while simultaneously preserving the patient's respect and independence. We teach them to use and encourage total communication. Finally, we suggest that they prepare for some failures despite their best efforts. We make these suggestions because few things are sadder than bad parenting emerging in a husband—wife relationship: "Talk for the nice speech therapist. You said your name today, I heard you. So did my sister. Say Harry." Harry's silence testifies that he knows what he is doing.

Making adjustments. Family members usually find it easier to adjust their own communicating if they are first educated about what patients can cope with and if they are reassured that patients are neither demented nor socially unaware although illness, confusion, despair, or perseveration may sometimes make it appear that they are. They can be helped further if they know that nothing very exotic need be done. In our experiences, families and even staff members (until they are taught) usually do too much rather than too little. The noises one typically hears in the halls of a rehabilitation unit suggest that somewhere deep within, someone is trying to reason with a deaf, prepubescent stone. Well-intentioned intelligent persons often talk too loudly, too slowly, and with exaggerated mouth movements, as if impaired communication could be overcome by a show of plodding force. We recommend instead that speakers slow down, shorten their sentences, make sure that only one person is talking at a time, and that the patient is focused on that speaker. We next urge them to watch for signs about how well they have done. If their efforts are inadequate, the patient will let them know by a head shake or a baleful look. Repetition, augmenting speech with gestures and props, being careful to isolate and otherwise highlight the main idea of a communication, and trying to get the patient to confirm that each part of an idea has been understood may also be useful. When all of this fails, the family can be reassured that it is proper to drop the topic and return to it later.

Assuming the burden of communication. Assuming the burden for communication requires something far harder than adjusting one's speech rate, being careful to repeat, and coming armed to each visit with a cord of topics to fuel nonstop talking. Normal speakers must accept that many of their utterances will be answered by frustration and silence or a few unintelligible noises. Such acceptance is hard, because most people seem to believe that it takes two to talk and that they are good at holding up their end. When the severely apraxic speaker does not reply, it is as unsettling as gulping a glass of milk expecting it to be cola. But accept it they must and go on talking until physiologic recovery and treatment make it possible for a patient to join in. Their willingness to do so is usually enhanced if the clinician can convince them that a patient's frustration is inevitable and impersonal, and that the patient is processing many things, and is profiting from their efforts.

Using a hierarchy of cues. And as patients recover and their interest in communication quickens, families usually relax and are ready to learn additional ways of assisting. Perhaps the best of these are (1) learning a hierarchy of cues for helping patients complete a message, (2) learning how to recognize when such a cue is necessary, and (3) learning to select the appropriate cue. Cueing hierarchies supply families with alternatives to looking on in prayerful helplessness or interrupting the patient to supply the word or complete the idea. No one cue or hierarchy is right for all patients, but several cues are possible with most, and these can be ordered as each patient's behavior dictates. Often it is enough to have a patient stop and start over. This cue's potency can sometimes be increased by reminding the patient to get an idea firmly in mind before resuming. If more help is needed, listeners can paraphrase what they think a patient has said. Patients usually will confirm if a paraphrase is on target, and occasionally they will even be able to do a bit of repetition or expansion on their own. A more powerful cue is provided by the cloze technique of supplying a context and a blank to be filled in: cup of _____; crime of _____; loaf of _____; jug of _____. Phrases can also be elicited by this method. Providing the first sound of a word either aloud or silently, while urging the patient to join in, can also trigger not only that word but the entire phrase. Listeners can also advance the conversation with questions such as "Were you saying something about your sister Corrine's husband?" Sometimes it may even be helpful for a listener to write an interpretation and have the speaker confirm it.

Learning when to intervene and with which cue may be the family's most difficult task. They must first be able to distinguish impotent from productive attempts to communicate, and then must be able to select the weakest cue that will help the patient while simultaneously preserving his or her independence. Discrimination and cue selection come only with experience and training. Clinicians learn to recognize what a patient does that is efficient. They also learn how to help without making the patient totally dependent. When they have learned these two things, they can invite the family to observe treatment and can instruct the family before, after, and during sessions. Once the family has watched the clinician, the roles can be reversed and the clinician can watch the family as they talk to the patient. This kind of family education is idealized; it is also ideal. Families who learn the steps between silence and seizure of all of the patient's communication opportunities and when to take what step can be important forces in the patient's communication.

Encouraging total communication. Encouraging total communication is perhaps the best of all methods for avoiding failed communications. Total communication results from speaker's supplementing speech with writing, drawing, gesturing, and even a communication board. In the acute stage of severe apraxia these other modalities may be as impaired as speaking is, but their combined use may be just potent enough to get a message across. Gestures are especially useful because they may well be the most preserved of all of the performances. Families can help patients expand their gesturing by learning to ask leading questions, such as "How big is it? What does it look like? What do you do with it?" They can also reenforce the patient's total communication by gesturing, using props, writing, and even drawing to communicate their own ideas. We do not want to imply that training in total communication resides totally with the family. Not at all. The clinician is the teacher. The family merely helps, but their involvement sometimes motivates a particular patient to try harder. The motivation probably comes from the patient's feeling less obvious and abnormal and therefore more willing to try.

Accepting some failures. Despite everyone's best efforts, many conversations during the severe, acute period will simply abort. The patient will be unable to make others understand. Sometimes accepting this inevitability, especially if done with as little disappointment and frustration as possible, is a great relief to everyone, including the patient. Doing something is not always best. It is probably important, however, at least for most patients, that broken communications not be left floating in the air like unpleasant odors. The family needs to say, "We didn't get it, did we; sorry; next time, maybe; we'll keep trying; let's drop it for now; in a week when you're talking better you can show us the error of our ways." Having said these things, the family needs to remember them, and return to the topic when that seems appropriate. Above all, they must show that they care, and they must keep on trying.

Observation of Treatment

Sometimes the best counseling occurs after the family has observed treatment. The family gets to see the patient's deficits and strengths, and to see the same happy, perseverative, inconsistent, frustrated, or anxious reactions to specific tasks and other people that they might previously have thought were directed only at themselves. They can observe the clinician cueing the patient and bailing out of failed communications. They can see that even the professional is not always successful. Clinicians can follow up these observations and new perspectives by answering questions and helping families to use what they have seen. Vaguely understood goals and procedures can be transformed into robust reality. Perhaps best of all, the family can see that something is being done. But, regardless of its benefits, observation is never automatic nor is it clandestine—at least in our clinics. Both patient and family are given a choice as well as an explanation about why we think watching is a good idea. Observation goes off without difficulty, especially if we have the luxury of having another colleague sit with the family to tell them what is happening and why. Indeed, we almost never separate observation and explanation. As all experienced clinicians know, however, some family members cannot watch, at least at first. They should not be made to.

Understanding the Other Changes

As baffling and frightening as the communication deficits are the other changes. Hemiplegia, fatigue, and the catheter testify that things are no longer the way they were. Tears flow easily. A break in routine, even a change in room or roommate, causes anger. Television is no longer interesting. Night brings confusion. Sometimes the family arrives and the patient turns toward the wall; the grandchildren bound into the room and the patient cries. One day the patient is able to share and the next day not. All experienced clinicians could add to this list. Unless the family has had a long history of family illness, or unless they are counseled, they will not know how to respond to such symptoms. Nor will they know whether such symptoms are temporary or permanent. We explain the cause and course of the emotional symptoms but only in collaboration with the physician and physical and occupational therapists. We tell the family that fatigue, depression, anger, and lability are usually muted by time and improvement in health, walking, and talking. If the physician reassures us that the patient is medically stable and improving in health, if the physical therapist predicts the return of walking, and if we predict some speech return, we advise the family and patient that their worst days are behind them and that the future will be better. Predictions about bladder control, visual field cuts, hemiplegia, and other physical disabilities are to be made by physicians and other health care professionals.

What the Patient is Told

We tell patients the same things that we tell families; but we tell them in different ways and at slower rates. We are especially careful to explain to patients why we spend so much time talking to their families. Family counseling done with patient's knowledge but without their participation is like whispering; it causes anxiety and sometimes even fear. Therefore, we try to tell them that we are teaching their families a cueing hierarchy, and then we show them some of the cues and prepare them to expect similar cues from their families. When we cannot talk to patients and families together we are careful to tell them the same things separately. If we plan to emphasize total communication including talking, which is normal, and gesturing or drawing, which are less so, we tell patients why. We warn them that their families will be encouraging them to do what we ask. We explain all of our methods and how our treatments fit with others that they are receiving. We describe our expectations, prognosis, and how we will measure recovery. We define the criteria for ending treatment. Finally, we reassure them that they have the last word; what they object to we will abandon. We often get the feeling that much of what we tell them they already know. As often as not we tell patients things only so that they will know we know too.

The Rest of the Rehabilitation Team

Teaching about comprehension. Teams have garnered more aphorisms than almost anything else in rehabilitation, and most clinicians either try to create one or join an existing one, perhaps because the "whole person" seems to need the symmetry of the "whole team." In our experience, teams are important but only if they communicate rather than merely convene. We begin most of our team encounters with listening to the points of view of others. The speech pathologist's time to talk often comes when someone says, "The patient is understanding everything." We usually hear this statement just before or after finding out at bedside testing that the patient can point to the window—when that is the first command—but then continues to do so even though the target shifts to nose, door, or bed; is as willing to agree that Moscow is his or her hometown as that Milwaukee is; will hand over reading glasses in response to "Give me your glasses so I can wash them," but cannot point to them when asked to point; and that much of the environment does not make sense. Our colleague on the team—often without knowing it—is really saying that "The patient understands something." Indeed, most patients—even global ones—understand some whole body commands; some gestures; and some low-level, stereotyped, predictable rituals of hospitalization. We do not speak Japanese but could probably get by for a few days of hospitalization in Japan, especially if we hid our monolingualism behind a cloak of friendliness and illness, and especially if we were lucky enough to meet only those who were too kind or too busy to try to peek up our cloak. This is not intended to be critical of health delivery systems (and certainly not of the Japanese). It is, however, a reminder that hospital communications are basic ones, and hospital workers are all clinicians intent on seeing the best in each patient.

That is as it should be, but in our view, team members will be of greatest use to the patient if simultaneously with the best they also see the rest—the things the patient cannot do. To help interested staff members understand how much a patient understands, we use both test scores on a variety of standardized tests and demonstrations of functional or pragmatic understanding. We consider such education crucial if only to prevent a well-intentioned staff member's sending the severely apraxic patient off to physical therapy unescorted only to have the patient end up sitting an hour with patients awaiting barium enemas. So that team members understand the formal and functional testing they observe or see reported, we begin their education (where appropriate) with the reminder that different conditions demand different abilities. We next describe and defend the selection of our tests. We admit that not even Pinocchio had to point to his nose on request, and that we are not saying patients understand nothing when we record their failures on pointing tasks. The importance of the pointing tasks is that the same patient who fails to point usually fails to understand more complex, realistic information such as the risks associated with arteriograms and the benefits to be had from selling the summer cottage. We end by contrasting formal tests with informal, pragmatic tasks; and where possible we demonstrate each patient's different responses to different tasks, including those that resemble what nursing service does each day. Obviously, such teaching can never be condescending, and it will not be if clinicians remember that some of the most useful information about a patient's ability to comprehend can come from other team members.

Teaching about the interaction of modalities.   The speech pathologist can also contribute to those team members who have not been taught previously that reading, writing, listening, and speaking are usually involved—albeit differentially—in the majority of left-hemisphere, brain-damaged patients. Patients who cannot talk usually cannot sign their names or write sentences—especially at first—and usually they cannot read well enough to get more than the vaguest idea about what their sympathy cards say. Without such education, the difficulty with writing is likely to be blamed on the patient's having to use the nondominant hand because of the right hemiplegia, and the reading problem may go unnoticed entirely. After all, doesn't the patient spend part of every day in the hall reading a magazine? We also reassure team members that we will treat all of each patient's deficits (if we plan to) and will inform them as each patient is able to do more. We end by telling them what they can do to help make a patient the best possible communicator.

Teaching teams how to help.   The question that may meld teams more tightly than any other is "What can we do to help?" Unfortunately, this question's frequent companion is "How about an alphabet or a word board?" Communication boards have a strange following. Almost everyone knows about them, and most seem to assume that communication boards are ideal for most speechless patients. Unfortunately, they are not. Few patients with left-hemisphere damage, regardless of speech diagnosis, can use them. Admittedly, the apraxic patient is a more likely candidate than the aphasic one, but even the apraxic talker may have difficulty. Merely placing a board in a speechless patient's room is no more effective than placing a notebook or a parrot there. We explain that a period of diagnostic treatment is necessary to determine if the patient can use a board. In the interim, the staff can be helped to recognize what things really do help.

We tell our colleagues that the best therapy they can give is to assume most of the burden for communication, thereby freeing the patient to heal.

We discourage questions delivered in a booming, sing-song voice and we counsel against even the gentlest of enticements to have patients imitate, count, sign, or recite. Instead, professionals are instructed to elicit responses to simple, one-step yes/no questions and to accept a head shake, a gesture of the hand, or even an unintelligible but differentiated grunt. We also teach the same cueing hierarchies for helping patients respond that were described in the section on family counseling, and we add the reminder that the patient needs to be as independent as possible, even during periods of great difficulty. Finally, if need be, we reassure them that merely taking time to listen rather than babbling is as welcomed by the patient as steak instead of mystery meat, and as healthy.

If family and staff know what is required of them, and if they understand what the speech clinician is trying to do, they are then free to create a friendly, stimulating environment. While communication often improves without such friendliness and stimulation, it flourishes with it.

Preparing to Practice

The cause of apraxia of speech, be it tumor, stroke, multiple sclerosis, trauma, or something else, will be unfamiliar and arcane to most patients and their families. Equally unfamiliar and mysterious will be apraxia of speech's treatment. Many people seem to expect that a pill, potion, or operation will remove the cause and alleviate the speech deficit. Others seem to believe that the apraxia can be overcome by force of will or by time. Therefore, if hospitalization and treatment are to be bearable, the speech pathologist needs to preface treatments with explanations. We begin with the explanation that our goal is to help patients regain as much speech as their systems will allow. We explain that time is not the nonpareil clinician and that improvement can be faster and more complete with hard work under clinical supervision. Treatment, we tell them, also makes recovery more orderly and less lonely.

We usually find ourselves working hardest to convince both patient and family about our stimuli and methods. Because we believe that improvement depends upon successful practice, we usually have severe patients begin treatment by imitating short, simple stimuli such as sounds in isolation and in CV and VC syllables. If imitation is insufficient, we try to elicit sounds and syllables with methods such as phonetic placement. We also have them count, or try to; and sing; and recite—anything to elicit speech. When we find something they can do, we have them repeat it time and again. Without forewarning, severe apraxic patients may think that such stimuli and methods are infantile. Also, unless they have been counseled, they most surely will worry that they have fallen into a displaced school teacher's clutches. Certainly, the whole experience contrasts sharply with what most people have come to expect of a hospitalization costing several hundred dollars per day. So we reassure patients that we recognize that their intelligence and insight are intact and that speech therapy is not school for grownups. We convince them, or try to, that successful practice creates better speech, that practicing short stimuli makes longer ones easier, and that imitation and phonetic placement may make it easier to talk spontaneously. If treatment has to begin with sounds and nonsense syllables, we reassure patient and family that such sounds and syllables are the raw material of intelligent, functional speech. Before one can say, "Make mine milk," it is necessary to say /m/, /k/, and the rest. When they object to ten or a hundred repetitions of the same response, we explain how treatment effects generalize. We reassure them that it is unnecessary to practice all sounds or all words, because intense practice with a few makes the rest easier to say.

Finally, we try to get patients not only to understand but to laugh. Drill need not be deadening. Apraxia of speech treatment needs—indeed demands—creativity and humor. A grin is the equivalent of a hundred repetitions. We try to elicit a few grins each session.

Treatment Methods

Diagnostic Treatment

The first treatments are usually diagnostic because one can seldom predict what is buried under severe apraxia. For us these diagnostic therapy sessions have three short-term goals: (1) finding the noises, sounds, words, or phrases patients can say and the most efficient methods for helping them say them; (2) determining how easily they can switch from one stimulus to another; and (3) determining if they can associate movements and their meanings. Therapy's major long-term goal, better functional speech, comes with reaching these three, and especially the first. Numbers (2) and (3) are especially important indicators of how quickly a patient is going to respond to treatments and of how much aphasia coexists with the apraxia. If patients can switch from one stimulus to another and can recognize the meaning of utterances the clinician is getting them to say, their prognosis is good, and any coexisting aphasia is probably not sufficiently severe to block the return of at least some functional communication.

Once the appropriate stimuli and methods have been selected and diagnosis and prognosis confirmed at least tentatively, the real work begins. If patients are to become functional talkers, they and their clinicians will have to work diligently and systematically. Diligence must either arrive with the patient or result from the clinician's counseling and perhaps a few demonstrations of success. System comes with selection and ordering of stimuli and methods. Stimulus selection and ordering were discussed in Chapter 8. Selection and ordering of methods are discussed here.

Imitation

One of the least invasive treatment methods is imitation, so we begin with it. The patient merely watches and listens as the clinician provides a model and then tries to produce as faithfully as possible what has been seen and heard. In our experience this method seldom works spectacularly with severely apraxic talkers unless they are experiencing significant spontaneous recovery and improving somewhat each day. For severe, stable apraxic talkers, on the other hand, the first and second imitative responses may be adequate, may even be good enough to bring tears or a gleam to the patient's eyes, but subsequent imitations are likely to be defeated by perseveration and struggle. These patients need more: more cues, for example, or more rhythmical presentation of stimuli than are present in most imitative paradigms. The moderately apraxic talker is the best candidate for an imitative program, and a full discussion of the method is reserved for the next chapter.

Phonetic Placement

As described by Van Riper and Irwin (1958), *phonetic placement* comprises a number of procedures:

1. descriptions of how a movement or sound is to be made;
2. development of associations, e.g., dam the air to make a /p/, make the air hiss for an /s/;
3. use of graphs, drawings, models, or other visual aids that demonstrate a movement or sound; and
4. manipulation of the patient's articulators.

An elaborate discussion of phonetic placement is Young and Hawk's (1955) book on the moto-kinesthetic method now renascent with Vaughn and Clark's publication (1979) on intra- and extraoral facilitation procedures. Interested clinicians will want to read these two works, because our discussion of phonetic placement will be brief. Experienced clinicians become masterly manipulators and describers. They learn when and how hard to push, rub, and stroke. They learn how to whittle tongue blades and mold plastic, which in turn help mold a patient's articulators, and their descriptions create trenchant pictures of what the speech mechanism should do. Since these methods were developed by speech pathology's pioneers, we will not describe all of them here. We will summarize selected techniques for teaching manner, place, voicing, and oral–nasal distinctions, however, and will then describe our first treatment session with a severely apraxic speaker.

Teaching manner distinctions. Manner distinctions—especially plosive and fricative—lend themselves to placement techniques. Plosives require total occlusion (we describe it as damming or trapping the air);

fricatives require partial occlusion (we describe it as hissing or the slow escape of air). Both require that patients be able to exhale predictably, however, and so with severe patients we often begin by teaching a predictable exhalation. It is usually enough to exhort them to blow while we simultaneously push inward against their bellies.

Because the apicoalveolar region is the only one plosives and fricatives share in American English (there being no bilabial or postdorsal, postvelar fricatives) we begin teaching the fricative-plosive distinction with /s/ and /t/. Once the patient can produce a predictable voiceless airstream, the clinician can shape the /s/ by having the patient close his jaw or grit his teeth, exhale forcefully, and produce a "narrow, high-pitched sound" like air escaping through a small opening. The flow of air can even be traced along the patient's cheek. If the resulting air stream is too diffuse, it sometimes helps to pull back on the corners of the patient's mouth. This movement, which resembles what one does to show one's teeth or make an /i/, helps change the quality to that of an /s/. To dam the air for the /t/, the patient's tongue tip can be guided to the alveolar ridge and held there. The patient can next be instructed to fill his mouth with air. Finally, the patient can be instructed to explode the air by rapidly and forcibly withdrawing the tongue from the alveolar ridge as the clinician simultaneously releases the upward pressure. Our movement which accompanies the direction to "explode" is usually a quick upward push against the bottom of the mouth followed by a quick release. The idea of a dam for /t/ can also be suggested if the clinician simultaneously urges the patient to say a /t/ while delivering a sharp upward tap under the jaw as the patient exhales air. The patient's mouth must be slightly open at the beginning of this maneuver, and at first, jaw and tongue may elevate together as the speaker attempts /t/. As quickly as possible the clinician should teach the patient to move the two independently, a dissociation that can sometimes be hastened if the clinician restrains the patient's jaw or if the patient is fitted with a bite block (see Figure 1) that sets between the upper and lower teeth, stabilizes the jaw, and prevents its total elevation. Once the dissociation of tongue and jaw movements is learned, the clinician's restraint or the bite block can be retired.

Teaching simultaneous manner and place distinctions. If /s/ and /t/ can be established, other sounds differing in both manner and place can be introduced. We usually begin at the front of the mouth. The /f/ can be gotten by molding the patient's lower lip over the lower teeth and then gently having him raise his jaw so that lip and upper teeth touch. The /Θ/ often follows the effort to get the patient's tongue slightly out of his mouth so that the teeth can gently contact it above and below. The /p/—or an approximation of it that can then be shaped—often results if the clinician first uses his hands to compress the patient's lips while simultaneously urging him to

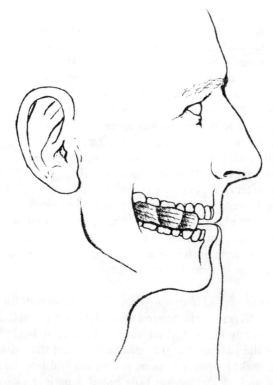

Figure 1. Diagram of a bite block being clenched between lower and upper teeth to stabilize the jaw.

build up air pressure in his mouth and then abruptly forces the patient's lips apart while simultaneously urging him to make a /p/ or popping sound.

Back sounds are harder; fortunately, they are also fewer. The /k/ sometimes comes if the clinician first has the patient open his mouth slightly, and then presses down on the tongue tip with a tongue blade while simultaneously pressing quickly upward against the floor of the mouth. To supply the upward push, the clinician places two fingers under the chin and far enough back so that an upward or lifting movement forces the tongue toward the roof of the mouth at about the position the tongue contacts the palate for a normal /k/. Patients are sometimes helped as well by being told to try breaking the /k/ contact by forcibly pushing air out of the mouth. Any approximations of the target can then be molded by repetition and analysis of each response.

Teaching voicing distinctions. The voiced −voiceless distinction is a hard one for apraxic talkers. While an apraxia of phonation and subsequent voicelessness is possible, it is more frequent in our experience that laryngeal activity is mistimed so that voicing is premature, late, or capricious, being correct sometimes and incorrect at others. But regardless of the cause or severity, phonetic placement may help establish the fundamental voice–voiceless contrast. By jiggling the patient's larynx, for example, the clinician can sometimes elicit voicing, especially if the jiggling is accompanied by a description of the "buzzing" that a turned-on larynx makes. By contrasting the buzz with a silent blow the clinician can sometimes get the patient to begin developing images that will speed learning of the voice–voiceless contrast. Once that distinction is learned, a considerable number of American English speech sounds may begin to reappear. While we have suggested that voicing distinctions are difficult and have discussed them after those of place and manner, it may be that an individual patient will be better able to make the voiced–voiceless contrast than those of manner or place. Diagnostic testing will reveal such a patient's existence. Once discovered, those proclivities can be accommodated. A clinician's aim is to help each patient improve; it is not to follow the stated or tacit assumptions of a book on treatment.

Teaching oral–nasal distinctions.   The best stimuli for establishing the oral–nasal difference will depend upon the patient's abilities and what he or she has already learned, if anything. We usually begin with /m/ and /ɑ/. We remind the patient that the /m/ is a hum and that /ɑ/ is merely the noise a person makes when he opens his mouth and lets the sound come out. If the /m/ and /ɑ/ distinction fails but if a patient can make apico-alveolar sounds, /n/ may be a good stimulus to contrast with the /ɑ/ or with some previously established oral consonant. If a patient's palate does not respond to repetition of oral–nasal pairs or to descriptions about where the air is to go, the clinician can sometimes train that palate by squeezing the patient's nares each time an oral sound is being produced nasally. Patients often automatically adjust their palates in response to this manipulation. We almost never teach /ŋ/ until the patient is only moderately or mildly apraxic, and by that time simple imitation is usually sufficient.

Phonetic Derivation

Occasionally, sounds that do not respond to other methods can be taught by phonetic derivation (Van Riper & Irwin, 1958). Phonetic derivation, called progressive approximation by some, involves teaching sounds or movements patients cannot make by modifying sounds or movements that they can. Derivation materials can be either nonspeech or speech postures and movements. For example, if a patient can say an /s/ but not a /ʃ/, the /ʃ/ can be derived by having the patient begin with an /s/ and add lip protrusion and rounding. As but one more example, an /f/ can sometimes be derived from a simple, lower-lip biting maneuver. This derivation of /f/ is an example of the general procedure of breaking a sound down into its phonetic components, which are then practiced before being recombined to yield the target sound.

While it needs to be probed experimentally, it may be that in some circumstances learning the phonetic components of speech sounds makes learning the sounds themselves more efficient. If for example, a patient learns to produce a predictable unvoiced air stream, that skill may generalize to all voiceless fricatives so that /ɵ/, /f/, /s/, and /ʃ/ come in quick succession. But while it is true that a sound may appear only after it has been broken down, it is equally true that it will endure only if practiced as part of an integrated sequence. We suggest that components be combined quickly, and that a sound obtained only with the help of another sound or movement be practiced on its own and in a variety of sequences as quickly as possible.

As will be obvious from subsequent examples of phonetic derivation techniques, imitation, phonetic derivation, and phonetic placement overlap and are powerful allies. Their idealized distinction is useful to us, however, for two reasons. The first is that imitation and phonetic derivation are less invasive than some forms of phonetic placement, so we try imitation and derivation before the invasive forms of phonetic placement. Second, phonetic derivation's integrity as a distinct technique provides a methodological framework for justifying the use of nonspeech gestures and even non-English speech sounds in treatment. Common examples of the derivation method (albeit mixed with elements of other methods) follow.

Deriving /f/. To make an /f/, a speaker rests the upper teeth against the lower lip, lowers the tongue, closes the velopharynx, and directs a stream of air through the constriction formed by teeth and lip. The two components most easily taught separately are labiodental valving and exhalation of a steady breath stream. In relearning the valve, we may have the patient practice applying considerable biting force of upper teeth against lower lip without doing anything else until the labiodental contact comes predictably. The hard bite may initially be useful as a cue about how the sound starts and may be retained in memory as an aid to self-correction during connected speech. Before we ask a patient to direct a flow of air through the labiodental constriction, however, we try to teach more normal biting pressure; otherwise the patient quickly becomes red-faced and any sound that manages to escape is unintelligible.

A total placement program for /f/—if imitation and derivation have failed—starts with a reminder to the patient of /f/'s importance in differentiating "four" from "bore" and so on. Next, the patient is told that the sound will be broken down into two parts—biting the lower lip and exhaling an unvoiced airstream. These two parts are then described in terms appropriate to the speaker's understanding. Then, one or the other part is demonstrated by the clinician. Demonstration is followed by getting the patient to imitate. We usually begin with imitation of the labiodental contact. If the speaker can imitate our movement, we encourage him or her to add the unvoiced airstream. If imitation of the contact is impossible or if the patient can muster only a gross approximation of it, we begin direct manipulation of the lip and jaw. We mold the speaker's lower lip over the lower teeth and then help raise the jaw. If the speaker persists in folding over too much of the lip, we inhibit part of the movement. If the speaker seems committed to stuffing the jaw entirely into the mouth, we inhibit this exaggeration as well. We continue to mold and shape until we get the best possible labiodental contact.

Sometimes speakers adjust contact if they are instructed to direct an unvoiced airstream through the valve. If the resulting /f/ is grossly distorted, some speakers make changes automatically. Others do not. Some cannot even get the knack of forcing air through the valve. They seem to "get stuck" once they have inhaled and gotten ready to blow. Among the clinician's choices at this point are to (1) concentrate on teaching an unvalved, voiceless airstream and to reintroduce the valving only after a predictable airstream is forthcoming, or (2) have the patient valve lightly and then try to force an airstream through the valve by pushing gently inward on the patient's belly.

As a result of these manipulations some patients begin closer and closer approximations of /f/. Others continue to have difficulty. For example, they may begin reflexively puckering as they attempt the unvoiced airstream. A puckered /f/ is neither pretty nor easily integrated into connected speech. It may help to emphasize exhaling rather than blowing. If puckering persists, even after the patient is advised against it, the clinician can inhibit the pucker by applying lateral pressure against the mouth's corners. The noises produced during all such manipulations may be only gross approximations of the target, or may be reasonable approximations produced in ways that will be impossible to integrate into connected movements, or may be reasonable approximations produced with relatively normal movements and postures. The first two conditions require analysis of where the patient is going awry, correction of the error(s), and drill of the acceptable valve. Reasonable approximations require only fine tuning. Once a patient is producing predictable /f/s, the usual practice of fading clinician participation begins, and the speaker is made to rely increasingly on self-generated cues to correct production. Finally, the /f/ can be practiced in words, although it is sometimes helpful to return to the sound in isolation for short periods at the beginning of each session even though a speaker seems to be gaining considerable functional control of the sound in words and even in sentences.

Deriving other voiceless fricatives.   Other voiceless sounds can be taught with similar strategies. The /θ/ can be derived from a predictable tongue protrusion. The /s/ may come when the patient learns to direct an air stream through a tightly closed jaw and tensely spread lips (as in producing /i/). An additional cue to /s/ is to tell the patient that its sound is "high," which seems physiologically to correspond to a very narrow breath stream created by grooving the tongue. Initial tension accompanying the jaw or lip postures can be relaxed with practice. Once /s/ is stable, a tolerable /ʃ/ can be obtained by teaching the patient to pucker while producing an /s/.

Deriving voiceless plosives. The voiceless plosives—which may be harder than the voiceless fricatives to teach—require that the patient learn to develop a dam or tight seal and release the air abruptly from behind it. To derive a /p/ we begin by having the patient blow. To this is added the idea of a dam or seal which is then quickly released to "explode" the air to the outside. Alternatively, the patient can sometimes get a /p/ by first pretending to make a bubble or by actually making a popping sound with the lips. Sometimes, suggesting that the explosion should be quiet or light will help inhibit a voiced cognate. If one or all these derivations are joined by placement techniques such as molding the patient's lips or helping to elevate the jaw, the /p/ is usually forthcoming. Once the /p/ is learned, a /t/ may come if the patient is first directed to touch the tongue to the roof of the mouth to make a dam. A clicking sound may also be the first step in deriving a /t/. If these methods fail, the clinician may have to resort to placement methods. In our experience, the /k/ either comes with imitation or requires phonetic placement. We have not found a target from which the /k/ can be derived, although we are sure other clinicians have.

Deriving voice. Severe patients often have an apraxia of phonation, making exotic derivations necessary. Humming, animal sounds, grunts, chewing (with delight), or coughing may get the larynx "on." If these activities are accompanied by the clinician's constant urgings for the patient to concentrate on the sound and feel of voicing, predictable voicing usually results. If not, combining phonetic placement and derivation by manually jiggling the larynx while encouraging production of a noise or a buzz may get voice. Another device that combines placement and derivation is to apply rapid, forceful (but careful) plunger-like movements inward against the belly muscles. If no sound is forthcoming with any of these methods, or if sound (once it appears) is not modifiable, or if the patient cannot predictably report whether the larynx is on or off, treatment is doomed. It is usually the globally aphasic speaker rather than the severely apraxic one who has these problems, however. Apraxic speakers learn to turn on the larynx and, once having learned voicing, give evidence of the readiness to begin coordinating voice with other phonetic components to produce a variety of vowels and consonants.

Deriving vowels. The /ɑ/ is usually the easiest to derive from any vocalization. The speaker has only to open the mouth and let the sound out. The urge to elevate the tongue can be inhibited with a tongue blade. Once the /ɑ/ arrives, the clinician can sometimes elicit an /i/ by instructing the patient to begin producing /ɑ/, then to elevate the jaw and spread the lips. Similarly, the /u/ or /ou/ may result if the patient begins with an /ɑ/ and then elevates the jaw and rounds the lips. Movements back and forth among these sounds can be strengthened by the clinician's manipulations of the patient's jaw and lips and by drill. The object is to help the patient make contrasting vowel movements, and then to use these to generate the voiced consonants. Other vowels such as /ɪ/, /æ/, and /ɛ/ can wait. In our experience, these vowels are nearly impossible to teach in isolation, but may begin to appear spontaneously in words.

Deriving voiced consonants. Once the patient has learned some vowels, it may be reasonably easy to derive the voiced consonants by using VC or VCV syllables. Certain vowels seem to have greater influence over some consonants than over others. The /u/, for example, may be more help to /g/; the /i/ may be best for /d/; and the /ɑ/ for /b/. Simple clinical tests will tell the clinician about these differential effects. Regardless of which vowels are used, a VCV context rather than a simple VC one may be necessary to keep voiced sounds from becoming voiceless, as they sometimes want to do when placed in the final position.

Voiced consonants can also be derived from their voiceless cognates, once vowels, or at least phonation, have appeared. The /v/ can come from using the voice of /ɑ/ plus the posture of /f/, the /z/ from /s/, the /ð/ from /θ/, the /b/ from /p/, the /d/ from /t/, the /g/ from /k/, and so on. Voiced fricatives seem more responsive than voiced plosives to this kind of phonetic derivation, however. Both voiced fricatives and plosives sometimes result, however, merely from having the speaker begin with a voiceless cognate and then make that voiceless sound louder and more tense.

Merging Phonetic Placement and Derivation

Phonetic placement and phonetic derivation can be merged in practice as long as the clinician has more than a nodding, undergraduate knowledge of physiologic phonetics. Slight changes in the height of jaw or tongue, a slight change in tension or in configuration of the lips, or a slight movement of the tongue's contact forward or backward may be just the necessary modification necessary to turn a barely acceptable sound into an acceptable one or to turn an awkward posture into one that can be used in connected speech. How many times have we taught static gestures which produce beautiful isolated noises that are impossible to work into connected speech? Speech is enough like gymnastics without requiring the tongue to perform doubled up or doubled over. A good phonetician/clinician will be aware of connected speech's requirements, even while shaping sounds in isolation.

Placement and derivation may be severe patients' best hope, unless they are those rare patients who can imitate words and even phrases, despite being essentially speechless when they try to speak spontaneously. We have seen such patients, especially acutely, but not often. More frequent is the patient who seems to have completely forgotten how sounds are to be made. With training that combines placement and derivation (and simple imitation), however, memory can return quickly, and the patient may begin to say treated sounds in untreated environments and may even begin using untreated sounds. If such progress is to make connected speech more functional, however, it is important that each patient be able to associate the sounds with their meanings. For this reason, we constantly associate sounds with their written forms, and we remind the speaker that sounds make differences in meaning as when "mean" becomes "bean." Language, then, is part of even placement and derivation methods.

Analysis of a Session

Severe patients, like the one to be described, usually thrive when imitation, placement, and derivation are combined. We videotaped the first session of a patient whose only speech consisted of profanity and variations of the words, "yeah" and "no." In the first session, we taught him several sounds including the /b/. We tried to teach /b/, first with imitation. But no matter how fervidly we demonstrated the /b/, he produced only an /ɑ/, and telling him to put his lips together before he started did not help. After less than a minute of imitation plus explanation, we changed to phonetic placement. We first guided his lips together, held them in that position, and directed him to build up air in his mouth. When we felt increased pressure behind his lips, we told him to pop the air by quickly releasing the bilabial contact. We aided this release by briskly forcing his lips apart. The model we gave him to imitate was /bɑ/, and we told him to make the entire CV utterance as loud as he could. The vowel and the idea of loudness were to make voicing more likely. His first few attempts were silent bilabial movements resembling those of a goldfish as it looks outward from its bowl at the human looking in. So we reminded him of the voicing, jiggled his larynx, and told him to concentrate just on the vowel while we helped him get the /b/ by manipulating his lips. He finally got it. The whole procedure took less than five minutes. He still needed hundreds of repetitions to improve his control, but very quickly we could begin reducing the number of cues required to elicit the sound.

The fabric of phonetic placement decorated with swatches of imitation and phonetic derivation was also evident in the same patient's relearning of /g/ in the initial position of a CV syllable. Practice began with imitation both because it is less invasive and because some other sounds, including an initial /s/, had responded to imitation. The patient watched and listened several times as the clinician said a series of /gʌ/s; however, his own attempts were all /dʌ/s. We urged him to watch more closely while we exaggerated the articulatory movements. Nothing. We explained that a /g/ is made by humping the back of the tongue to dam the air which is then exploded. We repeated the model. Still the /d/ came. We explained that the tongue tip must stay down while the back is humped to trap the air. Still a /d/. Then we had him try again while we pinned his anterior tongue to the mouth's floor with a tongue blade. The /g/ became /ɑ/ because the patient did not hump any part of his tongue. Next, we placed our fingers under his chin right in front of his larynx, held his tongue tip down, and simultaneously exhorted him to produce a /g/ each time we made a quick upward movement of our fingers under his chin. The first /g/ was not pristine, but it was not /d/.

These examples are typical of our practice with the severely apraxic talkers. We begin by introducing as few cues as possible. We do not begin immediately with a tongue blade or our hands. Blades and hands on the face or tongue and the stretching, tugging, and urging that accompany them may well send so much peculiar information into the patient's system that performance deteriorates. On the other hand, the severe patient may only get the sound if the clinician gets it by manipulation, so it is advisable not to waste time with noninvasive methods if they are effete. Once a patient begins producing any sound under the clinician's guidance, the cues responsible for causing the sound to appear can be faded, to be reinserted at intervals if the response weakens. After a sound has begun to appear, a single gesture may be enough to elicit the target as when touching under the patient's chin elicits a /g/ or a movement towards the lips elicits /p/.

Rhythm

Some sounds and syllables may be arousable only with rhythm. Often, it is enough for clinician and patient to produce a syllable such as /la/ repeatedly to any strong rhythm, even to the rhythm of a popular song. When used alone, the method of combining speech and strong, repetitive rhythms may be nothing more than clinical legerdemain—a trick. However, if the speaker is taught monitoring of the resulting production; if the sounds or syllables can be transferred into words, and the words into phrases; and if the strong rhythms can be faded or made more like normal prosody, rhythmic presentation of stimuli may work when other more prosaic methods have failed. The greatest challenge to this method is transferring the gains. Sounds seem to like the security that rhythm brings, and some seem unable to appear in any but a stereotyped, rhythmic environment. Nonetheless, even stubborn sounds can sometimes be lured away from the stereotyped rhythmic pattern that initially aroused them by a concerted systematic effort.

A few words on singing. We should not allow staff, family, or patients to believe that good singing means good talking. In our experience singing and speaking are usually separate activities—Keith and Aronson's patient (1975) was an exception—and singing a popular melody, while it may buoy a patient's spirit, usually does not improve speech. Regardless of what patients can sing, if they are to talk, talking must be practiced. This does not mean we reject Melodic Intonation Therapy (MIT) (Sparks & Holland, 1976; Berlin, 1976). MIT is not singing. To intone "bacon and eggs" is much different from singing "Will You Lie By Me In A Field of Stone?" Our own methods of eliciting speech with rhythm owes much to MIT, but our steps are far less elaborate, and we seldom use rhythm as the sole or even primary method. A method of combining rhythm and stress to improve articulation will be described in the next chapter.

Reading

While written stimuli are generally less potent for severe apraxic patients than for moderate and mild ones, it sometimes happens that an apraxic talker's articulators respond better during aloud reading than at any other time. Certainly, the hypothesis can be tested with each new patient. We routinely do just that by having a patient both imitate and read selected words and phrases.

The goal of a reading program with the severe patient is to have successful reading register as a set of cues which allows the patient to go on talking after the written cues have been faded. Our method has the patient read a selected number of responses aloud several times. When these responses seem stable, or if we want to see just how stable they are, we then have the patient speak what was on the card but only after the card has been turned over so that the stimuli are no longer in view. The task can be made harder by reducing the time the speaker sees the card or by increasing the time between the seeing of it and the saying of it.

When reading is good, it may be so because written stimuli, unlike auditory ones, can be placed before the patient for as long as necessary. Whether the superiority of read stimuli says anything about the underlying neuropathology of apraxia of speech, we do not know. We can tell quickly if it has a place in the treatment regime, however. A more extensive discussion of reading also appears in the next chapter.

Key Word Technique

In the *key word technique*,[3] a patient learns how to say sounds in many environments by practicing them first in a few key words. The method is

---

[3]Irwin and Griffith (1973) report a program of articulation training for children using key words. The interested reader may wish to consult their chapter and the data on which it is based.

akin to phonetic derivation because the goal is to help the patient transfer control of a target in a word that can be said to that same target in words that cannot. Drill of such meaningful utterances may spin magic for the severely apraxic patient just as for any other, and it may be that short, real words will be the quickest vehicle back to some functional utterances for some apraxic talkers. A man whose wife's name is Bess may regain control of the /b/ sooner if he practices "Bess" than if he is made to practice innumerable /bʌ/'s. That key words exist, and that they can be useful therapeutically, is evidence against the unfortunately common assumption that longer utterances are inevitably harder than shorter ones for the apraxic talker.

The method begins with efforts to find words that the patient says accurately and automatically. The next step is to repeat those words repeatedly to see if the patient can control them when they are less automatic. If so, the next step is to help the patient learn the cues associated with correct production. For example, if the patient whose wife's name is "Bess" says the /b/ in that word, the clinician can help him identify how the /b/ is made and how it feels and sounds when made correctly. But control must come to reside in motor centers, not language ones. So—to continue the example of "Bess"—the patient is urged to hold the /b/'s implosion stage for varying periods, to feel the lips pressing against one another, to release the sound on signal, and to endure endless descriptions and repetitions.

In the acute stage the patient may or may not quickly transfer his learning to other words. If he does, those words can be further stabilized and then made part of longer utterances. If he does not, the clinician will need to introduce specific stimuli to aid the transfer. The /bɛs/, for example, can be changed to /bis/, or /bɑs/, or /bɛt/, or /bɛd/, or /bɛn/, and so on. If the sound refuses to come loose from the key words, and if "Bess" is the only word in which the /b/ appears predictably even after much practice, the patient's prognosis is poor and depends upon how much progress is being made with other words and sounds. Such a person may be telling us that he is really a globally aphasic talker rather than an apraxic talker.

We do not mean to imply by the order of this chapter that we save the key word technique until others have failed. Not at all. Because it is noninvasive we try it early. We also try several other methods more or less simultaneously in hopes of finding out which methods most efficiently elicit which sounds. We often find that different targets respond to different methods.

Transition

The methods already described can move the severely apaxic speaker along recovery's road. But methods are not the only influences on how the patient will do. Others include how hard the clinician and patient work, how frequently practice is scheduled, how rigidly the criterion of correct or adequate is defined, and how many facilitating conditions (such as slow rate) the clinician introduces. If the patient is acutely apraxic, physiologic recovery will usually exert its considerable influence as well. We have seen severely apraxic speakers move so rapidly that the clinician makes daily revisions in the treatment plan and spends more time trying to keep up than in leading. For such patients, the movement from sounds and syllables to words and phrases and from placement and derivation to less invasive and mildly more exciting methods is quick, relatively effortless, and very rewarding. The severe, chronic apraxic speaker, on the other hand, is a greater challenge.

TREATING THE SEVERE, CHRONICALLY APRAXIC PATIENT

Chronic, severe apraxic talkers can be exciting discoveries. Seen on the orthopedic ward after having broken a hip, or on the medical ward during a diabetes workup, they give the impression of some understanding and of being in the world and of it. Their identification is seldom easy, however. A number of otherwise dissimilar patients may fit the profile of profound speech involvement, preservation of some understanding, and retention of social competence. They may be severe Broca's aphasic speakers or from the mild part of the global aphasia distribution. They may come from a malignant, depressed environment that has driven them toward silence or they may have merely abdicated. Hospitalization may merely have revived them temporarily. Or they may be severely apraxic. Diagnostic treatment can usually reduce these alternatives to one while simultaneously demonstrating the patient's prognosis for speech or total communication.

Counseling

Willing Suspension of Disbelief

Because chronic patients and their families have lived with disability, they have different counseling needs from acute patients and their families. Chronic patients may struggle impotently and give up prematurely. Families may have begun talking and doing for them. Everyone will need to learn new ways of coping and acting. Because physiologic recovery's influence (and perhaps that of previous treatment) was inadequate, they must accept that the newest therapy may do no more. Nonetheless they and the patient must commit themselves to that treatment. And there is the rub. Commitment without hope is impossible. When clinicians tell patients and families (as they must) to hope but not hope too much, they owe them probity and the best that is in speech pathology's methodology. That methodology must first of all be diagnostic.

Diagnostic Treatment

Goals of Diagnostic Treatment

If the patient and family agree to a willing suspension of disbelief, the clinician's task is diagnostic treatment. This treatment's first goal is to find out how much speech the patient can learn, how rapidly, and with what amount of generalization. The methods already described—imitation, phonetic placement, phonetic derivation, rhythm, reading, and key words—are appropriate to this task. Its second goal is to find out if the patient uses or can learn to use augmentative or alternative modes of communication. Evidence that the patient can either learn to talk or to use augmentative or alternative modes of communication justifies a period of intense treatment regardless of how long the patient has been severely apraxic; assuming—again—that the family and patient are willing.

Diagnostic Speech Training

Reasonably simple designs such as the multiple baseline design (Hersen & Barlow, 1976) in which several targets are selected and then treated sequentially reveal whether or not a patient can learn and whether the learning generalizes. The clinician begins by testing the stability of a variety of targets such as selected plosives, fricatives, and vowels in isolation; in syllables; or in words and sentences (if possible). Highly variable targets—adequate one time and absent the next—or targets which begin improving as soon as the clinician pays even scant attention to them are of little use. Stable targets present diagnostic treatment with a proper test. Only if otherwise stable targets improve with treatment, and if that treatment generalizes to untreated items, can clinicians be sanguine about their methods and about each patient's potential.

General Versus Specific Treatment Effects. The patient who improves spectacularly after only one or two sessions deserves special mention. Such patients usually have never been in treatment or have not had treatment for a long time. Once treatment begins, however, a number of treated and untreated stimuli seem to improve more or less equally. We warn patients and families about this phenomenon, and clinicians would do well to be leery of it themselves. These early effects can be beguiling, and can lure family, patient, and clinician into commitments and expectations that may well be shattered by subsequent events. We encourage families to temper their enthusiasm and clinicians to curb discussions about long-term treatment until the patient's real potential has been measured—until specific rather than general treatment effects have been determined. Too often we have seen patients say their first words in the speech pathologist's office only to have those become their only words.

Early gains may be general and significant because untreated, chronic patients fail to exploit a significant return of physiologic support for speech. In a sense, they may not have looked under the bandages to discover that the wound has healed. It is more likely, however, that such patients will have felt recovery's itch, will have tried to talk, and will have retreated back into silence upon discovering that recovery was far from complete and that speech was totally inadequate. Regardless of the reason, the majority of untreated, chronic apraxic speakers have some modest amount of unused physiologic support for speech that lies dormant until treatment rouses it. Most of the gains resulting from the activation of this previously unused support will be present after the first two or three diagnostic sessions and usually, at least in our experience, are insufficient to make speech more functional. The crucial test of whether patient and clinician should commit to long-term speech treatment is whether or not the patient shows specific learning, transfer, and maintenance. We take as long as a month to make these decisions. If the patient learns, if the learning transfers, and is maintained, treatment as already described can continue. If the patient fails to learn speech or if learning is excruciatingly slow, the clinician should probably begin diagnostic treatment in the other modalities. Indeed, diagnostic training in the other modalities can proceed simultaneously with speech training if the patient and clinician have time for it.

Diagnostic Training in Other Modalities

Some severe apraxic talkers can be taught to write, gesture, use a communication board, and draw even when they can talk only a little or not at all; they can sometimes do these things with greater facility than global, Broca's, or even Wernicke's aphasic patients.[4] Such abilities may not expose themselves spontaneously (without treatment), however; thus the need to design diagnostic training.

The methods are similar to those for measuring speech learning and generalization. Clinicians want to know if patients can learn to write single words and telegrammatic statements; if they can learn gestures to make wants and needs known; if they can point to letters, words, and pictures on a board; and if they can draw pictures to communicate ideas. Clinicians will want to design their diagnostic sessions so that they can discover simultaneously whether or not untreated utterances become easier to write, untreated gestures begin to appear, the patient can begin using the board creatively, untaught drawings appear spontaneously, and whether learning of all responses in all modalities is maintained. While maintenance is essential to the decision to continue treatment, generalization is not. For example, one patient taught us not to despair even if every written word has

---

[4]Many severe and moderate Wernicke's aphasic patients are excellent total communicators, however.

to be taught. Prior to treatment, he could not write even single words, but he began relearning individual words with only a few minutes practice on each. He was like a man learning to identify faces who began his learning with Paul Broca and Fred Darley. Recognizing one did not help him recognize the other, but once he had seen both, he did not forget either one. Patients who fail to generalize can either stay in treatment longer (although protracted treatment is generally not our preference) or they can be taught how to communicate the necessities and then be released. A clinician's goal for patients who generalize can be more ambitious. Such patients can be helped to generate original messages; they do not need to rely on only what the clinician has selected to teach.

Sometimes a candidate's appropriateness shines through the severest apraxia. At the behest of relatives, a patient once appeared in our clinic eight years after his stroke. He had no functional speech beyond "yeah" and "no," and while those two words can get one in and out of most activities, the family and the patient wanted more. When he left the hospital approximately eight weeks later, he could write a little, draw a little, gesture elaborately, and use a language board. How did we know he would be a candidate for such training? He learned to write words after only a few minutes practice and retained them with only occasional reminders. He easily made up gestures in response to questions such as, "How would you show someone you were tired?" With almost no prompting he could point to pictures on a language board in response to questions. He liked to draw even though his creations were functional rather than aesthetic. He relished communication in all these modes.

Acting on the Diagnostic Findings

The minimum requirements for continuing any kind of treatment are improvement on treated items and maintenance of that improvement. If treatment generalizes across items or across modalities, so much the better. If the patient does not learn in any modality, the clinician's only course is to stop treatment. Depending upon what a patient learns, the clinician must decide whether or not to teach speech or total communication (which may or may not include speech along with other kinds of communication behavior). Counseling will be necessary whether the clinician thinks treatment should end or continue beyond the diagnostic period. Patients and families need to know their options and what they can expect. Finally, they need freedom to make their own decisions.

Counseling When the Patient Will Not Improve

Some patients should not be made to endure treatment even if they can learn, and therapy's rigors and frustrations should always be spared those who do not learn. Because a belief in miracles, the unexpected, and the impossible keeps many of us sane, most families enter diagnostic treatment with great expectations. Trying to spare them disappointment accomplishes little, however, so if we decide after a trial of treatment that the patient cannot improve, we tell them so. We remind them, too, that our judgement is only the way it seems to us—that we could be wrong. We heard Norman Cousins' (1976) warning that people silly enough to believe an expert can seal their own fates. We have also heard of families and patients spending so much time and money pursuing future recovery that they lose the present and themselves.

Altering the Patient's Environment

Because environments can sometimes be changed even when patients cannot be, we have other treatment obligations toward those who cannot improve. We do not wish to imply that the following suggestions be reserved only for patients and families where improvement is otherwise impossible. Most apraxic talkers, regardless of how good they are, will do better in a supportive, therapeutic (not to be confused with clinical) environment. However, changing the environment is especially important for the severe chronic talker who cannot learn.

First, it may be helpful to discuss the patient's strengths and guide the family toward activities that utilize those strengths. Watching and walking are better than listening and sitting; raising flowers is better than discussing horticulture. One can fill the beer cooler and sweep up even when making change is impossible. One can draw to an inside straight even if unable to rub it in. These are only a few of hundreds of activities available to individual patients. Some of these the families will have discovered; the clinician can help with others. In addition to helping families plan activities that help, we try to have them recognize and limit activities that hinder. Constantly blaring televisions ("for company and stimulation"), a steady stream of gregarious friends for dinner ("Remember the time we . . ."), babysitting the grandchildren ("Grandad loved them before his stroke, and they can help him with his homework"), and constant encouragement to resume a hobby ("Look, here's something he once made.") may not be therapeutic.

Clinicians can help in other ways as well. Families can be released from any guilt about the patient's illness or failure to improve; in particular, they can be reassured that they should not be providing treatment. They can be encouraged to make decisions about jobs, insurance, and changed lives rather than waiting until they are sure that the patient is not going to recover; and they can be shown ways of including the patient in such decisions. They can be reassured that a miraculous recovery is probably not around the corner, and they should be advised against chasing every newspaper report of a cure for nervous system damage. Finally, family members may need a reminder to care for themselves while preserving a realistic amount of independence for the patient. Time away from the patient may be helpful to everyone, patient included.

All of these suggestions have as their aim making the present more compelling than the past. Because other professions are less able to communicate with the communication disordered, such counseling is sometimes left undone unless a speech pathologist does it. This counseling need not be long term, and therefore expensive. One or two sessions with periodic follow-up phone calls or visits may well be sufficient. As important as learning how to do such counseling and remembering to do it is recognizing when it is unnecessary. Patients and families are resilient. Most do well without us. Some do better with us. Being able to tell the difference is clinical acumen.

Counseling When the Patient May Improve

Deciding If It Is Worth It

If the clinician decides that the patient can improve, the patient and family should be provided with the data on which that decision was based. In addition, they deserve a reasonable assessment of the cost in time, money, and emotion; and a specific prognosis—how many words, and how clearly uttered; how much writing; how many gestures, and under what conditions. If total communication rather than speech is going to be taught, they will need to understand what total communication is. They will usually have no trouble accepting speech drills; however, they may balk at suggestions about writing, gesturing, or using a board unless the rationale is explained and unless they can be convinced that atypical communication is better than silence or head nodding. Regardless of whether the clinician's goal is speech or total communication, clinician, family, and patient have to ask seriously if efforts, even moderately successful ones, are worth it. During treatment, patient and family sit suspended—decisions are delayed, everyone waits and watches. Such suspension may not be good and must be balanced impassively against treatment's benefits. Progress, when it comes, often does so in dribs and drabs, and even successful communication will be painfully short of normal.

Increasing Independence and Risking Failure

If chronic, severe patients are to profit from treatment, they and their families will need to do more than merely accept treatment's rigors and incomplete results; they will have to begin changing the way they treat one another. We frequently see chronic apraxic persons who have surrendered to their conditions. They try to get by with a few head shakes, and refer all questions to someone else. Some (few, we hope) even abandon themselves to that unholy trio—the wheelchair, the television, and the bed. If efforts to improve speech or make patients into total communicators are going to be more than performances for the delight of clinicians, patients, and observers, patients must first begin reclaiming their independence in other ways. They must be willing to let people know what is on their minds and to initiate communication even though it means risking failure. Explaining the importance of independence, advising the family about ways of coping with the inevitable frustrations, demonstrating treatment methods and their effects, and completing specific carryover assignments involving families and patients will all help. The greatest boost, however, will come from improvement. Most patients in our experience do not give up their dependence until they know they have a chance of successful independence, and even then they do so only with people they trust. Because severely apraxic talkers who begin therapy during the chronic period can almost inevitably expect some failures to communicate, the family needs to learn that they have to stimulate or cue in all appropriate modalities. Such cueing will no doubt be a lifetime obligation. Family and patient need to learn not only how to do it, but how to endure it.

If speech alone is to be taught, clinicians can use methods discussed earlier in this chapter. Total communication requires other, different methods.

Learning Total Communication

Strengthening Each Mode

Once the counseling has been done and the patient has accepted total communication, which may or may not include speaking (depending upon the patient's abilities), treatment can begin. The first step is to improve each mode of communication as the patient's individual performance dictates. Earlier, we mentioned a patient whose speech was limited to "yes" and "no." Diagnostic testing showed him to be capable of relearning how to write. We began by making a list of the words he could use to make his life easier. Some of these he wrote approximations of without treatment; others had to be relearned. He began by copying words whose meanings we were sure he knew—Maalox, toilet, TV, uncle. We then had him copy after a delay, and then write from dictation. Finally, we had him practice writing the words as answers to questions: "What stomach medicine do you take?" "Why are you fidgety?" Ward personnel were given a list of the words he could write, and everyone urged him to write appropriate words on the ward, even if they were words not yet practiced. Finally, the most useful ones were written on his communication board (we probably should have had him do it) so he had only to point to the word he wanted. Drawing was taught in the same way. We began by deciding what he needed to communicate that drawing could help him with. We then started with copying, added delays, and finally encouraged volitional drawing. In our experience, patients are quick to draw once they are encouraged; and even severely involved patients can draw at least rudimentary objects.

Using a Communication Board

A patient can be taught to use a communication board with traditional behavioral methods. We begin by having the patient merely point to objects or activities on a Cleo (CLEO, Living Aids, see Figure 2) or some other board. If seeing the whole board is confusing, we limit the choices to two or more items. As competence improves, we expand the number of choices. Pointing to objects and activities by function follows pointing to them by name. First, "Show me the bed." Next, "Show me the one you sleep in." We next reenforce a board's functional use by having the patient respond to such questions as, "If you were in your wheelchair, and not able to lie down but wanted to go to sleep, what could you point to?" The questions length and complexity would be adjusted to accommodate the patient's understanding.

As experienced clinicians recognize, the next step—initiating communication with the board—is the giant step. In our files we have data on several patients who could handle all clinician-dominated steps with ease but never made that next step (perhaps because it's a leap or part of a separate journey altogether). We have not found foolproof ways of helping them transfer what they have learned under our control to their own, independent use of the board. We involve family and ward personnel in the treatment. We show them what the patient can do and how the board can be used to make meanings. We elicit their support in encouraging the board's use. We load the board with relevant items. We put the board on the ward and practice on the ward. We keep our fingers crossed.

Putting All of the Abilities Together

Once patients have a number of responses such as writing, gesturing, and perhaps even speaking available, they will no doubt need practice in selecting and using these for the most efficient communication. In our experience one of the best programs for teaching this total communication is Promoting Aphasic Communication Effectiveness (PACE) (Davis & Wilcox, 1981). The program has an elaborate conceptual basis but is simple and effective in action. Clinician and patient take turns communicating the identity of objects, actions, and ideas. Emphasis is on communication rather than on normal speech-language performance. To reenforce total communication, the patient is provided with pencil and paper and is encouraged to gesture, speak, and do anything else that helps. In its simplest form, patient and clinician take turns selecting from a pile of pictured objects placed face down and then communicating what they have selected. Stimuli in need of additional work can be reinserted into the stack

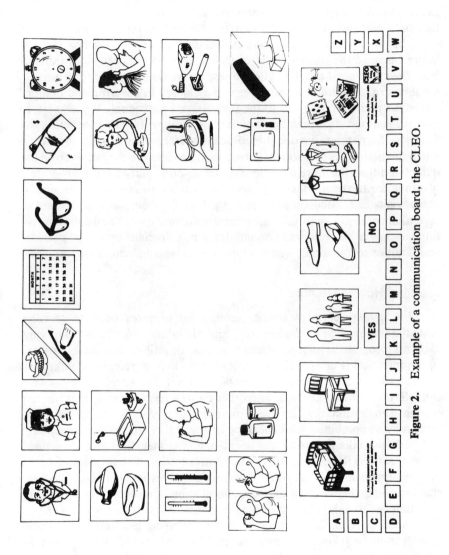

Figure 2. Example of a communication board, the CLEO.

237

and very difficult ones can be dropped. Among this program's other virtues is that it allows for easy involvement of the family. With the proper encouragement a wife can as easily gesture the identity of a cup of coffee as say it, and with the proper counseling patient and family can come to accept that such gestures are normal and better than silent resignation.

The more people the clinician can involve in the patient's program the better because the ultimate test of this program's success is its transfer from the clinic to where the patient lives. If a patient is bound for a nursing home we request and are usually given a chance to describe and demonstrate the patient's program to the institution's personnel. We also try to find at least one staff member who will be responsible for continuing the program. Sometimes we do; sometimes not. If a patient is going home, so much the better. As previously noted, we try to involve the family from the outset and transfer more and more of the responsibility for the program's continuance to them. Once a patient has learned to communicate needs, clinic visits can become progressively less frequent, and patients and caretakers are left to continue the program on their own. Total communication can never be complete communication. Clinicians owe it to patients and families to call a halt when returns begin lagging behind investments.

Learning How to Gesture

We have reserved a special section for gestures because of their potential importance to the severely apraxic talker. We are not implying that this program is distinct from that just described for teaching total communication. For speechless patients who cannot relearn to talk, gestures as well as other modes may replace speech. For severe patients who can talk only a little, gestures and other modes may augment their limited speech. In addition, for all severe patients the possibility exists that gestures may be combined with speaking in a way that will improve speaking and perhaps make gesturing less necessary. The method is called gestural reorganization (Rosenbek, 1978) after Luria (1970). The first step in gestural reorganization—that of establishing good gestures—is also the first step in making them part of total communication. If total communication is the clinician's goal, clinician and patient may want to stop after gestures have been learned. If the additional step of using gestures to improve speech is to be taken, clinician and patient move on to the appropriate procedures for doing that. Methods for both steps will be described.

Choosing a Gestural System

Ekman and Friesen (1972) describe two kinds of gestures: (1) emblems or gestures with "a direct verbal translation usually consisting of a word or two, or a phrase" (p. 357) and (2) illustrators or movements which accompany the rhythm and stress of speech. Emblems, or gestures that can be substituted for speech, are more appropriate than illustrators for the severe patient and AMERIND (Skelly, 1979) has much to recommend it as a system of emblems for therapeutic use. Based upon American Indian sign language, AMERIND signs have the advantages of being intelligible even to naive persons and of having been modified for performance with one hand. Easy intelligibility means that families and patients need not learn a unique or arbitrary system, an advantage that speeds up treatment and may well make it more acceptable. That they can be performed with one hand makes it possible for even a severely hemiplegic patient to use them successfully. All signs are described and displayed in Skelly's 1979 text. They allow patients who learn all or a portion of them to communicate a considerable amount of information about their needs and psyches. We owe her not only for the signs but for much of the theory and methodology of gestural reorganization.

Method for Strengthening Gestures

Even apraxic speakers with mild aphasia will need training if gestures are to become functional as communication in the absence of speech or provide the basis for speech reorganization. Collins and Wertz (1976) have developed a method of gestural training which appears below in a slightly edited form. The method is traditional in that each step requires less of the clinician and more of the patient. The seven steps are not a prescription. Some patients do not need to take all seven; others need more and smaller steps; yet others can profit from the seven steps but not in the order of their presentation here.

In Step One, the clinician demonstrates each gesture[5] and determines that the patient recognizes its meaning. If the patient does not, the meaning is taught. Gestures that are not learned are dropped. We usually work with from two to ten gestures at a time, although especially good patients may be able to work simultaneously on more. In Step Two, patient and clinician perform simultaneously. At first the clinician may have to shape the patient's hand and otherwise direct it to the proper position in space. When the patient can begin to perform with less clinician assistance, treatment can advance to Step Three, imitation. The patient looks, and then performs. The amount of delay is increased in Step Four. We have no rigid rules about how much delay or about what the patient should do while waiting. We do know that a session of 1-minute or even 30-second delay intervals would be excruciating and probably inefficient, so we seldom use more than 15 or so seconds of delay. Step Five requires the patient to

---

[5]Specific gestures are not described in this book. Readers are referred to Skelly (1979) and are encouraged to consider other gestural systems as well.

perform gestures upon spoken or written request, depending on which modality is more potent. Step Six is a crucial carryover step because the patient performs in response to a question or other appropriate stimulus. Taking this step is sometimes as disastrous (and surprising) as breaking through the ice after having walked more than halfway across a frozen lake. We say this because many patients move briskly through the first five steps only to sink on Step Six. If a patient does have difficulty, extending the practice at Step Six or returning to previous steps may both help. Because patients are notorious for doing everything we ask when we ask it, but little or less when we are not present, we suggest a seventh, or transfer, step. Activities for Step Seven vary, but usually include monitored use of the gestures outside the clinic and with people other than the clinician. We give the people who communicate with the patient a list of the gestures, we have them observe treatment and learn the gestures, we watch them treat the patient, and we set specific goals for using the gestures outside of the clinic. These steps are summarized in Table 1.

Treatment remains at each step until the patient can respond predictably, and it retreats to a previous step when a gesture shows any signs of breaking up or weakening. The clinician should not allow a gesture to lose precision as treatment progresses or as more gestures are added. We usually work on several gestures simultaneously even though some of them may be at different steps.

Table 1.
Steps in Teaching Gestures as an Alternative Mode of Communication

Step	Procedure
I.	Clinician demonstrates the gesture and determines that the patient recognizes its meaning.
II.	Clinician and patient perform gesture simultaneously with the clinician assisting the patient as necessary.
III.	Patient performs gesture imitatively.
IV.	Patient performs gesture imitatively after delay.
V.	Patient performs gesture in response to auditory or written stimulus, depending on which is more potent.
VI.	Patient performs the gesture in response to questions and other appropriate environmental stimuli.
VII.	Transfer.

Gestures and Total Communication

If gestures are to be a part of total communication, treatment time can be shared with work on other response types. Work on several kinds of responses can sometimes proceed simultaneously by selecting similar stimuli for gesturing, writing, for display on the communication board, and even for drawing. Working on the same stimuli in several modes is not mandatory, however. If total communication is the goal, the clinician may want to find out what the patient does best in each mode and encourage selection of the best mode for each individual communication. Gestural reorganization or using gestures as the basis for improved speech will be discussed in the next chapter.

SOME DATA

Severe, chronic apraxic patients are often ideal for study because they are usually invariable. Also, changes resulting from treatment are easy and relatively inexpensive to measure because the units for study are often but not inevitably sounds or syllables. But even severe, acutely apraxic patients can yield convincing treatment data because, despite their often rapid change, the knowledgeable clinician can select stimuli for treatment and study that spontaneous recovery cannot overtake during the period of that study. If such responses change with treatment, the clinician's methods are vindicated.

One Man's Change

L.S. was 61 years of age when he suffered a left-hemisphere cerebrovascular accident causing a right hemiplegia and speechlessness. Strength in the arm and leg began returning within a few hours. Speech did not. When we saw him nine days after his stroke he was ambulatory but nearly speechless, and he could not imitate anything but /ɑ/. He could follow one- and two-step commands, however, and could write his name and a few other words. While he had obvious aphasia, the inordinate severity of his speech deficit suggested that he would evolve into an apraxic speaker and that we should start treating that apraxia.

To begin with, two vocalic sounds, /i/ and /u/, and two diphthongs, /oʊ/ and /ɑɪ/, were selected for treatment and placed in a multiple baseline design. In such a design a number of targets are first tested and then treated in order. The four sounds were tested in VC and CV syllables presented imitatively. In treatment, the clinician said each target sound slowly and with exaggerated posturing, and then guided the patient's articulators toward the proper shape as he tried to say it. Once treatment of /i/ began, baseline testing of the other three continued, as did progress testing of the /i/. So that the reader is oriented to the ways of reporting multiple baseline designs, data points to the left of the dotted line in Figure 3 represent imitative performance of the vowels in CV and VC words during no treatment or baseline testing sessions. Data points to the right show performance on those same stimuli after 20–30-minute treatment periods. All test responses were scored with a multidimensional scoring system from tapes by someone other than the patient's clinician. In this and all subsequent figures, data points represent the mean score for a set of ten stimuli; the higher the score, the better the performance.

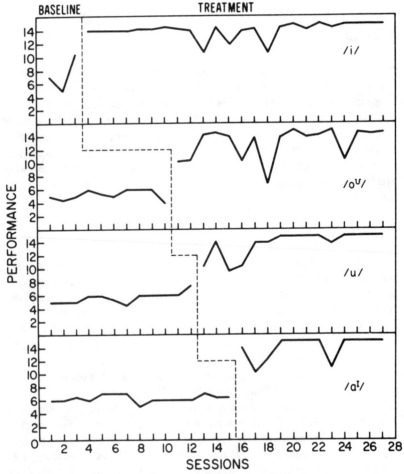

Figure 3. Treatment data for two vocalic sounds and two diphthongs.

The most convincing treatment data in such multiple baseline designs are those showing changes only after treatment. As can be seen, /i/ and /u/ were anxious to be off under spontaneous recovery's urging, and did not wait for us. The /oʊ/ and /ɑI/, on the other hand, were content to wait, perhaps because they were harder. Their jump in performance after treatment attests to treatment's potency. This is not to say that they—like /i/ and /u/—would not have improved without our help. They would have. The data show only that treatment can hasten recovery even during the acute stage.

The reader is not to conclude that these four sounds are the inevitable first targets for the severely apraxic. Indeed, we would not have taught /oʊ/ and /ɑI/ except that we were interested in testing our treatment's adequacy and wanted, therefore, some difficult sounds that spontaneous recovery would be slow to mend. By combining these two dipthongs with /i/ and /u/ we had a group of targets that served both the talker and the clinician.

In Figure 4 are displayed the data for word-initial /m/, /p/, /b/, /t/, and /r/ elicited imitatively from the same patient. We began treating these in the eighth session once the vowel program was well underway. The treatment was similar to that for the vowels except that the clinician could depend more upon imitation and less upon phonetic placement. The patient's health was improving and his responsiveness and familiarity with his native language along with it. Only the data for /t/ and /r/ show an unequivocal treatment effect. After considerable variability, he finally settled on a reasonably unyielding and wrong response when asked to produce these two targets during baseline testing; but after treatment, performance began to improve immediately. The /m/'s variability probably reflects interference from the treatment of homorganic sounds. It was sometimes produced accurately during sessions 4 and 5 of pretreatment testing, and once treatment began, it immediately improved, only to become more brittle as treatment began on /p/ and /b/. Such interference among homorganic sounds is but one force during treatment that the multiple baseline design can identify. Another is the generalization of treatment effects from one sound to another.

Data for /s/, /f/, and /Θ/ from the same patient appear in Figure 5. These sounds were treated briefly in isolation and then in words, and all baseline and progress testing were completed with untreated single words presented imitatively. The treatment was the same as for the plosives—imitation abetted by phonetic placement. Baseline performance was reasonably stable for all three sounds, and all improved once treatment began, although /f/ was slow to rise and was plagued by considerable variability. Taken together the data in Figures 3, 4, and 5 confirm the potency of traditional methodology for this severe apraxic speaker.

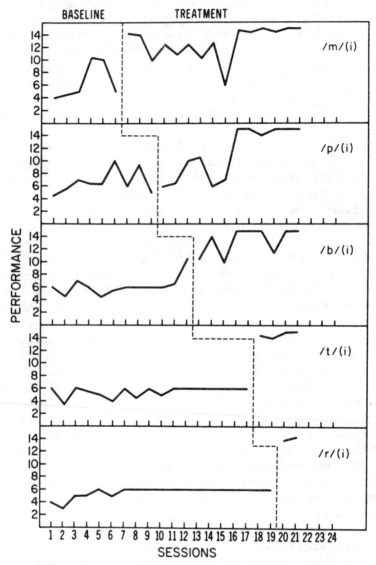

Figure 4. Effects of treatment for word-inital /m/, /p/, /b/, /t/, and /r/. Only /t/ and /r/ show an unequivocal treatment effect.

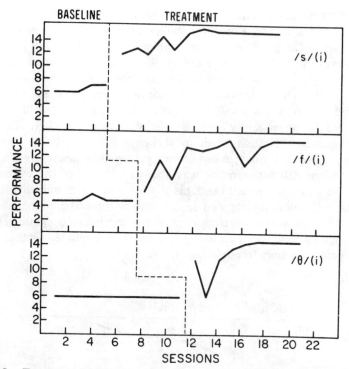

Figure 5. Treatment data for word-initial /s/, /f/, and /Θ/. All three show the effect of treatment.

A Metaphor for Speechlessness

E.B. White's *The Trumpet of the Swan* (1970) describes Louis, a trumpeter swan unable to speak from birth, who lives first a silent and then a sylvan life armed with trumpet, blackboard, and chalk. These he used to communicate; the trumpet being for other swans, the blackboard and chalk for humans. The story is a metaphor. The swan prevails over a human handicap—a speech defect. The severely apraxic speaker can also prevail. Like Louis, severely apraxic patients can communicate even if they cannot talk. The story of Louis no more diminishes the adult apraxic patient's predicament than does any other animal metaphor of the human condition—*Animal Farm,* or *Pogo,* for example.

Despite hours of treatment during three months, one of our very severe chronic apraxic patients never gained volitional control over even one word. Speech drill was agony. In the clinic his articulators could sometimes be coaxed, cajoled, or dragged into the correct shapes for short words but he could never say these words without the clinician's help. The

agony of many such patients when seen chronically is that they regain only
limited and exorbitantly expensive speech and are better off being taught
total communication as soon as the clinician is sure they will never talk
again. As early as the second week of this patient's treatment we began
simultaneous speech and total communication training because it was
obvious, although not inevitable, that he would never speak again. He
relearned how to write words after only a few minutes of drill on each,
words that he subsequently approximated outside of the clinic. Learning
for three groups of 20 such words are shown in Figure 6. Before treatment
he would reject each word; in our scoring system that meant he got a score
of 5 for each. After training he was able to write all of the words. But
because he was using his left hand, his scores were 14s, or mild distortions,
rather than 15s, or completely correct. It is to be remembered that even his
distorted written words were intelligible. He also became a good gesturer
and learned to draw. Both gesturing and drawing developed on their own.
The clinician had only to encourage them.

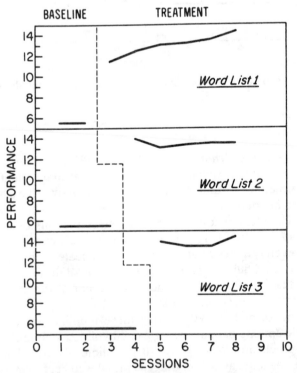

Figure 6.   Treatment data for three lists of 20 words. All three
lists responded to treatment.

Earthbound Realities

Success usually is less complete, as exemplified by the next severe chronic patient. He had a left-hemisphere CVA one year prior to beginning our treatment. He was seldom intelligible to anyone but his wife, who seemed to understand at least some things, although her bringing him to treatment says that she too was having trouble. He could not say some sounds at all, but others he could manage in short words and phrases. The most difficult sounds we treated with a variety of methods, including phonetic derivation. For example, initial /r/ was learned only by having him glide from /u/ to /r/. Learning is shown in Figure 7. For initial /z/, phonetic derivation was less successful. Figure 8 shows that after one session of practice in moving from /s/, which he could produce, to /z/, which he could not, he seemed to be learning. After that one session, however, he lost the /z/ and never regained it while we persisted with derivation methodology. We got it back by changing methods. We began stimulating the larynx by holding it between our fingers and jiggling it. Simultaneously we guided his jaw into a "clenched teeth" position. We simultaneously urged him to imitate our /z/. This time he learned and retained the /z/. Besides highlighting a method's strengths and weaknesses, the withdrawal design—like the

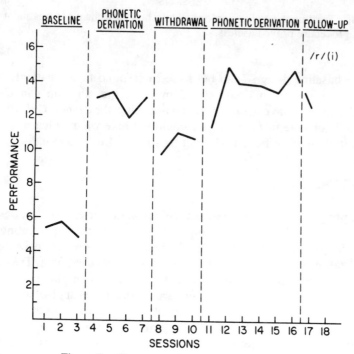

Figure 7.   Treatment data for word-initial /r/.

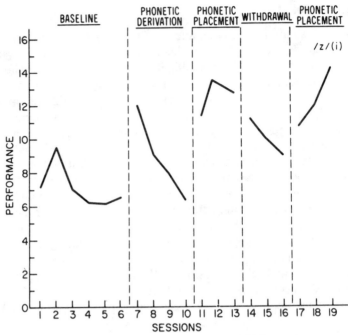

Figure 8. Treatment data for word-initial /z/, showing a change in treatment when the first procedure proved useless.

multiple baseline design—can be made to respond to the patient. If the patient is failing as this patient did initially, the clinician can change methods, perhaps save the patient, and not abuse the design. Unfortunately, we did not save this patient. He could not take what he learned in the clinic with him when he left. He quit treatment after two months.

ENDING TREATMENT

It is tempting but dangerous to treat severe patients for years. They deserve better. Behavioral criteria can support a decision to stop treating. By testing the patient at intervals the clinician will know when learning and generalization have ceased. When they do, so should treatment. Treatment stops also when the patient has had enough, when the patient has recovered, or when family and patient are making the best of what remains to them. However, many severe patients, even chronic ones, improve significantly and move into the moderate and mild ranges of severity. The clinician follows with different methods, methods described in the next two chapters.

10

Treating the Moderately Apraxic Patient

Moderately apraxic speakers have an excellent chance of recovering functional speech, especially if they move into the moderate range during the first month. Regardless of how quickly they move, they thrive under treatment's influences unless they have a significant coexisting aphasia. They also allow for the rewarding practice of speech pathology for other, related reasons. Most of their errors are predictable in locus and type, so clinicians have bountiful material for task continua. As a result, therapy can be orderly. They can usually hear their errors and may even be able to predict them, so clinicians do not have to monitor their every utterance. Generally, they hold a strict criterion—sometimes stricter than the clinician's—of what is adequate, and they work to reach it, so clinicians do not need to spend hours teaching them to evaluate their performance. Most of them are dedicated and ready to practice long after their clinicians have adjourned for refreshments. What, then, has the clinician to do? The clinician's duty is to nurture each patient's skills and attitudes in a rich loam of counseling, appropriate stimulus selection, and efficient methodology.

COUNSELING

Some patients do not arrive at the moderate part of the distribution with the knowledge or the psyches to put their considerable skills to the best use. This does not belie the earlier praise of these patients. It merely reflects our impression that very little in life prepares one for living with the results, however transient, of brain damage. Little, that is, except another's clinical experience. It is the clinician's experience, transmitted at first through counseling, that will prepare the patient and family for treatment, for living with apraxia while treatment is progressing, and for coexisting with the residuals of apraxia when treatment ends.

The amount of counseling will depend on what moderate apraxia represents for each individual. If it is a stage entered systematically after weeks of physiologic recovery and treatment, little counseling beyond that accomplished during the severe period will be necessary. Patients in this condition know what improvement feels and sounds like and know how to achieve it. Patients who enter the moderate range quickly, perhaps before seeing a speech pathologist, and patients who have been confined to the moderate range for what (at least to them) seems a long time, may require extensive counseling if they are to accept treatment's initiation or endure its continuation. The problems to be discussed in the next section may or may not be sources of pain or unease for any given patient. We describe them because they usually come up sometime during our treatment of most apraxic speakers, especially moderately involved ones.

Variability

Good and Bad Days

Good and bad days may be cloaked by the severely apraxic patient's disability, but they exist as naked reality for the moderately involved. Counseling can help patient and family recognize and accept the inevitability of this variability. Patient and family can be shown that getting up on the wrong side of the bed plagues apraxic and nonapraxic alike. Brain damage merely exaggerates the normal condition, making it more likely that the apraxic person's left foot will touch the floor before the right. Some bad days just happen; others are caused by frustration, anger, depression, angst, and fatigue. Those that just are, must simply be endured. Specific causes, on the other hand, can sometimes be managed. If a spouse's failure to visit or a night nurse's maliciousness is causing the negative feelings and hence the variability, the staff, family, and patient can work together to make changes. Weekend passes reduce depression; rest reduces fatigue; activities other than therapy and watching television may act as a general-purpose balm. During treatment on bad days, the clinician can surreptitiously retreat to simpler stimuli, to less rigid criteria, to more breaks, and to more encouragement. When speech is difficult or even impossible during such times, the patient can be reassured that silence is okay. Improvement is the best counselor, however, and most patients, while they may continue to grouse a bit, come to accept some variability as long as its magnitude begins shrinking with treatment and spontaneous recovery. For the family, things may not be quite so easy. They need to understand that the variability has nothing to do with them (if it does not), but that it is a ubiquitous result of brain damage. They also need reassurance that variability is reduced by time and treatment.

Influence of the Listener

Several times during treatment's course, the moderately apraxic speaker may complain that talking is easy in the clinic and hard everywhere else—with wife, business partner, hospital roommate, children, or minister. Again, the problem is one of variability. Patient and family need to be reminded that any speech, whether normal or abnormal, is influenced by situations. Few indeed are the speakers who are equally fluent in all conversations, and apraxic speech, especially while it is being treated, is even more vulnerable to the environment. Comparing what is happening as an apraxic talker relearns speech to other skill learning such as golf, tennis, crocheting, or making a mornay sauce may help them understand.

Clinician's Problems with Variability

Patients and families may not be alone in rueing variability. Clinicians, too, are sometimes disturbed, perhaps because they take the variability to be a sign that their treatment is failing to carry over. The clinician's worry, like that of the patient and family, is often unnecessary. Probably the data, if they ever come in, will tell us that improved responses do not go from clinic to street or living room until they have been practiced hundreds or thousands of times, and, even then, the transfer is likely to be slow. If a response is present in the clinic one day but absent on the outside the next, we need only conclude that more practice is needed. While it is being practiced, patient, family, and colleagues can be soothed by the observation that treatment generalizes systematically rather than immediately.

Time

Two conditions make counseling about time crucial for the moderate apraxic: the often rapid improvement from severe to moderate apraxia, and the patient's obsession to talk as fast as possible as soon as it is possible to talk at all. The first may cause a patient to feel that all progress comes easily, but it does not. Progress after the first few weeks is slow; patients will be happier once they learn and accept this. The second may be symptomatic of the attitude that better speech is something to be barged in upon. It is not. An apraxic tongue needs extra time to get where it is going. Normal, open-loop control of speech must be abandoned for slow, deliberate, closed-loop control. All lessons about time are easier to learn if the patient can accept one more thing: masquerading as a normal talker is not only impossible, it is harmful.

Long- and Short-Term Goals

Once lessons about time are learned, other activities come easier. In our experience, patients are better at goal setting if they are not thinking about either the way it was or the way they would like it to be. They have crucial goals to set. They need to establish manageable short-term goals—"I'm going to produce a better /r/ this week"—as well as realistic long-range ones—"I'm going to delay a decision about work for three months." Short-term goals are especially crucial for the chronic patient, because progress toward long-term ones is excruciatingly slow. Even acute patients should plan for today as well as for tomorrow if for no other reason than to keep them attending to the present. The point is this: long and even short-term goals are possible only if the patient has learned patience.

Beginning With Silence

Patients who have learned patience also find it easier to accept our advice that most conversations (and especially the important ones) must begin with silence. The silence is to make sure that the idea is firmly in mind. Apraxic articulators are unpredictable enough without allowing them to move about under the enervated impulse of an inadequately formed idea. The struggle to turn an inadequate idea into speech noises may make speech needlessly unintelligible and may even frustrate further thought. Even when patients accede to our demands for silence prior to talking, they may still err by trying to make up for the time spent in thought by racing through speech once they begin. They are reminded that speech, once begun, must contain pauses and slow, articulatory movements. We try to help patients understand that more time is lost responding to the listener's unceasing "Huhs?" than is taken up by careful planning and execution.

This advice, despite its sanity, is not enough. Both the silence required for planning and the reduced rate of speech movements required for the best possible movement do not come naturally nor do they result automatically from the patient's understanding or insight. There are several reasons why. Most normal speakers talk with surprising rapidity, so nothing about having talked normally prepares the patient to talk apraxically. In addition, an apraxic patient's language is still being processed or prepared for motor realization with normal or near-normal speed and with indifference to the neuromotor system's fate. Finally, patients usually have an understandable need to appear normal. Therefore, if patients are to learn how to use time to their advantage, counseling must be combined with drill. The patient must both want and learn to go slow.

Leaving Treatment Prematurely

One other potential misuse of time, at least in the speech pathologist's eyes, is for a patient to leave treatment prematurely. Inevitably, some patients are less impressed than their clinicians with speech's contribution to their quality of life. Many want to leave the hospital when they can walk without someone's holding on to their pajama backs. Even some patients who value speech above most other abilities seem confident that their apraxia is as likely to improve spontaneously as it is to improve with treatment. Some—the lucky ones—will be right. Others will not be. They will enter the chronic period with significant impairment and will have passed untreated through those first few weeks postonset when treatment may have its best chance of success. If the clinician feels that the patient's leaving will endanger further speech return, the obligation is to say so. Finally, however, a clinician must accept the patient's decision, regardless.

Decisions About the Future

What Patients Want to Know

As patients improve, they begin to talk more about the future. They begin asking, "Will I go back to work? Will I be able to help the children when they bring problems home? Will I hunt, sail, ski, bowl, or read again? Will my marriage endure?" Such questions need not send the speech pathologist scurrying down the hall to a psychologist or psychiatrist colleague. Often enough, the speech pathologist is not being asked for help but for attentive listening, reassurance, and a realistic prognosis for speech return. Given these things, the answers to all such questions are likely to come from the patients and their families. Patients, for example, seem to sense when their minds and speech are clear enough to allow a return to home and to work. They also return to friends and interests in response to a tattoo only they can hear. Clinicians need to be careful lest the noise from their answers drown out the sound of each patient's own music.

Contributions of the Team

On the other hand, when a patient and family obviously need help, such help probably should come from a team. This is not to say that six health care professionals bombard the family with advice. It is to say that the team first sit down and make a realistic assessment of the patient's chances for work, responsibility, and fun. The physician knows about the patient's health, medications, chances of survival, and about the probable quality of that survival. The social worker will know about the family's finances and insurance. The physical therapist can predict the amount of mobility and how functional the arm will be. The speech pathologist will know how well the patient reads, writes, and understands; how many people can be coped with; how the frustrations of not being understood are handled; and how much talking wears the patient out. If all of this information can be put together and coherently presented at a team meeting with family and patient, the family can then make enlightened plans. Knowing makes the future less threatening.

Preparing For Treatment

Most moderate patients have had counseling and treatment prior to entering the moderate range, and so nothing need be done to prepare them for therapy's rigors. Moderate patients beginning treatment for the first time, however, will need the same kind of preparation that was described in Chapter 9. In addition, moderate patients, even if they are chronic, can usually be reassured that improvement is likely. Often this is enough to prepare them for treatment, and the predicted progress, when it comes, will keep them prepared.

SPECIFIC TREATMENTS

The difference between treatments for severe and moderately involved apraxic patients is as subtle as when yellow green becomes yellowish green. Because of the subtlety, we probably could get only a few speech pathologists to agree upon its reality. So be it. For us, the distinction is useful as a way of highlighting differences among methods that might otherwise be obscured. In the chapter on severe apraxia, for example, we primarily discussed methods for teaching sounds and syllables and for developing total communication. In this chapter, we show how to stabilize sounds by expanding the number and type of environments in which they appear; we add more flesh to some methods already described such as gestural reorganization; and we introduce additional methodology, such as the contrastive stress drill.

Imitation of Contrasts

Treatment's cornerstone for the moderately apraxic talker is often simple imitation of carefully selected speech sound contrasts. This imitation is seldom in need of bolstering by phonetic derivation or placement as it is for the severely apraxic. Instead, the clinician can attend to manipulating stimuli and fading cues so that the patient says ever more difficult things successfully and independently. Imitation of contrasts was introduced briefly in the previous chapter. The discussion in this chapter is expanded, and the method is divided into three overlapping stages.

Stage One.   In Stage One, clinicians provide patients with auditory (listen to me) and visual (watch me) cues or with auditory cues alone, and patients imitate. Clinicians can supply the model once or several times. Patients can be told to respond immediately or after a delay. They can make one or more than one response without further intervention from their clinicians. If patients are unsuccessful even though they try to respond simultaneously with the clinician or immediately after the clinician has finished, the clinician can increase the cues' potency by speaking more slowly, by altering stress, by accompanying speech with rhythmical, non-intrusive gestures, and in a host of other traditional ways.

The typical activity in Stage One is for the clinician to select a single target and organize the practice material so that the target's environment rather than the target itself is altered. For example, if the patient is practicing an /s/, a typical list of stimuli might be "see, saw, say, sigh, so, sow, saw, and Sue." When these combinations can be produced several times successfully, they can be made part of a phrase. "I see, I saw, I say," and so on. Any number of words may be practiced each session. Each word may be repeated one or several times consecutively, although troublesome stimuli should probably be drilled more frequently than easy ones, because too much practice on easy ones may cause the patient to perseverate and retard the learning of more difficult responses. Some patients can respond several times quickly; others will need pauses between each stimulus. All patients, however, seem to have a limit on the number of responses—even successful ones—they can make before they begin making a flurry of mistakes. We take that flurry as a signal to stop or change tasks, and we try to anticipate a flurry and stop before mistakes force us to. Patients' speaking rates can be slow, normal, or varied, depending on how well they are doing; and they can be held to strict or lax criteria of correctness. They can drill a single target or several during each session. Targets can appear in initial, medial, or final position.

Even in Stage One where clinicians are exercising maximum control, the imitations need never be robot-like or mindless. Patients can be active participants. They can help set criteria of correctness, can listen to each of their responses and judge their accuracy, and can undertake self-correction. Finally, they should be encouraged to go beyond what the clinician is requiring as long as they can do so successfully.

Stage Two.   Imitating contrasts of a different sort dominates Stage Two. The patient contrasts the target with sounds other than the following or preceding vowel, as is most frequently the case in Stage One. A consonant target, for example, is contrasted with another consonant as when /s/ is contrasted with /t/. So, for example, instead of practicing "see, sigh, Sue," the patient would move back and forth between such pairs as "see–tea, sigh–tie, Sue–two." Similar contrasts could be required for targets in word-medial and word-final positions.

At first, the contrasts can be easy, as when the target is paired with a very dissimilar sound, an /s/ and /m/, for example, or a /g/ and /f/. As the patient improves, the contrasts can be made increasingly more difficult until the speaker is contrasting cognates such as /s/ and /z/ or /g/ and /k/. The toughest contrast is probably between a target and the sound or sounds most frequently substituted for it. Because the /k/ frequently becomes /t/ in apraxic speech, word pairs such as "state" and "stake" may be very challenging. Once such a contrast is learned, however, connected speech's intelligibility is improved substantially.

Because some apraxic speakers distort sounds as frequently as they substitute them, contrasts can also be between targets and sounds whose influence cause those targets to be distorted, or between targets and sounds that the distortions most closely resemble. To distinguish between these two is not caviling. For example, the influence of a /k/ on a preceding /t/ as in the word "talk" sometimes causes the /t/ to be produced too far posteriorly or with two contacts, one anterior and one posterior, with the result that the /t/ is distorted rather than replaced. This distortion is probably best treated with a /t/–/k/ contrast, just as if the /k/ were being substituted for the /t/ rather than merely resulting in its distortion. Apraxic speakers also frequently produce fricatives with a plosive quality and plosives with a fricative quality. These distortions usually result from a loss of precision rather than from assimilative influences as in the /t/ and /k/ example previously discussed. Drilling contrasts of plosives and fricatives made at approximately the same place in the mouth may reduce these errors. For example, /p/ and /f/ words such as pie–fie, poe–foe, poo–foo; /t/ and /s/ words such as tie–sigh; two–Sue; toe–so; and so on can be contrasted. Such contrasts are especially effective if the speaker is careful to speak slowly, at least for the first few repetitions.

Other apraxic distortions may be more subtle. Consider these examples of distorted /t/ drawn from several patients. One rounded his lips when producing /t/ even when the following vowel was not rounded. Another produced it with slight and inconsistent nasalization. Another used the whole of his tongue to make the valve. In none of these cases is another sound substituted for the target, and in some—such as the broad contact—the reasons for the errors are not easy to discover. So, what are the proper contrasts? Sometimes the distortion's essence is captured by a plosive–fricative, an oral–nasal, or a plosive–plosive contrast. At other times, no contrast may be appropriate until the patient has practiced the target in a variety of CV environments, as in Stage One or until the sound has been stabilized with phonetic placement or derivation methods. For example, before the patient who produced a /t/ with lip rounding could contrast /t/ and other sounds, we had to help him inhibit the rounding. This we did by pulling back on the corners of his mouth. Once he could inhibit the rounding with minimal help from us, we had him practice both rounded and unrounded /t/ in a form of negative practice, which is itself a form of contrast.

Despite the subtleties, each apraxic patient's pattern of errors usually gives the clinician ample material for contrasts. Consider these responses by an acutely apraxic patient to a list of 25 initial /t/ words presented imitatively. Ten /t/s were distorted, three were omitted, the /p/ was substituted for the /t/ eight times, and the /k/ was substituted twice. Twice it was correct. No literature guides clinicians to the best or most efficient use of such data, however, so they rely on experience and instinct. Since this patient could sometimes make a /t/ and could often approximate it with only slight distortion, we lingered at Stage One only long enough to remind him of what /t/ sounded and felt like and to give him some instruction about carefully planning and listening. It would have been a useful clinical experiment to have measured the amount of generalization from this Stage One drill, but we did not. Equally informative would have been data about the relative effectiveness of certain kinds of Stage Two contrasts. We might well have asked what would have happened to all of his errors if he had drilled only /p/ and /t/ contrasts. Again, alas, we did not. Instead, we moved immediately from Stage One to four contrasts in Stage Two: /t/ and silence as in /ti/ and /i/; /t/ and /p/ as in /taɪ/ and /paɪ/; /t/ and /k/ as in /ti/ and /ki/, and, because his distortions resulted from abnormal voice onset time, we added /t/ and /d/ contrasts as in /tai/ and /dai/. Furthermore, instead of practicing one set of contrasts and then another, we combined them all into lists such as /taɪ/, /aɪ/, /daɪ/, /paɪ/, /kaɪ/, /ti/, /i/, /di/, /pi/, /ki/, and so on. He rapidly got better. We do not know if some other organization of the stimuli would have been even better yet.

In Stage Two as in Stage One, clinicians can use linguistic and phonetic knowledge, creative spirit, and all of the rest that is unique to their métier. Most of all contrast training will require clinicians to be at their most protean. Targets will differ in their resilience, and contrasts in their difficulty; these differences will require different responses from the clinician. Sometimes, both sounds in a contrast can be practiced equally; sometimes one or the other will have to be emphasized. Some contrasts will have to be more carefully prepared for with special instructions or special stimulus presentation (shorter words, more common words, slower rate) than others. Initially, for example, certain contrasts may require a short period of phonetic placement or some other special technique before simple imitation can be relied upon. Some patients seem to need to concentrate on only one contrast, whereas others do better with several. Fortunately, each patient's responses are a sure sign of what is right, and clinicians willing to follow their patients will not go far astray.

Stage Three. Stage Two and Three blend as dawn into light of day, because in Stage Three the clinician merely makes the contrasts harder and tries to move the patient's speech ever closer to normal. One-syllable words can be replaced with polysyllabic ones. Words can be followed by phrases and sentences with identical (I see — I say), similar (I see — you say), or dissimilar (I see — who can say) constructions. Or, stimulus length can be maintained, but the stimuli can be made harder in other ways. For example, easy vowels in CV or CVC syllables can be changed for harder ones, as when "set" becomes "sit" and "tall" becomes "teal." The final consonant can be changed, as when "taught" becomes "talk" (the /k/ and /t/ are uneasy companions even in mild apraxia of speech). The target's position can be changed. If the patient can say the sound at the front of a word, it can be moved to the middle or the end. Patients who can respond correctly two times can be directed to respond three, four, or more times consecutively without the clinician's help. Criteria of adequacy can be made more stringent. Long pauses between repetitions can be replaced by shorter ones. Once a patient can work for 30 seconds before needing a change in stimulus type, the clinician can try to require 45 or 60 seconds.

The patient's speaking rate often has the heftiest influence on articulatory accuracy. Slowly talking apraxic speakers often reach otherwise inaccessible targets, so difficult contrasts are usually practiced first with a slow rate. As contrasts get easier or to make easy ones more challenging, the patient's rate can be increased systematically. Drill of specific stimulus pairs ends only when they can be produced at an optimum rate, the fastest rate that still allows articulators to get where they are going with a minimum of struggle. Each speaker's optimum rate may or may not be within the normal range.

Rhythm and stress can also be altered in Stage Three. Practice can begin, for example, with equal and even stress and progress toward normal. An expanded discussion of the therapeutic uses of rhythm and stress is forthcoming.

Having the patient work with multiple contrasts also effectively increases difficulty. This permutation was described briefly in Stage Two but is more properly a Stage Three maneuver. For example, if the target is initial /t/, the patient can alternate among several words beginning with sounds that substitute for the /t/. A typical drill might have a patient alternately produce tame, fame, same, aim, dame, and name. The patient cannot simply alternate between two movements as when only a single pair of stimuli is practiced. Luck and perseverance will seldom result in a correct response. Usually, some sounds in a list such as the one above will be more difficult than others, and these can be practiced more. On the other hand, if one response is especially strong, it may be wise to practice it less. Weaker responses often cannot compete with their stronger brethren. An especially demanding drill at this stage is to have patients select and produce the words or phrases in any order they choose. The clinician's task is to report what has been produced.

Implicit in all these bits and pieces at Stages Two and Three is that the apraxic speaker is challenged by greater independence. Anything that requires patients to plan, produce, monitor, and correct will make them more independent. Anything that increases independence is good treatment, whether or not it appears in this section or in this book.

Why Imitation of Contrasts Works

Imitation has a chance of working, because in apraxia of speech, imitation is not dissociated from spontaneous speech as it is in conduction and transcortical motor aphasia. The patient, therefore, can transfer control from imitative to spontaneous talking. Imitation also works because it allows the clinician to provide the patient with predictable, stable, and multiple cues. It may provide the clinician with greater control over what the apraxic patient does than any other method. Finally, imitative performance stands between automatic acts, which the apraxic patient can sometimes do, and volitional – purposive ones, which he or she usually cannot, and it is nearer to the automatic.

In 1968, Darley said that imitation was especially difficult for the apraxic patient. Despite the warning, imitation continues to be a prominent and successful treatment for the apraxic talker. The apparent conflict between what Darley said and what clinicians do is not real. Darley was describing the apraxic patient's response to imitation used diagnostically, which may often be more threatening than therapeutic. Imitation done therapeutically is different because the clinician describes, exhorts, cuddles, molds, and models. Indeed, therapeutic imitation is no more simple imitation than morality is an unblemished driving record.

To limit a program to imitation, even with embellishments, is unwise, however. Patients do not learn to talk by following even the most enlightened leader. Methods must take them further into independence. The contrastive stress drill may be just the vehicle.

The Contrastive Stress Drill

In its simplest form, the contrastive stress drill (Fairbanks, 1960) is a question-and-answer dialogue between clinician and patient. The clinician selects or creates a short phrase made up of one or more sounds that the speaker needs to drill. Drill begins with the patient's using the preselected phrase as the answer to a set of questions. Presumably, the contrastive stress drill is therapeutic because stress (phonetic or linguistic, not emotional) can facilitate improved articulatory movements (primarily stressed speech units are apt to be better articulated than those with lesser amounts of stress). The primary stress in the patient's answer is determined by the clinician's question. For example, if clinicians want the patient to drill initial /b/ they can put a "b" word such as "bought" in a sentence and, by asking the right question, elicit natural, primary stress on that target word. If the practice sentence is "I bought one," and clinicians want primary stress on "bought," they have only to ask, "Did you sell one?" If the patient understands the task, the response will be, "No, I *bought* one." Stress comes more naturally in response to a question than to a command such as "Stress the verb" or "Stress the word 'bought'."

The contrastive stress drill may be one of the most potent techniques for stabilizing apraxic articulation and improving prosodic profiles. We emphasize stabilization rather than restoration because the method is useless with a sound the patient cannot produce in at least some environments. The world's finest stress fails to carry a tongue to the right position unless that tongue was already on its way or at least knew where it was going when the stress was introduced. Unless a tongue knows its target, stress only leads to louder and longer errors.

Constructing A Contrastive Stress Drill

The contrastive stress drill must be built according to rules. First, we construct the drill around one or a limited number of target sounds or sound combinations. The rest of the sounds making up each sentence should be ones the patient can say easily, or at least relatively so. For instance, an /s/ might appear as the only target in a set of ten or so sentences as in these examples: I bought some, I said it, sit down, I got some, I saw you, I saw her, I see, who said, you don't say, we sell it. To load a sentence with more than one difficult sound or cluster is to increase the chance of failure. This warning introduces the second rule. Each target should be a sound or sound combination the patient can produce normally or near normally at least sometimes, because contrastive stress is unable to make sounds appear which the speaker has little or no control over. Because our own patients have surprised us so often, we hesitate to define operationally "at least sometimes," except to say that the target should be present in other than a few stereotyped or automatic responses. It should be present, for example, in some words the patient uses volitionally and appropriately or, at very least, the patient should be able to imitate the target as part of a word or sentence. If in doubt about the appropriateness of a target, try it. The patient will tell you.

Third, word and total utterance length should be controlled. If either is too long, the patient may forget what is to be said or be unable to sustain the necessary vigilance and motor control to say it. Because we begin contrastive stress drills when the patient can say CV, VC, and CVC words, our early drills use only single-syllable words. These are usually organized into two-, three-, and four-word sentences. As the patient progresses within a session or across sessions, words and utterances can be made longer.

Fourth, the target and the words in which it appears must be knowingly rather than capriciously located. This means purposefully placing the target in word-initial, medial, or final position, and purposefully placing the word containing the target at or near the front, middle, or back of the utterance. Location will make good responses more or less likely depending on the clinician's diligence and the patient's symptoms. Although we cannot prove it, our feeling is that the apraxic patient's difficulty with initiation makes a more posterior placement reasonable, epecially at first. For example, the /s/ in "Sue" might better be practiced in "I met Sue" before being tried in "Sue met me." Similarly, a final or medial position /s/, as in "face" or "basement," might be better than an initial /s/ as in "savior."

Finally, the nontarget sounds, as already suggested, should be ones the patient has excellent—although not necessarily perfect—control of. Such a construction will reduce mistakes and allow the patient to concentrate on the target. Even moderately apraxic patients are easily derailed by a string of challenges. They need some easy movements, at least at first.

Step One: Imitation. Practice usually begins with imitation. The clinician provides the sentence with equal and even stress and increased articulation and pause time. "I'll say it slowly and evenly and you say it after me." For the target sentence "I say it," containing initial /s/ as a target, the clinician would begin with a slow, evenly spaced and stressed /ɑɪː seɪː ɪtʰ/, and the patient would imitate as closely as possible. The dots show increased articulation time for the vowels. The h represents strong aspiration of final /t/. The space between the words is exaggerated and equal to show increased and equal pause time between words. While this step may be unnecessary to correct articulation, we usually begin with it to guarantee that the patient understands and will be able to remember the sentence. Also, if a patient fails even with equal and even stress, the clinician will know to change all or a portion of the utterance.

Step Two: Questions and answers. The next step (the first step for some patients) is to introduce the question-and-answer dialogue beginning with an explanation of why and how the method works. In appropriate terms, we tell the patient that articulation is facilitated by primary stress, and primary stress can be made to occur predictably and naturally in response to a question. Once some patients have heard the explanation, they are able to begin practicing. The clinician has only to say, for example, "The sentence we're going to drill is 'I saw it'; I'll ask you a question, and you give me those three words in answer." Others require further priming, which the clinician provides by modelling both question and answer. For example, the clinician might say all of the following: "The sentence is 'I saw it.' I will ask you (the patient) 'Did you *hear* it?' and you reply, 'No, I *saw* it'." Or, if a patient needs some but not quite so much help, the clinician can ask the question and then answer it simultaneously with the patient. The patient may also be helped if the clinician models both an answer with appropriate stress and one with inappropriate stress.

Once the patient has the idea of the drill (and this does not take long in most instances) the real business begins, which is to drill the target in the stressed position. At first, the patient can be made to repeat the same stress pattern over and over. For example, the patient may respond several times consecutively with "I *saw* it" to the question, "Did you *hear* it?" Later, to prevent perseveration and boredom and to improve overall articulatory accuracy and stress profiles, the clinician can ask a series of questions about the same sentence. For example, instead of asking, "Did you *hear* it?" the clinician can ask "*Who* saw it?," to which the patient must respond, "*I* saw it." Or, the question can be, "You saw *what*?," to which the patient replies, "I saw *it*." For the same reasons—preventing perseveration and boredom and improving overall articulatory accuracy and stress—we practice a set of at least five to ten short target sentences. If the patient does best with only a single repetition of each sentence before moving on to the next, then we present the stimuli that way. If several repetitions of the same sentence get increasingly better responses, we use several repetitions before moving on to the next sentence.

If the patient's naturally occurring stress is ineffective in facilitating articulation, the patient can be taught to alter pause time by placing a longer pause before the target word. The patient can also be instructed to use that pause to "get set" for the target. Other ways of making the contrastive stress drill easier while preserving its essential features are to select easier words, change the target's location in the word or sentence, slow the utterance down overall, and practice individual words before reinserting them in the drill. If a patient does not learn the contrastive stress drill, or only makes contrasts unpredictably and irregularly, the message probably is that too much aphasia is interfering, and the drill should be abandoned.

Step Three: Making the drill more difficult. As the patient's control of the target improves, the drill can be made more difficult. One way is to change criteria: to be counted a success, the target must sound more normal. Another way is to change stimuli. A single target in the utterance can be joined by others. Or a target can be introduced over which the patient has somewhat less control, or the target can be moved around in the utterances. Final voiceless plosives, for example, can be moved to word-initial position or voiced ones to word-final position, because these sounds in these positions are notoriously hard for apraxic speakers. Also, the target's environment can be made harder. For example, if an /s/ is harder in the presence of /t/, then a /t/ word can be placed before or behind the target. Responses can be speeded up. The sentences can be made longer. The clinician can try to weaken the patient's hold on the utterance by distraction. Anything. The idea is to have a good time, to challenge the patient, to create independence, and to make the drill a communication between two people.

Step Four: Going beyond contrastive stress. Once a target or set of targets is improved, the drill can be expanded and modified. Words that previously had been practiced only in sentences provided by the clinician can be elicited in unique responses by using carefully chosen questions and special instructions so that the patient understands the game. For example, the patient can be told to use "saw" in a self-generated sentence. Since this may be a hard step, the clinician can guide the patient's creativity by suggesting themes; for example, "Tell me about a TV show you saw last night." Or questions can be made to elicit the target sound(s) in untreated words. This technique can sometimes be facilitated if the clinician provides a few examples while urging the patient to supply others. Once a few new words have been identified, the clinician can help the patient organize them into sentences. For example, if the target is /s/ and the patient recalls a previously untreated word such as "sore," a sentence might be prompted by, "Tell me something about a sore head." Once unique responses have begun to emerge, they can be turned into drills. The patient says, "I have a *sore* head," and the clinician replies, "You have a *wrinkled* head?" The patient replies, "No, I have a *sore* head."

One danger is that patients, blithely creating sentences, may use combinations that are too difficult. The target may be okay, but the rest may be too hard. Clinicians can help them with such difficult sentences by intervening with some face-saving comments, by instructing them to slow utterances down, or by helping them to simplify sentences by omitting some words and perhaps substituting some others. If sentences remain difficult, they can be taken all the way back to imitation before being returned to the question-and-answer dialogue. Patients usually understand the necessity of such manipulations.

Final extensions of the contrastive stress drill include asking the patients questions calculated to elicit a variety of responses and having them ask their clinicians questions. These and other steps are usually saved for mild patients and will be described in detail in Chapter 11.

Why Contrastive Stress Works

Questions about why things work tug at our sleeves as we go through what are often the prosaic activities of daily clinical practice and urge us to go in search of explanations. Thus aroused, we are better clinicians, for we begin to look beyond technique. We are also more likely to blunder, because finding out why something works, especially if that something is a behavioral method, is infinitely harder than merely measuring its effect. Nonetheless, off we go.

Kent (1976a) has said that rhythm acts as a kind of "substratum for virtually all perceptual and motor activities" (p. 89), a position supported by Lenneberg (1967) and others. The contrastive stress drill may provide a stress–rhythm substratum that, for the apraxic patient, resembles the rhythmic basis of normal motor speech control and one that "supports" or even "summons" articulatory movements. Even if this substratum is itself altered by the same trauma that caused the apraxic articulatory errors (as it most surely is), it may quickly improve with practice and once again be ready to perform its supportive function. Companion hypotheses about why the stress–rhythm substratum is able to be used therapeutically to improve apraxic articulation are that it may be somewhat more resilient to trauma and somewhat quicker to respond to physiologic recovery. A related hypothesis is that areas of both left and right hemispheres, and perhaps subcortical structures as well, serve stress and rhythm. Regional cerebral blood flow and positron emission tomography studies may make these hypotheses testable.

A less heady explanation of contrastive stress' effect is that the drill merely slows the patient's speech down and disrupts any tendencies to use open-loop control over movement. Probably, however, it is not merely slowing articulation time that helps the apraxic talker, because they are notoriously slow movers without our help (Kent & Rosenbek, 1983). The effect on pause time may be more important. Increased pause time gives the articulators a breather between movements and the brain a chance to plan for upcoming movements. It can also be posited that increased concentration on stressed elements prevents the tongue from stumbling along erratically in what amounts to a barren landscape without highlights. Stressed syllables become landmarks. These speculations could be tested by comparing the effects of manipulating articulation time, pause time, attention, and location of stress.

Regardless of why a contrastive stress drill works, it has advantages in addition to improving intelligibility. First, it adds variety, and apraxia of speech drills cry out for variety. Second, it resembles more normal conversation, because it is a series of questions and answers rather than a series of imitations. Finally, it moves the patient toward carryover, because it is more like what people do when they talk. No doubt the second and third interact; because the patient is practicing answers in the clinic, answers come easier outside.

Reading as Treatment

Reading's influence on apraxic speech is variable from patient to patient. Some apraxic patients cannot read aloud. Others can, but the resulting speech is no better than in a variety of other conditions. Some read aloud better than they talk in any other condition. Most present a mixed pattern: some stimuli are better read; some are better performed with some other stimulation; some stimuli are indifferent. All of these patterns may change as the patient does. Nonetheless, reading drills may be salutary for some stimuli at some time in treatment for some patients. When it works, reading has the additional advantages of being good homework, of providing variety, and of helping reduce any coexisting aphasia. We have developed a four-step reading program. The steps may be reordered, some may be omitted, and all may be integrated into a total behavioral treatment that includes imitation and a variety of other methods.

Step One: Diagnosing reading's salutary effect. The first step is diagnostic and involves comparing the patient's speech adequacy for spontaneous, imitated, and read stimuli. This step may have been completed as part of the total evaluation. If not, all sounds and sound combinations the clinician is planning to drill should be tested several times in each of the three conditions with a variety of word and phrase lengths. These data are expensive, especially if one goes looking for tiny differences. We do not. Clinical significance is what we want, and clinically significant differences are not hidden in a standard deviation to be discovered only by a *t*-test. They are obvious to the eye and ear. If reading aloud facilitates the apraxic patient's speech, the clinician will know it and can use it.

Step Two: Reading aloud. In Step Two, the patient simply reads stimuli aloud at whatever rate and with whatever number of repetitions the clinician decides are necessary. The stimuli can be written large or small, in print or cursive, and they can be prepared beforehand or on the spot. While it may be therapeutic for apraxic speakers to read without listening to or feeling the speech they are producing, we never risk such passivity with the chronic apraxic talker and seldom even with the acutely apraxic speaker. Rather, patients are helped to hear and feel each response and to compare consecutive responses to each other, to normal, and to the best of which they are capable. No rules, at least no rules known to us, govern how long patients stay on Step Two. We usually have them remain on it only until a response is stable and the best of which they are capable, and then we move on to Step Three. If a response falters, we return to Step Two. Movement between Steps Two and Three may be made several times for each response, and certainly several times each session. The aims are to keep patients successful and moving constantly toward independence.

Step Three: Fading cues.   Reading cues are faded in Step Three. This can be accomplished by requiring a response after briefer and briefer exposure to the written stimulus, or following longer and longer delays between seeing the stimulus and saying it. The difference between these two procedures may be significant, although we do not know, since we either mix the two or use progressively longer delays. When using increasing delay intervals, patients are urged to keep responses in their heads and to mull them over in any way that helps. Preparing during the delay rather than nodding off, and getting off to a good start once a delay is over, are crucial. In Step Three as in Step Two, the patient is forced to analyze each response and how it was made. It does little permanent good to return a perfect cross-court volley or to execute a perfect jibe if one does not know how it happened, and the same is true in apraxic therapeutics. If a response falters, and well it may even after several consecutive good repetitions, patient and clinician can temporarily return to Step Two, can lengthen exposure of the written stimuli, or can decrease the delay between when a stimulus is read and when it is said.

Step Four: Increasing independence.   Next, reading cues can be faded even further by showing patients the stimulus only once and then having them produce it several times consecutively. Independence can also be increased by turning the exercise into a contrastive stress drill. A potential complication is that patients will stumble when moving from Step Three to Step Four. Some can make a response even after a long delay, but are unable to do as well when forced to make consecutive responses. To enhance a patient's chances of moving errorlessly from Steps Three to Four, the clinician can take a more active role in cueing any responses that appear to be suffering. To integrate the contrastive stress drill into the reading paradigm, the clinician can merely ask patients appropriate questions and direct them to respond with the statement they have just read. The response can remain in the patients' view as they try to say it, or it can be removed. What finally is to be accomplished in Step Four is that the patient begins using the utterance with no cues. How reading and contrastive stress are combined, or when, is secondary to this goal of increased independence.

Why Reading Helps

Probably no one knows this with certainty. It may be merely that the visual stimulus is less fleeting than the auditory, in which case the modality differences per se are less significant than is the total time of exposure. Another related possibility is that memory is taxed less in the early stages of a reading program, and the speaker as a result is freer to concentrate on motor movements. Perhaps the visual or graphemic representation has a more powerful effect on the apraxic speaker's motor programmer than does the auditory representation, because apraxia of speech is an auditory–vocal disorder and visual input avoids a portion of the damaged auditory–vocal loop. Perhaps the hypothesized translation of visual-to-auditory equivalents plus the visual processing system's greater integrity has a summing effect so that a stronger message arrives at the programmer.

How thin is the air around the word "perhaps." Perhaps it is best to leave the whys to others and retreat to the valley where the clinical struggle is usually waged. For in that valley the why is often less important than the effect. So long as something works, discovering why can await the slow accumulation of clinical data.

Gestural Reorganization

An increasingly popular treatment (Rosenbek, Collins, & Wertz, 1976; Rosenbek, 1978; Simmons, 1978; Nailling & Horner, 1979; Ostreicher & Hafmeister, 1980) in which speech and gestures are combined may be especially useful for the moderately apraxic talker. According to Luria (1970), such a treatment, which we have come to call *gestural reorganization,* and which he would call an example of *intersystemic reorganization,* provides an alternative neurobehavioral basis for speech performance. The idea—if not the nomenclature—is an old one. For decades, clinicians have been pairing something patients can do with something they cannot do as well in hopes of improving what they cannot do. For the typical apraxic talker, simple limb gestures are likely to be more intact than are speech gestures. The idea in gestural reorganization is that the more robust limb gestures are paired with the somewhat punier oral gestures in an attempt to improve the oral gestures.

Gestures have been divided into two general types: emblems and illustrators (Ekman & Friesen, 1972). Emblems have meaning and can replace a word or phrase. AMERIND (Skelly, 1979) is a system of emblems. Illustrators, according to Ekman and Friesen, "are those acts which are intrinsically related on a moment-to-moment basis with speech, with phrasing, content, voice contour, loudness, . . ." (pp. 358–359). They identify eight illustrators; we are interested therapeutically in two—

"baton: movements which accent or emphasize a particular word or phrase" and "rhythmic movements: movements which depict the rhythm or pacing of an event" (p. 360). In our experience, emblems are for speechless apraxic patients and for patients with Broca's aphasia; illustrators are for apraxic speakers with some ability to talk. The program to be described uses illustrators, because it is for moderately apraxic patients. Because gestural programs are newer and more experimental than the other programs described in this book, we have added a few words on gesture and brain damage.

Gesture and Brain Damage

Left-hemisphere brain-damaged adults with aphasia (Cicone, Wapner, Foldi, et al., 1979) and without (Mateer, 1978) have difficulty with gestures. Researchers (Goodglass & Kaplan, 1963; Duffy & Duffy, 1981) disagree about whether the deficit is apraxic or aphasic. Goodglass and Kaplan (1963) suggest that a gestural deficit is apraxic when it is present both upon request and on imitation, and aphasic if present upon request and absent on imitation. Their research seems to have demonstrated that the gestural deficit resulting from left-hemisphere damage is more often apraxic than aphasic. On the other hand, the research of Cicone et al. (1979) seems to suggest that gestural deficits following left-hemisphere damage are aphasic. Their findings lead them to posit the existence of a central processor common to speech and gesturing which, when damaged, leads to both aphasic speech and aphasic gesturing. Continued research will doubtless demonstrate that the gestural impairment may be either apraxic or aphasic, depending on the site of the lesion. All of this is less important therapeutically, however, than is a series of observations that the gestural deficit in left-brain-damaged patients is not absolute (Kimura & Archibald, 1974; Mateer & Kimura, 1977); that it is not as severe as the speaking deficit; that patients with apraxia of speech can learn to gesture (Skelly, 1979); and that gesturing helps them talk. Our confidence in gesture's therapeutic potential spawned the present eight-step program.

Step One: Explaining the program's purpose. Patients need to understand gestural reorganization (without being burdented with either the term or the neuromythology) because they do not automatically embrace our suggestions. Even for the cooperative, motivated ones, a future of tapping and talking may seem peculiar. There is nothing arcane in this. Many, perhaps most, stroke victims do not want to appear abnormal, or do not want to appear any more abnormal than their hemiplegia has already made them. Initially, therefore, they may spurn any suggestion to gesture for fear that it will add to their abnormal appearance. Of necessity, then, we devote considerable energy to helping each person understand that the hands or feet can help the tongue along. We also reassure each person that the gesturing will not necessarily be permanent. Sometimes this turns out to be a lie, but by the time the lie is discovered, the patient usually does not care. So as not be be too misleading, we also warn them that they may have to rely on the gestural accompaniment for a long time in some especially difficult conversations. If appropriate, we compare the gestures to other aids—glasses, hearing aid, cane, a brace—that have more respectable histories as permanent prostheses. We end with a flourish by trying to convice them that it is better to be understood than to be anonymous. If they consent, we then demonstrate what the gestures can accomplish and begin a period of diagnostic treatment.

Step Two: Diagnostic treatment. We begin by finding a simple, repetitive gesture or gestures (for variety) that the patient can do predictably. The gestures selected are usually different for each patient. Some people tap with an index finger, some drum with some or all of their fingers, some squeeze index finger and thumb together, some clench a fist, some tap a foot, some tap a palm against one of their thighs. The dexterous ones use a variety.

Unless patients have hemiplegia, we also measure their ability to gesture with right and left sides. Whether the gesture is performed by the left or right side or bilaterally is of more than superficial interest. The data (Rizzolatti, Bertoloni, & Buchtel, 1979; Botkin, Schmaltz, & Lamb, 1977; Summers & Sharp, 1979) are convincing that speech and right-hand gesturing, drawing as they do on the left hemisphere, can degrade each other. Having patients use their left hands may not be the solution, however, because most patients are right handed and perform even simple gestures better with that hand than with the left. When hemiplegia fails to solve the issue, patients can be tested. Their responses will show what is best.

At this step, the clinician's task is to find out if a gestural reorganization program seems reasonable. First one must determine each patient's ability to imitate the tapping of a few simple rhythm and stress patterns. We usually begin with three equally stressed, equally spaced taps (/ / /). If the patient can do it immediately or after a few trials, we vary the pattern slightly by altering the stress (u / /) or the rhythm (/ / /). When the patient can perform at least one of these patterns predictably, we introduce a speech task to be performed simultaneously with the gesture. Depending on the speaker's severity we use counting, a simple nonsense syllable such as /lɑ/, or a simple phrase such as "I like you." If the patient shows promise of being able to learn predictable gesturing and of pairing it with speech, treatment moves on to Step Three.

Step Three: Stabilizing the gesture. Several activities are possible at this step, depending on how well a patient does. We usually begin by tapping a simple pattern on the patient's arm or on the arm of a chair. Once we have provided the model several times, we have patients try to imitate. If they have difficulty, we urge them to tap along with us, and we will even take their hands in ours and guide them if need be. Once patients can imitate, we increase the delay interval between the model and the reproduction, and we introduce other patterns. Anytime tapping begins to degenerate we retreat to previous activities such as taking a hand in our own. Patterns can also be made simpler by slowing their overall rate or by shortening them. As gesturing improves, overall rate, complexity, and length can be increased. The greatest danger at this step is moving too rapidly. Gestural reorganization's potency depends on good gestures. Doing two things simultaneously is difficult when both things are normal; when one or both are impaired, combining them can be disastrous.

Step Four: Beginning to pair gesture and speech. Clinicians begin this step by selecting and ordering an easy set of speech stimuli. Next, they provide the gestural and speech models for each stimulus with therapeutically appropriate rhythm and stress. They can provide the model once or several times. We prefer tapping out the model on the patient's body as this heightens the effect, but clinicians can tap on furniture or on their own bodies as appropriate. After a few repetitions by the clinician, the patient is instructed to talk and tap simultaneously with the clinician. The list of stimuli can be practiced in any appropriate order.

If the drill is successful, all that is needed is repetition. Failure requires adjustments. The rate can be slowed. The gesture can be changed or the patient can use a different hand. The patient can do the talking while the clinician both taps and talks, or the patient can do the tapping while the clinician does both. The stimuli can be modified. In extreme cases, clinician and patient can return to Step Three.

Several issues cannot be dictated but, rather, will have to be decided after clinical experimentation. The gesture can be combined with each syllable of an utterance or with each word; or with only some of the words, perhaps the nouns or nouns and verbs; or only with the target word. How hard shall each gesture be? If speech is to be produced with equal and even stress, each tap is as strong as its neighbor. If it is to be practiced with more normal stress and rhythm, the taps can be stronger on the primary stressed items and weaker on those receiving less stress. Similarly, polysyllabic words requiring a tap on each syllable might first be practiced with equally strong taps on all syllables, followed by taps of varying strength corresponding to the word's natural stress pattern.

Step Five: Fading cues. This step differs only in hue from the one before. In Step Five, the clinician provides the model and then begins fading the simultaneous cues. In its most efficient form, it becomes simple imitation with the patient going it alone either once or several times after the clinician has provided a model. Simple imitation, however, may need to be preceded by the gradual fading of simultaneous cues, especially during those early sessions when gestural reorganization is first being introduced. For example, the clinician's gestures can become less firm or the clinician who has been tapping on the patient can stop that and begin tapping on a piece of furniture. The number of taps accompanying an utterance can be reduced. Instead of using one tap for each word, the clinician can provide a tap only for the first word, or the most important words, or the most difficult ones. Simultaneous verbal cues can be faded similarly. The clinician can speak softer or more rapidly or can model fewer of the words in each utterance. At times it will be enough to provide just the first sound of certain words.

From this point on, the clinician needs to cue only if a response's integrity begins to suffer and then only enough to repair the response while preserving at least some of the patient's independence. It may be cue enough to have patients think more carerfully about the first word, for example, or to remind them about slowing the rate by increasing pause time. The usual victim of carelessness at this step is the gesture; therefore, many of the cues to be faded last will be those that help patients gesture accurately.

Step Six: Gesture and contrastive stress.   In this step the patient taps as an accompaniment to answers to the clinician's questions. This step may well require nothing more than some instruction: "This time I'll ask you to answer a question using the sentence we've just worked on, and I want you to tap out the rhythm while answering." If necessary, demonstration can follow these directions. If the patient is unsuccessful, the clinician may have to go through all of the early stages of the contrastive stress drill as previously described. Maintaining the integrity of both gesture and speech is crucial.

Considerable variety can be introduced during this step if a patient is good. The stress and rhythm can be altered by varying the questions or by special instructions for the patient to speed up or slow down. The stimuli can also be changed for greater challenge. More instances of the target, more targets, longer utterances, a different phonetic environment for the targets, and different sentence types can all be introduced as long as their introduction is orderly. If responses sag, treatment can retreat to previous steps or the stimuli can be altered. Again, sloppiness of either gesture or speech must be guarded against throughout.

Step Seven: Greater volitional −purposive control.   Now patients are more independent. The practice can be of original questions and answers, perhaps beginning with words they have already practiced but in previously unpracticed sentences. Next, they can be directed to use unpracticed words as answers to questions prompted by each patient's biographical data or by read or heard material. The clinician must be especially assiduous here lest a patient try to resort to being normal. Another, more frequent problem is that such practice will be more than the patient can handle because language skills, and therefore the sentences generated, will outrun motor skills. If particular words or targets show themselves to be difficult during such drill, they can be strengthened by a return trip through previous steps. By now, the therapy should be a friendly tramp anyhow, with both patient and clinician ready to back up, to take side trips, to stop and rest, and to change the present or the next day's goals in response to how things are going.

Step Eight: Fading the gesture. Some patients quit using the gestural accompaniment; others do not. Significant spontaneous recovery usually causes the gesture to fade more or less automatically. When it does not fade although the clinician thinks it could, the clinician can help the patient leave the gesture behind. Nothing more sophisticated is required than practice with a progressively higher proportion of responses without accompanying gestures. More difficult than helping the patient abandon the gesture is prohibiting the patient from doing so prematurely. Even when patients are doing well and can get along without gestural accompaniment in most situations, we remind them to fall back on gestures when talking is tough, as when they are giving their histories to a new physician or explaining why they failed to yield to a school bus. The gesture need not be faded for the treatment to be a success, however. Gestures, like hearing aids and glasses, can become permanent prostheses. One of our patients continued to tap several years after his stroke. No one seemed to mind.

Why Gestures Work

Luria (1970) says that apraxic speech can be "reorganized" by pairing it with some more intact set of responses or behaviors. In our gestural program, speech is paired with simple, repetitive gestures. The assumptions of the program are that apraxia of speech is a disruption in the auditory–vocal loop on which normal speech primarily depends, and that limb gestures, which are more intact in the apraxic speaker, are added to that loop, thereby improving speech performance without actually repairing the loop. The same general mechanism may be at work when a Parkinson patient's shuffling gait is improved if he or she is careful to step on each of a set of parallel black strips placed at intervals in his direction of movement. Reorganization carries with it the unfortunate implication of altered neuromotor activity, and perhaps even a new neural substrate for motor speech performance. Such an explanation is too grand and goes well beyond what we know or can test. It may be sufficient to reason that gesturing takes the patient out of an open auditory–vocal loop and forces him to perform less automatically and with closed loop control.

Another explanation for gestural reorganization's success may be that gestures simply distract from speech and that speech comes more easily after being forced into the background. This explanation, which washes up lagan-like on the shores of all therapies, originally belonged to stuttering therapy. We do not find it compelling. It seems unlikely that the tremendous concentration on both speech and gesture required by gestural reorganization would allow anything—especially speech—to slip into the background.

A third explanation is that the gestures slow speech and heighten stress and rhythm profiles. According to this view, the effect of gesturing is a secondary one. Nailling and Horner (1979), for example, argue that gestures stabilize the pace of speech and that it is this stability which is therapeutic. There seems little doubt that a predictable, replicable stress and rhythm profile improves speech for a variety of patients, including apraxic ones. Research comparing different methods may allow us to test this and other hypotheses. If the gestures work because they impose predictability, then they should be no better than simple contrastive stress. Studies comparing the two methods are necessary, as are studies comparing gestural reorganization and other less exotic methods.

If one is willing to abandon explanations about loops and neural reorganization, it may be enough to conclude that (1) gestures can be used to disrupt the apraxic talker's premorbid fast rate and open loop control, and (2) they can become a vivid reminder of treatment's lessons. Typical patients have been talking all their lives. A treatment that helps them merely talk again may not be as effective as one that includes a cue about what one has to do to talk better. Gestures can be that cue.

Reorganization Using a Pacing Board

Helm (1979) described the use of a "tactile pacing apparatus" (p. 351) with a palilalic patient. The pacing board (see Figure 1) she described is about 13 inches long, 2 inches wide, and is partitioned by dividers into eight sections, each a different color. The board is lightweight and portable, but its greatest value may be that a program using it is superior to simple gestural reorganization. Its general use is simple: the patient is taught to touch each of the squares in accompaniment to each unit of speech. Instead of tapping against a table top, leg, or something else, patients touch a different square as they say each portion of a target utterance.

Step One: Learning to use the board. Treatment begins with the patient's learning how to tap or even rub each segment of the board predictably, first with a pattern of equal and even stress, and then with a

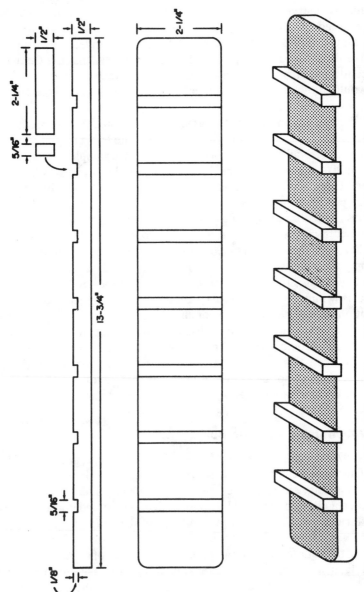

Figure 1. A pacing board (Helm, 1979) useful in helping the apraxic talker control speech rate and rhythm. (From Helm, N: Management of palilalia with a pacing board. *J Speech Hear Disord,* 1979,44, 350—353, with permission.)

variety of stress and rhythm patterns. The best way seems to be for the patient to move a finger along each segment until it bumps the divider. If the patient is not hemiplegic, the clinician may want to try both left and right hands to see which is better. Movement to Step Two should wait until the patient can make predictable movements along the board.

Step Two: Adding speech. This method is identical to that described for gestural reorganization. The clinician chooses appropriate stimuli such as single words or phrases made of short words, and then teaches the patient to say one word or one syllable simultaneously with contacting one of the board's segments two words, two segments; three words, three segments, and so on. At first, the patient may need considerable help. The clinician may even take the patient's hand and direct it and do all of the other things described in gestural reorganization. The goal is to make the patient independent in combined speaking and use of the board before leaving this step for the next.

Step Three: Expanding the program. If using the board is accompanied by improved articulation and perhaps improved stress and rhythm as well, the program can be expanded. Stimuli can be made harder or longer and the patient's reliance on the clinician and even on the board can be reduced. Stimuli that lend themselves to contrastive stress drill can be practiced according to the guidelines for that method previously described. Instead of merely answering questions, however, the patient can accompany answers with appropriate movements on the board. As part of increasing a patient's independence, clinicians can fade their participation and can even instruct the patient to reduce the number of taps on the board that accompany each utterance, until only key words are accompanied by contact with the board. Usually the last tap can be saved for the word containing the target. If a person never gets free of the board, the board has not failed. Like other prostheses, it may be the permanent companion of intelligibility.

Gesturing With and Without the Board

Using the board may be superior to simple gesturing because of the board's uniqueness. If nothing else the different colors of each of the board's portions make it and the drill memorable, thereby helping the patient internalize the lessons of therapy. When asked, "What are you supposed to do when you talk?," the patient may be more likely to answer, "Slow down" if practice has been with the board than if it has been with unassisted gesturing. Certainly, using the board makes it more likely that the correct answer will be forthcoming than if the clinician merely provides advice and admonition. A problem is that the board may not allow the latitude for more normal stress and rhythm profiles that simple gestural reorganization does. In our experience, patients tend to use the board in a methodical, stereotyped way unless they are carefully taught. The stereo-typed pattern may be ideal at first, but later on the clinician may have to force variation.

Why the Board Works

The same hypotheses about why simple gesturing works are probably the same ones that explain the board's effect. It may bring about a form of Luria's (1970) intersystemic reorganization. Certainly, the board intro-duces into the act of speaking a unique, vivid cue. Perhaps it breaks into open-loop control. Perhaps it has its effect by imposing a slowed stress and rhythm profile on the patient's speech. It remains to be determined if apraxic patients get more benefit from this than from other methods. Clinical research into the relative efficacy of specific techniques is invious territory. One can only hope that explorers willing to make some tracks can be found.

SOME DATA

Moderately apraxic patients are easy to study, especially in the chronic stage, because they are lawful. Even their variability is predictable. They are also rewarding to study because they usually improve unless they have an equally severe coexisting aphasia which limits their ability to generalize and to hold gains. A patient with equally severe apraxia and aphasia usually does well in the clinic and poorly outside, regardless of how much practice has been provided. We will present data on one such patient, but not before we show more satisfying treatment data from patients who learned to talk in and outside of the clinic.

The Same Things Over and Over

R.B. was admitted to therapy three years after a left, middle cerebral artery thromboembolic episode had left him with a mild aphasia, a severe apraxia of speech, and a dense right hemiplegia. He could understand what was said to him even when it was complex; he continued to read for pleasure although more laboriously than before his stroke; and he could write words and sentences, but only with great difficulty. His mild coexist-ing aphasia was most evident in writing. His speech prior to treatment was intelligible only to his wife and only if she knew the topic. His speech was characterized by trial and error groping, by myriad sound substitutions and

distortions, by severe dysprosody and struggle; and by predictable variability. He had no dysarthria, although his speech sounded, except for the
substitutions, like a spastic dysarthria.

His therapy was almost exclusively the imitation of contrasts which,
as he said during a videotaped interview, required him to "do the same
things over and over again." Typical of how he learned are his data for
word-initial /l/ in Figure 2. The /l/ was contrasted with /d/. The improvement during treatment and the decline during withdrawal attest to a treatment effect. Treatment was reinstated; the response stabilized, and now
appears in corrected speech.

Among the thngs R.B. taught us was that baseline testing should be
concealed. Figure 3 shows what he did with the initial /str/ when he inferred
from two baseline sessions that it was next to be learned. Before the third
session, he practiced on his own. Unfortunately, we did not ask him about
his method.

These are selected data. Clinicians should not think that we worked
only on these sounds or that we worked on them in the order presented.
With R.B., as with our other patients, we first chose for drill those sounds
which could make the most difference in his intelligibility. Nor was our

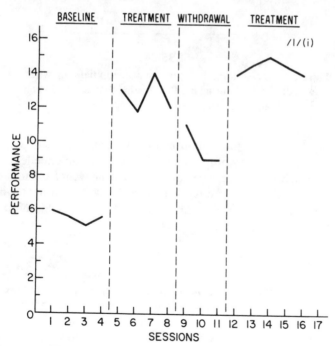

Figure 2.   Treatment data for word-initial /l/.

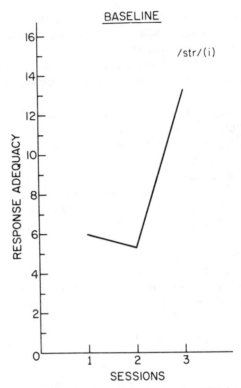

Figure 3.   Accelerating baseline for word-initial /str/ when speaker discovered during baseline testing that /str/ had been placed in single-case design.

methodology limited to the imitation of contrasts. As with our other patients, we used a variety of methods. R.B. gave us an excellent opportunity to use nearly our entire repertoire, because he went from unintelligible to intelligible under most circumstances. He left treatment when he could tell most people what was on his mind. He had a lot on his mind, as his family and friends now attest.

Tap and Talk

L.S. was introduced in the previous chapter. The progress we described for selected vowels and consonants continued and the patient became, by the end of treatment, a moderate to mild apraxic talker. He was able to talk functionally to all but the rudest or most imposing of listeners. When he was talking well, his apraxia was mild; when he was talking under pressure, he moved back into the moderate range. To save himself during the difficult times, he would resort to the gestural reorganization that we had originally introduced as soon as he had moved out of the severe range. In his case, gestural reorganization was combined with imitation of contrasts and the contrastive stress drill. In other words, he practiced everything to a gestural accompaniment. His gesture was simple: he merely tapped out a rhythm using any available flat surface—chair, table, his other hand. At the time our data were collected, he was still variable, but the data for word-initial /st/ (Figure 4) suggest a treatment effect nonetheless. Even more convincing are observations from an alternating treatment design in which tapping and simple imitation were compared. While the data points are limited, the clear trend of the data in Figure 5 is for sentences accompanied by gestures to be more adequate as measured by a multidimensional scoring system than sentences unaccompanied by gestures. He never abandoned the gesture completely, although he did switch from his left to his right hand—a switch that may have interesting implications. He still resurrects the gesture when he is under pressure; he likes it.

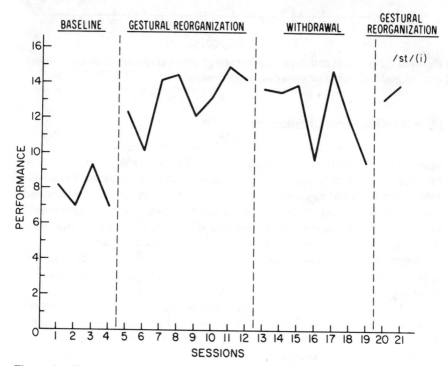

Figure 4.   Treatment data for word-initial /st/ treated with a program of gestural reorganization. The response is variable but improving.

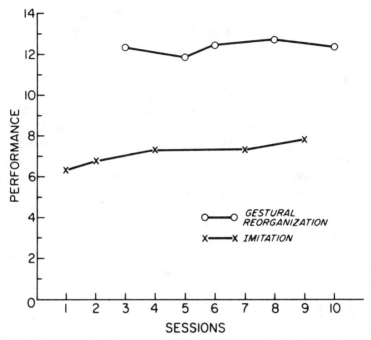

Figure 5.   Treatment data from an alternating treatments design show clear superiority of gestural reorganization over simple imitation.

I Get No Kick From Champagne

H.K. suffered the acute onset of right-sided weakness and speechlessness eight days prior to beginning speech treatments. When we first saw him, he was severely aphasic and apraxic, but he could understand far more than he could say. With spontaneous recovery's help, he regained some speech and understanding during the next two weeks. At one month duration, his spontaneous progress had slowed sufficiently so that data from a variety of single-case designs could show a treatment effect.

Imitation of contrasts was the treatment of choice, even when he was severely involved. As he entered the moderate range and after spontaneous recovery had ceased to be a daily influence on his speech, we tested our methodology using a series of withdrawal designs. As can be seen in Figure 6, training on initial /st/ generalized to the final position, but training on initial /tʃ/ did not. In this he resembled the patient (R.B.) described in Chapter 8 and in this chapter. On the other hand, H.K. is an informative contrast to that speaker, because his progress is more variable. Whereas that speaker's curves (see Figure 8-7) show only a little variability and

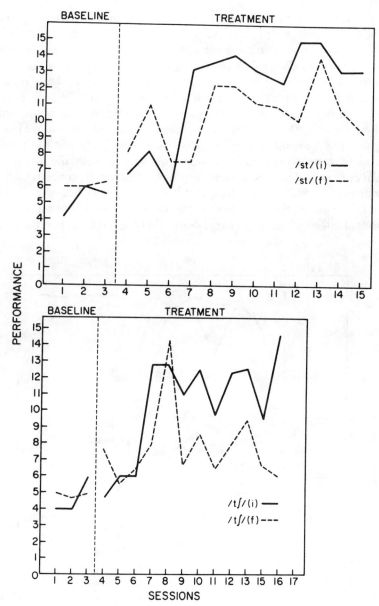

Figure 6. Treatment data showing a modicum of generalization from treatment of word-initial /st/ to word-final /st/ but no generalization for word-initial /tʃ/ to word-final /tʃ/.

quick learning, H.K. shows considerable variability and slower learning. But learn he did.

We also used him to find out if gains from an imitative program would generalize to reading. Specifically, we wanted to know if practicing initial position /s/ in an imitative program would make it easier to read /s/ words aloud. The data in Figure 7 shows that it did. The /s/ in reading responded immediately, but was generally more variable from day to day. Once we knew that treatment would generalize in that direction, we were more confident about assigning reading lists for his practice outside of the clinic.

Fourteen months after the onset of his aphasia and apraxia, we placed this patient in a modified alternating treatment design to test the relative potency of simple imitation and imitation with vibrotactile stress and rhythm cues superimposed on auditory ones (Rubow, Rosenbek, Collins, & Longstreth, 1982). We called our design modified because, strictly defined, it requires that the same behavior be treated with two different methods. Instead of using the same words (behavior) in our two treatment

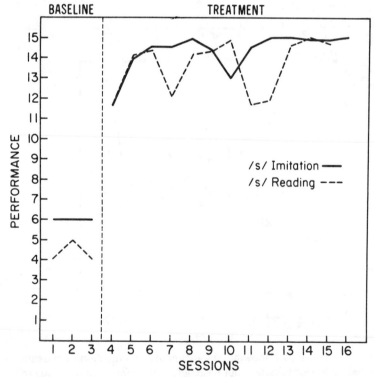

Figure 7. Treatment data showing generalization from an imitative program to reading.

conditions, we randomly assigned a group of plosive words to the simple imitation treatment and a group of fricative words to the imitation plus vibrotactile condition. Prior to treatment, all words in both groups were equally hard for the patient—he could never say them correctly. The words treated with simple imitation improved from an average of 5.0 to an average of 6.9 as measured on a 16-point rating scale. Performance on the fricative words treated with imitation plus vibrotactile stimulation changed from an average of 5.0 to 10.8, a change of 5.8. This change was clinically significant and suggests that vibrotactile stimulation may have a place in apraxia of speech treatments.

I Do Not Prefer Hand Signals

Not all moderately apraxic patients improve. R.S. came to the clinic two years after a left-hemisphere thromboembolic episode that left him mildly hemiplegic and moderately apraxic and aphasic. Because his entire speech-language system was involved, we treated both his apraxia and his aphasia. The apraxia treatments were to begin with gestural reorganization, because he gave the impression clinically of needing something to pace his articulators. In a note he wrote during our eloquent explanation of gestural reorganization's virtues he said, "I do not prefer hand signals." It took us only a little longer to drop the gestural program than it did for him to tell us how he felt about it.

Instead, we used a program that combined reading and imitation of contrasts. We had him work simultaneously on several initial position consonants in words and short phrases. Each stimulus was written on a card, and he practiced switching from one to the other. He learned the treated words and was able to transfer the learning to untreated ones. If we were to show data on his learning of single sounds in short words, the program would look like a success. The data would be deceiving, however, because R.S. was unable to say these sounds in connected speech outside the clinic. This is not to say that he was speechless, only that his extra clinic speech would never tip anyone off that he was in speech therapy.

We staffed him several times in an effort—ultimately futile—to decide why we were failing. He was a smart man, he wore a goatee and had several inventions to his credit. He could write a little and understand the activities of daily living. His judgment was good, unless one wants to fault him for staying in treatment for three months. He had a bilateral hearing loss but wore an aid. He did not have dysarthria. He did have a significant amount of aphasia. After a series of similar patients, we have come to the conclusion that aphasia determines apraxia of speech treatment's apogee. The less the aphasia, the greater the likelihood and amount of recovery from apraxia of speech. He had too much aphasia.

MOVING OUT OR ON

Moderately apraxic speakers can make selected listeners understand at least some things, so such a patient is not doomed even when progress stops. The alert clinician recognizes when a moderately involved patient is done improving and tries to beat the patient to the suggestion that treatment should end. Because most patients have an easier time accepting their apraxia, regardless of its severity, than do their clinicians, ending treatment for the patient who has ceased to improve is usually relatively easy if the clinician only pays attention to the patient's desires. Regardless of its ease, however, an end to treatment should usually be gradual rather than abrupt. Sessions can be spaced at longer intervals, or periodic follow-up visits can be scheduled. Before the last session, patient and family can sit down with the clinician and take stock of what will be possible, fun, and even therapeutic. They can also be told that they are free to return anytime with questions, problems, or new potential.

If moderate patients are improving, they may well pass into the mild range without knowing it, because the boundary between moderate and mild is as indistinguishable as that between reality and fantasy. But noticed or not, the passage is a fortunate one. Mildly apraxic speakers' chances of speaking near normally in at least some environments are good, especially if they enter the mild range within the first two or three months, or if they can tolerate additional, intensive treatment.

11

Treating the Mildly Apraxic Patient

Probably no two randomly selected speech pathologists could agree on the number and types of errors that distinguish a mildly apraxic speaker from a moderately apraxic one. On the other hand, judges can agree on which patients are mild, moderate, and severe, using a 7-point rating scale (Hoit-Daalgard et al., 1980). This agreement is important because expectations, counseling, and (to a small degree) methods for the mildly apraxic speaker are slightly different from those already described. We thought that the distinctions were great enough to warrant a short chapter on the mild patient's treatment.

COUNSELING

Mild patients present a special counseling challenge, because they are so different from each other. Some sense that something like the way it used to be may again be possible—work, club membership, church, coaching a softball team, functional speech. Others despair, because of what they perceive as their significant communication handicap, of ever returning in more than a nominal way to their previous style of life, especially if that life required talking to patients, clients, or customers. Others recognize that their communication may be adequate but that their strength and health will not be. Others withdraw from the world despite having adequate communication, strength, and health. If they cannot be perfect, they will not be. So the clinician is protean and prepares for several possibilities.

Certain problems arise frequently enough, however, to allow for general discussion.

Masquerading as Normal

Laughter may be harder for the mildly apraxic talker than for others, because the need to masquerade as normal may be greater. Unfortunately, such a masquerade requires too much energy, too much avoidance, and too many costume changes. Worst of all, it is seldom successful and it is never necessary. Naive listeners are not fooled by even the cleverest disguise and are more likely to be amazed by what they see as the patient's recovery and courage than they are to be embarrassed or offended by residuals. So we encourage our patients to err boldly and to take risks with communication. Make a toast at your son's wedding, sing, deliver a eulogy, go back to work, dictate a letter, sing in the choir.

Preparing to Self-Correct

Even mildly apraxic talkers make errors, and sometimes if the stresses are great such speakers may be nearly speechless. Clinicians need not warn them of this; they know it. Clinicians can help them accept the inevitability, however, and they may even be able to teach patients a few tricks to reduce the frequency and negative effects of such failures. To reduce error frequency, we urge patients to use closed-loop control for all but the most automatic utterances. We also teach them to recognize good and bad influences on their speech and to keep bad influences to a minimum. We urge them to self-correct even if it takes extra time. Finally, we encourage them to laugh—or at least smile—at each lapse no matter how severe.

Not easy tasks these, not even for the mild patient; but they can be accomplished. Supportive family and friends are the most help, but the clinician capable of showing patients how far they have come, how good they are, and how much they miss by hiding can be an influence as well. The greatest help, however, probably comes from continued improvement. If all else fails, however, and if the patient is constantly hiding and avoiding friends and any other kind of involvement, the clinician may want to consider referral. Mild patients are good candidates for the psychologist or psychiatrist because they can talk.

Decisions About the Future

During treatment or as it is about to end, the clinician may help with the patient's decisions about work or retirement, driving, social commitments, hobbies, nursing home placement, and the like. As a rule, we do not make any of these decisions, especially about driving. Coping with stroke or other illness is hard enough without the additional burden of being protected from responsibility or of having responsibility stolen away. We do listen, however. If more than listening is needed, we try to help. For example, if the patient is concerned about returning to work, we do common sense things like find out what the patient's job requires and then measure, as best we can, the patient's ability to meet those requirements. We may interview management and coworkers, review samples of previous work, and interview the spouse about how the patient was handling job stresses prior to illness. If the patient can work but not at the old job, we see if relocation or reassignment is possible. Often it is not communication but diminished endurance and reduced ability to cope that retire the patient.

Of all the decisions about the future, placement is often the hardest. Fortunately, most mildly apraxic patients return home, because they can talk and usually, they can walk. If a nursing home is being considered, however, the clinician can be a listener, someone to whom the family can talk about their fears and guilt. If they need help with selecting a home and financing it, they should be referred to a social worker or other professional. Immediately prior to the patient's going, the clinician may want to meet with nursing home officials to describe what the patient can and cannot do and how to help. Promising the family and patient that return visits to speech therapy will be scheduled and that a speech pathologist will always be available by phone to answer questions and help solve problems also makes it easier for the family to accept the reality of nursing home placement.

Occasionally, a patient and family only need encouragement about decisions they have already made. A clinician's support can be just the additional help patients and families need to do what they have decided to do anyhow. We usually end up telling patients and families that the best test of a decision's rightness is to act on it, and the best attitude about a decision is that it can be reversed.

PREPARING FOR TREATMENT

Mild patients seldom need much preparation. Chances are great that they will have had considerable experience with it already and that treatments for their mild conditions will not be radically different from those with which they are already familiar. The two distinctions between treating moderate and mild patients that may be differences worth preparing patients for are that they will be required to be increasingly independent and increasingly creative. As patients improve, they do more and their clinicians do less.

SPECIFIC TREATMENTS

The mildly apraxic talker normally has both consistent and variable errors of articulation and prosody. The consistent errors, as when an /r/ is always distorted, may require previously described methodology such as phonetic placement. The mild, variable errors, on the other hand, can be treated by extensions of methods appropriate to moderate apraxia of speech. These extensions require good language. Fortunately, because they usually have only a mild coexisting aphasia, mildly apraxic talkers can complete meta-linguistic tasks. They can experiment with speech, invent sentences and reword them, and play word games. They will be required to do this and more by the methods that follow.

Expanding the Contrastive Stress Drill

Contrastive stress drills, as already described for the moderately apraxic talker, are appropriate for the mild speaker as well. To make the drills more challenging, the words and sentences can be made longer, more targets can be added to each sentence, and more rare words can be used. The patient can also be directed to respond with a faster speaking rate or after longer delays or with fewer intervening cues from the clinician. Several specific variations are described below.

Variation One.   Unlike moderately apraxic talkers, mild ones may be able to concentrate their attention on the stress, rhythm, and total speech sound make-up of sentence length utterances rather than having to be mindful of specific sounds or syllables within an utterance. If so, stimuli can be constructed with more attention to meaning, variety, and usefulness and less to speech sound make-up. Also, such patients can practice a variety of stress profiles for each utterance because of being freed from having to put primary stress time and time again on only the word containing the target sound or sounds. In Variation One, then, the clinician asks a variety of questions about each utterance, thereby eliciting a variety of patient responses. For example, if the practice utterance was "Beethoven's deafness began while he was still young," a series of four questions could move the stress from "Beethoven" to "deafness" to "began" to "young." If rhythm, stress, or articulation in one or more of these answers is consistently wrong, the appropriate questions can be repeated. If compensations such as a pause before polysyllabic words or an intrusive schwa in consonant clusters are necessary to the patient's intelligibility, these too can be practiced. The aim is not necessarily to make even mildly apraxic patients normal, it is to make them as good as their neuromotor systems will allow.

Variation Two. Patients can create original sentences using target words, phrases, or ideas supplied by clinicians; or they can supply utterances they want especially to work on. Once a sentence has been created, patient and clinician can drill it, with or without modifications, depending on its adequacy. Sometimes, a patient's own sentence will be marred by slight syntactic and semantic errors or will be too difficult motorically. The clinician can alter syntax, supply missing words, change wrong words, and substitute easier ones. If the difficult portions of an utterance are retained, they can be lifted from the utterance, practiced individually, and then be reinserted.

Variation Three. The clinician can elicit responses by asking open-ended questions: "What state were you born in?" "Where do your children live?" "How to you prepare milk gravy to go with cold packed squirrel meat?" This activity may be easier than sentence creation, because it is not metalinguistic. If so, it should come earlier, for it is an excellent carryover activity.

Variation Four. Patients can do the asking. If a patient has difficulty, the clinician can guide the questions toward a set of targets by cueing the patient to ask certain kinds of questions; for example, "Ask me what my favorite game meat is." Variations Three and Four can be combined so that clinician and patient take turns asking and answering questions. Troublesome responses can be extracted and drilled under easier conditions.

Variation Five. The drills can be built from other materials, such as the plot of a show seen on television or a newspaper account of cannibalism. As in other variations, we retain reasonably rigid standards of adequacy lest speakers begin to rush, to make errors, or to listen less carefully. This variation may be difficult even for non-brain-damaged patients, so clinicians may need to focus patients on specific ideas or utterances.

Variation Six. Conversation can be the last step. The conversation should be controlled, however, because if simple conversation were therapeutic, speech pathologists would be out of business. Neither clinician nor patient can allow content to become more important than production. The temptation to do so will be great with several of these variations and especially great with this last one. We tell patients to talk during this phase as if each sentence had been practiced for a month. If clinicians can focus a conversation on previously practiced material, so much the better.

Reading

Mild patients may read quite well, making written material useful in and outside of the clinic. If used in the clinic, reading practice can be organized so as to increase the patient's independence as described in Chapter 10. Reading can also be combined with other methods such as contrastive stress. For example, the patient can be asked to read aloud a sentence from the newspaper. The content of the sentence or the sentence itself can then be practiced as a contrastive stress drill. Reading may also be useful to the patient as he or she begins practicing a series of polysyllabic words for the first time or as a way of strengthening difficult utterances that emerge from previously described variations of the contrastive stress drill. For homework, the patient can read lists of words or sentences in an order and at a pace which diagnostic therapy has found to be good. Such homework can be completed with or without supervision, depending on the patient's family and how well they all get along. Auditory and reading modes can be combined for homework by having the patient practice materials presented by a Language Master or equivalent device. The addition of the auditory modality increases the likelihood that patients will notice their errors, because they can check their productions against the original. Reading, if done both at home and in the clinic, bonds environment and clinic and improves carryover.

STRENGTHENING RESPONSES

The drills already described emphasize success. They are designed to move the patient toward volitional-purposive communication with only enough errors to speed learning. However, unless physiologic improvement has been nearly complete or treatment has been protracted and intense, treated responses will never be as hardy outside of the clinic as within it. Their strength can be improved, however, by a few relatively simple embellishments of traditional procedures. Such embellishments are not exclusively for the mild patient; they are included here as a convenience.

Interference

Patients can be helped to withstand outside pressures on their speech by learning to withstand a clinician's pressures. A variety of threats to a response's integrity can be built into a session. One group of such threats comprises things the clinician does while the patient is silently sitting waiting to make a particular response. Perhaps the greatest threat comes from the clinician's talking about a topic related to the response the patient is trying to "hold." For example, if the target is "Geese die from eating lead shot," the clinician can distract the patient with talk of ducks, hunting, and steel. If the patient has a coexisting aphasia, these related ideas will be especially disrupting. Somewhat less distracting would be for a clinician to talk about unrelated and unemotional topics such as the weather.

Perhaps even more disruptive is to require competing responses. While waiting to produce the target, "Geese die from eating lead shot," patients can be instructed to count, perform some other serial speech task, or even answer unrelated questions. Having done this, they can then be asked for the target. Also, if they make errors, clinicians can then introduce those errors into the retention interval. For example, if a patient distorts the initial /l/, as in "lead," by producing it with a plosive-like quality, the clinician can have the patient listen to or produce "d" words prior to saying the target utterance.

Speeding Responses

A character builder for treated responses is requiring that their rate be controlled—made faster or slower according to conditions or commands. Most apraxic talkers, regardless of their stage in treatment, seem to rush or at least to want to rush. One of our drills involves chicanery. We try to trick patients into forgetting their lessons about going slow enough so that they are maximally intelligible. We do this by beginning to speak faster ourselves; by diverting the patient's attention from production to content; by trying to elicit longer answers, which are naturally produced faster; and by appearing to relax the patient-clinician relationship. We usually begin such training with a warning about our intention. Also, anytime we dupe a patient into talking too fast, we interrupt the drill with a reminder. We also have them practice at varying rates, alternately slower and faster.

Sounds in Isolation

One criterion of successful treatment is that a patient learns to self-correct. Errorless speech is impossible even for the normal speaker, but the normal speaker almost never has difficulty self-correcting, although one of the authors recalls a lecture in which he said, "Dons and Jarley" three times, and could not self-correct until after a several second pause in which he silently spelled the names and rehearsed them—Johns and Darley. Successful treatment means teaching apraxic talkers to self-correct. In our view, one of the most efficient ways of improving self-correction is to have even the mildest patient practice sounds in isolation. The goal is not merely to say the sounds, but to analyze their quality and feel, and to create associations that will guide jaw, lips, and tongue through the right movements regardless of where the speaker is or who is listening. This is hard work. Sometimes, when we begin it, a previously successful patient experiences a flurry of errors. Educated patients can endure the flurry.

SOME DATA

Classically Apraxic

R.M. was in many ways the classically apraxic patient. He was 63 years old and in his usual state of good health when he developed right-side weakness and speechlessness. The weakness began to disappear within hours, and when we saw him ten days after his left-hemisphere thromboembolic episode, he was nearly normal on the right side and his speech was improving. Instead off being speechless, he could say a few automatic phrases and even answer some questions. Nonetheless, many of his attempts to talk ended in frustrated silence. Because we knew from nursing service that the silences were less frequent each day and because bedside testing showed him to have reasonable auditory and reading comprehension, we diagnosed severe apraxia of speech and mild aphasia and predicted substantial and rapid improvement. We counseled the patient that his worse days were behind him and explained that his inevitable recovery could be hastened by twice-daily treatments. He was willing. We knew that designing a single case study to demonstrate a treatment effect would require careful stimulus selection, because physiologic recovery was having its inexorable way.

We chose two kinds of therapy materials, because our treatment had two purposes. We wanted to restore the patient's faith in his articulators by giving him a variety of successes, so we had him spend about three quarters of each session practicing one- and two-syllable words replete with plosives. We wanted also to see if we could document the assumption—stated as fact by many professionals—that treatment speeds the acutely apraxic talker's recovery. To get the documentation, we created 20 difficult sentences such as "It is impossible to predict success," tested them for stability, randomly assigned 10 to a notreatment condition and 10 to a treatment condition, spent one-quarter of each session treating the appropriate 10 sentences, and periodically measured the change in performance for all 20 sentences.

Both kinds of stimuli were treated with extensions of contrastive stress. Both groups improved; the treated group improved most. Physiologic recovery no doubt accounts for some of the change in both sets. The better performance on the treated sentences—especially since they were harder, on the average, than the untreated ones—attests to a treatment effect. Whether it was because of the specific work done with the sentences or because of an interaction of effects from the sentence drill and the confidence building drill with the plosive words cannot be determined.

A few words before leaving this example. We do not ordinarily prescribe work with peculiar and difficult sentences. This patient was special. He moved rapidly into the mild range. His treatment lasted less than a month, and he was essentially normal at discharge. We spent a portion of each session with such difficult material only to test our attitude that even such naturally fortunate patients are doubly blessed by receiving even short periods of treatment.

Her Name is Wanda

It sometimes happens that patients arrive at the mild part of the distribution talking well overall but with a sound or sounds that are consistently distorted or even substituted for, especially when they are under pressure. The patient to be described, therefore, was not unusual because he had specific errors. What did make him unusual, however, was that the errors were intractable. We could not improve them. We include him in this chapter for balance. Even the mildly apraxic patient may not get better, or at least some of his symptoms may persist.

The patient was referred to us when his wife noticed that after a plateau of several months, beginning 18 months after his stroke, his speech was beginning to improve. The reported improvement after a several month plateau surprised us, but since we spend a portion of each day being surprised anyway, we agreed to evaluate this patient. The family planned to move close to our clinic if we decided we could help. He had considerable functional speech when we first saw him, and our evaluation showed mild apraxia of speech and mild aphasia. An extensive evaluation of his connected speech confirmed that he could not make an /r/ shape in any environment so when he introduced his daughter as Wanda, we called her Rhonda. Our error. Her name really was Wanda, fortunately for him. He also distorted the /l/ and /j/ inconsistently and made a variety of consistent assimilation errors. For example, "pancake" became "kamcake," and "popcorn" became "copcorn." The biggest offenders in the assimilative pattern were the /t/ and /d/, which often intruded upon any other plosives in their vicinity.

Treatment involved both specific and general speech and language training. His language improved significantly, the number of assimilative errors was reduced, and those that did occur, he got better at self-correcting. In many ways, however, the data on /r/, shown in Figure 1, are the most interesting. The /r/ was treated in isolation with strong auditory-

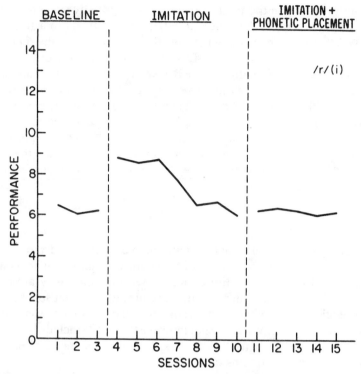

Figure 1. Treatment data for word-initial /r/ showing its intractability.

visual cues, exaggerated oral posturing, and greatly increased articulation time. We drilled it every day for a month. As can be seen, it was intractable and adding phonetic placement did not help, so we quit trying to change it. We mention this patient because his apraxia was mild, but we had to treat the /r/ as if it were being produced by a patient incapable of any but a few speech movements. He is instructive also because our failure with a part of his program is a reminder that mildness is not, a priori, a good prognostic sign.

DISCHARGE AND FOLLOW-UP

All patients eventually leave therapy, or at least intensive therapy. Often enough, departure is the patient's rather than the clinician's decision. More than once a patient has called us aside to tell us that today will be his last day. He hopes our feelings are not hurt. Regardless of who makes the decision, it can be accompanied by advice to prepare the patient and family for life without treatment. We usually warn families that speech may sag briefly after treatment ends; but that improvement, however slight, may well continue for months or years. We remind everyone that regardless of how well the patient talks, he will continue to vary and may at times be unable to say anything. Finally, we remind them that the planning, evaluation, and self-correction that got him to discharge will get him well beyond it, and that treatment's techniques and tricks can be used long after formal therapy has ended.

Seldom is treatment ended without at least one follow-up visit. Besides providing the clinician with invaluable data on the evolution of apraxia, follow-up gives the patient and family a place to go with unexpected problems and traumas. We also offer appropriate workbooks or a Language Master with the idea that the break from treatment is cleaner if a piece of the clinic goes home permanently or on loan. One needs to be careful about books and machines, however. Rather than being reassuring, they can cause guilt if patients fail to understand that they are free to use them or not. Regardless of how treatment ends, we let patients and families know we are available for future consultation. Seldom do we have takers, unless it is to return the Language Master that has been all but forgotten on the closet shelf. Mildly apraxic patients usually do not need us once they leave.

References

Abbs, JH, & Cole, KJ: Consideration of bulbar and suprabulbar afferent influences upon speech motor coordination and programming, in Grillner S, Linbloom B, Lubker J, et al. (Eds.): *Speech Motor Control*. New York: Pergamon Press, 1982, pp. 159−186

Agronowitz, A, & McKeown, M: *Aphasia Handbook for Adults and Children*. Springfield: Charles C Thomas, 1964

Alajouanine, T, Castaigne, P, Lhermitte, F, et al.: Etude de 43 cas d'aphasie post traumatique. Confrontation anatamo-clinque et aspects evolutifs. *L'Encephale*, 1957, *46*, 3−45

Alajouanine, T, & Lhermitte, F: Aphasia and physiology of speech, in Rioch DM and Weinstein EA (Eds.): *Disorders of Communication*. Baltimore: Williams and Wilkins, 1964, pp. 204−219

Anderson, T, Bourestom, N, & Greenberg, F: Rehabilitation predictors in completed stroke. Final Report. American Rehabilitation Foundation, Minneapolis, 1970 (unpublished)

Aten, JL, Darley, FL, Deal, JL, et al.: Letter: Comment on AD Martin's "Some objections to the term *apraxia of speech*." *J Speech Hear Disord*, 1975, *40*, 416−420

Aten, JL, Johns, DF, & Darley, FL: Auditory perception of sequenced words in apraxia of speech. *J Speech Hear Res*, 1971, *14*, 131−143

Aten, JL, & Lyon, JG: Measures of PICA subtest variance: A preliminary assessment of their value as predictors of language recovery in aphasic patients, in Brookshire RH (Ed.): *Clinical Aphasiology: Conference Proceedings*. Minneapolis: BRK Publishers, 1978, 106−116

Barlow, DH, & Hayes, SC: Alternating treatment design: One strategy for comparing the effects of two treatments in a single subject. *J Appl Behav Anal*, 1979, *12*, 199−210

Basso, A, Capitani, E, & Vignolo, LA: Influence of rehabilitation on language skills in aphasic patients: A controlled study. *Arch Neurol*, 1979, *36*, 190−196

Basso, A, & Vignolo, LA: Come se imposta rieducazione del linguaccio nell' afasia: utilita di una analisi qualitativa dell' eloguio patologico. *Europa Medicophys*, 1969, *5*, 140−160

Bauman, JA, Waengler, HH, & Prescott, TE: Durational aspects of continuous speech: Comparative measurements based on vowel and consonant productions by normal and apraxic speakers. Paper presented to the American Speech and Hearing Association, Washington, D.C., 1975 (unpublished)

Bay, E: Aphasia and nonverbal disorders of language. *Brain*, 1962, *85*, 411−426

Bayles, KA: Language and dementia producing diseases. *Commun Dis: J Cont Educ*, 1982, 7, 131–146

Benson, DF: Aphasia rehabilitation. *Arch Neurol*, 1979, 36, 187–189

Berlin, C: On: Melodic intonation therapy for aphasia by RW Sparks and AL Holland. *J Speech Hear Disord*, 1976, 41, 298–300

Birch, HG: Experimental investigations in expressive aphasia. *NY State J Med*, 1956, 56, 3849–3852

Birch, HG, & Lee, J: Cortical inhibition in expressive aphasia. *AMA Arch Neurol Psychiaty*, 1955, 74, 514–517

Blumstein, SE: Review of "Generative Phonology—Evidence from Aphasia," by M. Schnitzer. *Cortex*, 1974, 10, 206

Blumstein, SE: *A Phonological Investigation of Aphasic Speech*. The Hague: Mouton, 1973

Blumstein, SE, Cooper, WE, Goodglass, H, et al.: Production deficits in aphasia: A voice-onset time analysis. *Brain Lang*, 1980, 9, 153–170

Blumstein, SE, Cooper, WE, Zurif, EB, et al.: The perception and production of voice-onset time in aphasia. *Neuropsychologia*, 1977, 15, 371–382

Bogen, JE: The other side of the brain. I. Dysgraphia and dyscopia following cerebral commissurotomy. *Bull Los Angeles Neurol Soc*, 1969, 32, 73–105

Bolinger, D: *Aspects of Language*. New York: Harcourt Brace, 1975

Botkin, AL, Schmaltz, LW, & Lamb, DH: "Overloading" the left hemisphere in right-handed subjects with verbal and motor tasks. *Neuropsychologia*, 1977, 15, 591–596

Bowman, CA, Hodson, BW, & Simpson, RK: Oral apraxia and aphasic misarticulations, in Brookshire, RH (Ed.): *Clinical Aphasiology: Conference Proceedings*. Minneapolis: BRK Publishers, 1980, pp. 89–95

Brain, R: *Speech Disorders: Aphasia, Apraxia, Agnosia*. London: Butterworths, 1965

Brown, JR: *Mind, Brain, and Consciousness*. New York: Academic Press, 1977

Broida, H: *Communication Breakdowns of Brain Injured Adults*. Houston: College-Hill Press, 1979

Buck, M: *Dysphasia: Professional Guidance for Family and Patients*. Englewood Cliffs: Prentice-Hall, 1968

Buckingham, Jr, HW: Explanation in apraxia with consequences for the concept of apraxia of speech. *Brain Lang*, 1979, 8, 202–226

Burns, MS, & Canter, GJ: Phonemic behavior of aphasic patients with posterior cerebral lesions. *Brain Lang*, 1977, 4, 492–507

Butfield, E: Rehabilitation of the dysphasic patient. *Speech Path Therapy*, 1958, 1, 9–17, 60–65

Butfield, E, & Zangwill, OL: Re-education in aphasia: A review of 70 cases. *J Neurol Neurosurg Psychiaty*, 1946, 9, 75–79

Cairnes, CE: Markedness, neutralization, and universal redundancy rules. *Language*, 1969, 45, 863–885

Canter, GJ: The influence of primary and secondary verbal apraxia on output disturbances in aphasic syndromes. Paper presented to the American Speech and Hearing Association, Chicago, Illinois, 1969 (unpublished)

Chapin, C, Blumstein, SE, Meissner, B, et al.: Speech production mechanisms in aphasia: A delayed auditory feedback study. *Brain Lang*, 1981, 14, 106–113

Cherry, C: *On Human Communication*. Cambridge: MIT Press, 1966

Chomsky, N, & Halle M: *The Sound Pattern of English*. New York: Harper & Row, 1968

Cicone, M, Wapner, W, Foldi, N, et al.: The relation between gesture and language in aphasic communication. *Brain Lang*, 1979, 8, 324–349

Cleo Living Aids. 3957 Mayfield Rd., Cleveland, Ohio.

Clouzet, O, Pollak, A, Bianco, E, et al.: A neurolinguistic longitudinal study of a pure motor aphasia. *Acta Neurol Lat Am*, 1976, 22, 134–143

Collins, M, Cariski, D, Longstreth, D, et al.: Patterns of articulatory behavior in selected motor speech programming disorders, in Brookshire, RH (Ed.): *Clinical Aphasiology: Conference Proceedings.* Minneapolis: BRK Publishers, 1980, pp. 196–208

Collins, MJ, Rosenbek, JC, & Wertz, RT: Spectrographic analysis of vowel and word duration in apraxia of speech. *J Speech Hear Res*, 1983, *26*, 224–230

Collins, MJ, Shaughnessy, AL, & Becher, BJ: Acoustic analysis of vowel reduction in aphasia. Paper presented to the American Speech-Language-Hearing Association, Atlanta, Georgia, 1979 (unpublished)

Collins, MJ, Wertz, RT: Intersystemic reorganization in apraxia of speech. Paper presented to the American Speech and Hearing Association, Houston, Texas, 1976

Costello, J, & Onstine, J: The modification of multiple articulation errors based on distinctive feature theory. *J Speech Hear Disord*, 1976, *14*, 199–215

Cousins, N: *Anatomy of An Illness As Perceived by the Patient: Reflections on Healing and Regeneration.* New York: Norton Press, 1979

Crary, M, & Fokes, J: Phonological processes in apraxia of speech. A systematic simplification of articulatory performance. *Aphasia, Apraxia, Agnosia,* 1979, *1*, 1–12

Critchley, M: *Aphasiology.* London: Edward Arnold, 1970

Culton, GL: Spontaneous recovery from aphasia. *J Speech Hear Res*, 1969, *12*, 825–832

Dabul, B: *Apraxia Battery for Adults.* Tigard: CC Publications, 1979

Dabul, B, & Bollier, B: Therapeutic approaches to apraxia. *J Speech Hear Disord*, 1976, *41*, 268–276

Dahlberg, C, & Jaffe, J: *Stroke: A Doctor's Personal Story of His Recovery.* New York: W.W. Norton & Co., 1977

Darley, FL: *Aphasia.* Philadelphia: W.B. Saunders, 1982

Darley, FL: Treat or neglect? *ASHA,* 1979, *21*, 628–631

Darley, FL: Treatment of acquired aphasia, in Friedlander, WJ (Ed.): *Advances in Neurology, Volume 7: Current Reviews of Higher Nervous System Dysfunction.* New York: Raven Press, 1975, pp. 111–146

Darley, FL: The efficacy of language rehabilitation in aphasia. *J Speech Hear Disord*, 1972, *37*, 3–21

Darley, FL: Aphasia: Input and output disturbances in speech and language processing. Paper presented to the American Speech and Hearing Association, Chicago, Illinois, 1969 (unpublished)

Darley, FL: Apraxia of speech: 107 years of terminological confusion. Paper presented to the American Speech and Hearing Association, Denver, Colorado, 1968 (unpublished)

Darley, FL, Aronson, AE, & Brown, JR: *Motor Speech Disorders.* Philadelphia: WB Saunders, 1975

Davis, GA, & Wilcox, MJ: Incorporating parameters of natural conversation in aphasia treatment, in Chapey, R (Ed.): *Language Intervention Strategies in Adult Aphasia.* Baltimore: Williams and Wilkins, 1981, pp. 169–193

de Ajuriaguerra, J, Hecaen, H, & Angelergues, E: Les apraxies, varietes cliniques et lateralisation lesionelle. *Revue Neurologique,* 1960, *102*, 499–566

de Ajuriaguerra, J, & Tissot, R: Disorders of speech, perception, and symbolic behavior, in Vinken, P, Bruyn, G (Eds.): *Handbook of Clinical Neurology, Vol. 4.* New York: Elsevier, North Holland Pub. Co., 1969, pp. 48–66

Deal, JL: Consistency and adaptation in apraxia of speech. *J Commun Disord,* 1974, *7*, 135–140

Deal, JL, & Darley, FL: The influence of linguistic and situational variables on phonemic accuracy in apraxia of speech. *J Speech Hear Res*, 1972, *15*, 639–653

Deal, JL, & Deal, LA: Efficacy of aphasia rehabilitation: Preliminary results, in Brookshire, RH (Ed.): *Clinical Aphasiology: Conference Proceedings.* Minneapolis: BRK Publishers, 1978, pp. 66–77

Deal, JL, & Florance, CL: Modification of the eight-step continuum for treatment of apraxia of speech in adults. *J Speech Hear Disord*, 1978, *43*, 89−95

Deal, LA, Deal, JL, Wertz, RT, et al.: Statistical prediction of change in aphasia: Clinical application of multiple regression analysis, in Brookshire, RH (Ed.): *Clinical Aphasiology: Conference Proceedings*. Minneapolis: BRK Publishers, 1979, pp. 95−100

Denny-Brown, D: The nature of apraxia. *J Nerv Ment Dis*, 1958, *126*, 9−33

DeRenzi, E, Pieczuro, A, & Vignolo, LA: Oral apraxia and aphasia. *Cortex*, 1966, *2*, 50−73

DeRenzi, E, & Vignolo, LA: The Token Test: A sensitive test to detect disturbances in aphasics. *Brain*, 1962, *85*, 665−678

Deutsch, SE: Oral form identification as a measure of cortical sensory dysfunction in apraxia of speech and aphasia. *J Commun Dis*, 1981, *14*, 65−73

Deutsch, SE: Prediction of site of lesion from speech apraxia error patterns. Paper presented to the American Speech−Language−Hearing Association, Atlanta, Georgia, 1979 (unpublished)

Dimond, S: *The Double Brain*. Baltimore: Williams and Wilkins, 1972

DiSimoni, FG, & Darley, FL: Effect on phoneme duration control of three utterance-length conditions in an apractic patient. *J Speech Hear Disord*, 1977, *42*, 257−264

Duffy, RJ, & Duffy, JR: Three studies of deficits in pantomimic expression and pantomimic recognition in aphasia. *J Speech Hear Res*, 1981, *24*, 70−84

Dunlop, JM, & Marquardt, TP: Linguistic and articulatory aspects of single word production in apraxia of speech. *Cortex*, 1977 *13*, 17−29

Egan, O: Intonation and meaning. *J Psycholinguist Res*, 1980, *9*, 23−39

Eisenson, J: *Adult Aphasia: Assessment and Treatment*. New York: Appleton-Century-Crofts, 1973

Eisenson, J: Aphasia: A point of view as to the nature of the disorder and factors that determine prognosis for recovery. *Int J Neurol*, 1964, *4*, 287−295

Eisenson, J: *Examining for Aphasia* (Rev. Ed.). New York: The Psychological Corp., 1954

Eisenson, J: Prognostic factors related to language rehabilitation in aphasic patients. *J Speech Hear Disord*, 1949, *12*, 290−292

Ekman, P, & Friesen, WV: Hand movements. *J Commun*, 1972, *22*, 353−374

Fager, KL, & Deutsch, SE: Utterance length effects on speech segment durations in apraxics versus normals. Paper presented to the American Speech−Language−Hearing Association, Los Angeles, California, 1981 (unpublished)

Fairbanks, G: *Voice and Articulation Drillbook*. New York: Harper & Row, 1960

Fitts, PM, & Posner, MI: *Human Performance*. Belmont: Brooks-Cole, 1967

Fletcher, H: *Speech and Hearing in Communication*. New York: D. Van Nostrand, 1953

Freeman, FJ, Sands, ES, & Harris, KS: Temporal coordination of phonation and articulation in a case of verbal apraxia: A voice onset time study. *Brain Lang*, 1978, *6*, 106−111

Fromkin, V: *Tone: A Linguistic Survey*. New York: Academic Press, 1978

Fromkin, V, & Rodman, R: *An Introduction to Language*. New York: Holt, Rinehart and Winston, 1974

Fromm, D, Abbs, J, McNeil, M, et al.: Simultaneous perceptual-physiological method for studying apraxia of speech, in Brookshire, RH (Ed.): *Clinical Aphasiology: Conference Proceedings*. Minneapolis: BRK Publishers, 1982, pp. 251−262

Gazzaniga, MS, Bogen, JE, & Sperry, RW: Dyspraxia following division of the cerebral commissures. *Arch Neurol*, 1967, *12*, 606−612

Geschwind, N: The apraxias: Neural mechanisms of disorders of learned movements. *Am Sci*, 1975, *63*, 188−195

Geschwind, N: Disconnection syndromes in animals and man. *Brain*, 1965, *88*, 237−294, 585−644

Geschwind, N, & Kaplan, E: A human cerebral disconnection syndrome. *Neurol*, 1962, *12*, 675−685

Gloning, K, & Quatember, R: Some classifications of aphasic disturbances with special reference to rehabilitation. *Int J Neurol*, 1964, *4*, 296⁻304

Gloning, K, Trappl, R, Heiss, WD, et al.: Prognosis and speech therapy in aphasia, in Lebrun, Y, & Hoops, R (Eds.): *Neurolinguistics 4: Recovery in Aphasics*. Amsterdam: Swets and Zeitlinger BV, 1976, pp. 57–64

Glosser, G, Kaplan, E, & LoVerme, S: Longitudinal neuropsychological report of aphasia following left-subcortical hemorrhage. *Brain Lang*, 1982, *15*, 95–116

Goldstein, K: *Language and Language Disturbances*. New York: Grune & Stratton, 1948

Goodglass, H: Phonological factors in aphasia, in Brookshire, RH (Ed.): *Clinical Aphasiology: Conference Proceedings*. Minneapolis: BRK Publishers, 1975, pp. 28–44

Goodglass, H, & Kaplan, E: *The Assessment of Aphasia and Related Disorders*. Philadelphia: Lea and Febiger, 1972

Goodglass, H, & Kaplan, E: Disturbance of gesture and pantomime in aphasia. *Brain*, 1963, *86*, 703–720

Granich, L, & Prangle, G: *Aphasia, A Guide to Retraining*. New York: Grune & Stratton, 1947

Guilford, AM, & Hawk, AM: A comparative study of form identification in neurologically impaired and normal adult subjects. *Speech and Hearing Science Research Reports*. Ann Arbor: Univ Michigan, 1968

Halpern, H: Therapy for agnosia, apraxia, and dysarthria, in Chapey, R (Ed.): *Language Intervention Strategies in Adult Aphasia*. Baltimore: Williams and Wilkins, 1981, pp. 347–360

Halpern, H, Darley, FL, & Brown, JR: Differential language and neurological characteristics in cerebral involvement. *J Speech Hear Disord*, 1973, *38*, 162–173

Halpern, H, Keith, RL, & Darley, FL: Phonemic behavior of aphasic subjects without dysarthria or apraxia of speech. *Cortex*, 1976, *12*, 365–372

Hartman, J: Measurement of early spontaneous recovery from aphasia with stroke. *Ann Neurol*, 1981, *9*, 89–91

Heaton, RK, Chelune, GH, & Lehman, RAW: Using neuropsychological and personality tests to assess the likelihood of patient employment. *J Nerv Ment Dis*, 1978, *166*, 408–416

Heaton, RK, & Pendleton, MG: Use of neurophysiological tests to predict adult patients' everyday functioning. *J Consult Clin Psychol*, 1981, *49*, 807–821

Hecaen, H: Introduction a la Neuropsychologie. Paris: Larousse, 1972a.

Hecaen, H: Studies of language pathology, in Sebeok, TA (Ed.): *Current Trends in Linguistics 9*. The Hague: Mouton, 1972b, pp. 591–645

Hecaen, H, & Assal, G: A comparison on constructional deficits following right and left hemispheric lesions. *Neuropsychologia*, 1970, *8*, 289–304

Hecaen, H, & Gimeno, A: L'apraxie ideo-motrice unilaterle gauche. *Rev Neurol*, 1960, *102*, 648–653

Heilman, KM: Apraxia, in Heilman, KM, & Valenstein, E (Eds.): *Clinical Neuropsychology*. New York: Oxford Univ. Press, 1979, pp. 159–183

Heilman, KM: Ideational apraxia—a re-definition. *Brain*, 1973, *96*, 861–864

Heilman, KM, Schwartz, HD, & Geschwind, N: Defective motor learning in ideomotor apraxia. *Neurol*, 1975, *25*, 1018–1020

Helm, N: Management of palilalia with a pacing board. *J Speech Hear Disord* 1979, *44*, 350–353

Helm, NA: Criteria for selecting aphasic patients for melodic intonation therapy. Paper presented to the American Speech and Hearing Association, San Francisco, California, 1978 (unpublished)

Helm-Estabrooks, NA, Fitzpatrick, PM, & Barresi, B: Visual action therapy for global aphasia. *J Speech Hear Disord*, 1982, *47*, 385–389

Hersen, M, & Barlow, DH: *Single Case Experimental Designs: Strategies for Studying Behavior Change.* New York: Pergamon Press, 1976

Hoit-Daalgard, J, Murry, T, & Kopp, H: Categorical perception: Its relationship to severity of apraxic speech. Paper presented to the American Speech-Language-Hearing Association, Detroit, Michigan, 1980 (unpublished)

Holland, AL: *Communicative Abilities in Daily Living.* Baltimore: Univ. Park Press, 1980

Holtzapple, P, & Marhsall, N: The application of multiphonemic articulation therapy with apraxic patients, in Brookshire, RH (Ed.): *Clinical Aphasiology: Conference Proceedings.* Minneapolis: BRK Publishers, 1977, pp. 46–58

Hornstein, S: Amnestic, agnosic, apractic, and aphasic features in dementing illness, in Wells, CE (Ed.): *Dementia, Contemporary Neurology Service No. 9.* Philadelphia: Davis, 1971, pp. 36–60

Ingram, D: *Phonological Disability in Children.* New York: Elsevier, 1976

Irwin, JV, & Griffith, FA: A theoretical and operational analysis of the paired stimuli technique, in Wolfe, WD, & Goulding, DJ (Eds.): *Articulation and Learning: New Dimensions in Research, Diagnostics, and Therapy.* Springfield: Charles C Thomas, 1973, pp. 156–194

Itoh, M, Sasanuma, S, Hirose, H, et al.: Abnormal articulatory dynamics in a patient with apraxia of speech: X-ray microbeam observation. *Brain Lang,* 1980, *11,* 66–75

Itoh, M, Sasanuma, S, & Ushijima, T: Velar movements during speech in a patient with apraxia of speech. *Brain Lang,* 1979, *7,* 227–239

Jackson, JH: Remarks on nonprotrusion of the tongue in some cases of aphasia, 1878, in Taylor, J (Ed.): *Selected Writings of John Hughlings Jackson, Vol. 2.* London: Hodder & Stoughton, 1932, pp. 153–154

Jakobson, R: Aphasia as a linguistic problem, in Saporta, S (Ed.): *Psycholinguistics.* New York: Holt, Rinehart and Winston, 1961, pp. 419–427

Johns, DF: Treatment of apraxia of speech. Paper presented to the American Speech and Hearing Association, New York, New York, 1970 (unpublished)

Johns, DF: A systematic study of phonemic variability in apraxia of speech. Doctoral dissertation, Florida State Univ., 1968. Unpublished.

Johns, DF, & Darley, FL: Phonemic variability in apraxia of speech. *J Speech Hear Res,* 1970, *13,* 556–583

Johns, DF, & LaPointe, LL: Neurogenic disorders of output processing: Apraxia of speech, in Whitaker, H, & Whitaker, HA (Eds.): *Studies in Neurolinguistics 1.* New York: Academic Press, 1976, pp. 161–200

Judson, HF: *The Search for Solutions.* New York: Holt, Rinehart and Winston, 1980

Keatley, MA, & Pike, P: An automated pulmonary function laboratory: Clinical use in determining resp;iratory variations in apraxia, in Brookshire, RH (Ed.): *Clinical Aphasiology: Conference Proceedings.* Minneapolis: BRK Publishers, 1976, pp. 98–109

Kearns, KP: The application of phonological process analysis to adult neuropathologies, in Brookshire, RF (Ed.): *Clinical Aphasiology: Conference Proceedings.* Minneapolis: BRK Publishers, 1980, pp. 187–195

Keenan, JS: *A Procedure Manual in Speech Pathology with Brain-Damaged Adults.* Danville: The Interstate Printers and Publishers, Inc., 1975

Keenan, JS, & Brassell, EG: *Aphasia Language Performance Scales (ALPS).* Murfreesboro: Pinnacle Press, 1975

Keenan, JS, & Brassell, EG: A study of factors related to prognosis for individual aphasic patients. *J Speech Hear Disord,* 1974, *39,* 257–269

Keith, R: *Speech and Language Rehabilitation. A Workbook for the Neurologically Impaired.* Danville: The Interstate Printers and Publishers, Inc., 1972

Keith, RL, & Aronson, AE: Singing as therapy for apraxia of speech and aphasia: Report of a case. *Brain Lang*, 1975, *2*, 483–488

Keller, E: Parameters for vowel substitutions in Broca's aphasia. *Brain Lang*, 1978, *5*, 265–285

Kelso, JAS, & Stelmach, GE: Central and peripheral mechanisms in motor control, in Stelmach, GE (Ed.): *Motor Control: Issues and Trends*. New York: Academic Press, 1976

Kent, R: Models of speech production, in Lass, NJ (Ed.): *Contemporary Issues in Experimental Phonetics*. New York: Academic Press, 1976a, pp. 79–104

Kent, R: Study of vocal tract characteristics in the dysarthrias. Presented to the Veterans Administration Workshop on Motor Speech Disorders, Madison, Wisconsin, 1976b (unpublished)

Kent, R, & Rosenbek, JC: Prosodic disturbance and neurologic lesion. *Brain Lang*, 1982, *15*, 259–291

Kent, R, & Rosenbek, JC: Acoustic patterns of apraxia of speech. *J Speech Hear Res*, 1983, *26*, 231–249

Kertesz, A: *Western Aphasia Battery*. New York: Grune & Stratton, 1982

Kertesz, A: *Aphasia and Associated Disorders: Taxonomy, Localization, and Recovery*. New York: Grune & Stratton, 1979

Kertesz, A, & McCabe, P: Recovery patterns and prognosis in aphasia. *Brain*, 1977, *100*, 1–18

Kimura, D, & Archibald, Y: Motor functions of the left hemisphere. *Brain*, 1974, *97*, 337–350

Kleist, K: *Gehirnpathologie*. Leipzig: Barth, 1934

Klich, RJ, Ireland, JU, & Weidner, WE: Articulatory and phonological aspects of consonant substitutions in apraxia of speech. *Cortex*, 1979, *15*, 451–470

Kratochwill, TR (Ed.): *Single Subject Research: Strategies for Evaluating Change*. New York: Academic Press, 1978

Kreindler, A, & Fradis, A: *Performances in Aphasia: A Neurodynamical, Diagnostic and Psychological Study*. Paris: Gauthier-Villars, 1968

Langacker, RW: *Language and Its Structure: Some Fundamental Linguistic Concepts*. New York: Harcourt Brace, 1968

LaPointe, LL: Aphasia intervention with adults: Historical, present, and future approaches, in Miller, J, Yoder, D, & Schiefelbusch, R (Eds.): *Contemporary Issues in Language Intervention, ASHA Reports 12*. Rockville: American Speech–Language–Hearing Association, 1983, pp. 127–136

LaPointe, LL: An investigation of isolated oral movements, oral motor sequencing abilities and articulation of brain injured adults. Doctoral Dissertation, Univ. of Colorado, 1969 (unpublished)

LaPointe, LL, & Horner, J: *Reading Comprehension Battery for Aphasia*. Tigard: C.C. Publications, 1979

LaPointe, LL, & Horner, J: Repeated trials of words by patients with neurogenic phonological selection–sequencing impairment (apraxia of speech), in Brookshire, RH (Ed.): *Clinical Aphasiology: Conference Proceedings*. Minneapolis: BRK Publishers, 1976, pp. 261–277

LaPointe, LL, & Johns, DF: Some phonemic characteristics in apraxia of speech. *J Comm Dis*, 1975, *8*, 259–269

LaPointe, LL, & Wertz, RT: Oral-movement abilities and articulatory characteristics of brain-injured adults. *Percept Mot Skills*, 1974, *39*, 39–46

Larimore, HW: Some verbal and nonverbal factors associated with apraxia of speech. Doctoral dissertation, Univ. of Denver, 1970 (unpublished)

Lebrun, Y, Buyssens, E, & Henneaux, J: Phonetic aspects of anarthria. *Cortex*, 1973, *9*, 126–135

Lebrun, Y, & Hoops, R (Eds.): *The Management of Aphasia*. Amsterdam: Swets and Zeitlinger BV, 1978

Lecours, AR, Dordain, G, & Lhermitte, F: Recherches sur le langage des aphasiques: I. Terminologie neurolinguistique. *Encephale*, 1970, *59*, 520−546

Lecours, AR, & Lhermitte, F: The "pure form" of the phonetic disintegration syndrome (pure anarthria); anatomo-clinical report of a historical case. *Brain Lang*, 1976, *3*, 88−113

Lecours, AR, & Lhermitte, F: Phonemic paraphasias: Linguistic structures and tentative hypotheses. *Cortex*, 1969, *5*, 193−228

Lemme, ML, Wertz, RT, & Rosenbek, JC: The effects of stimulus modality on verbal output in brain injured adults. Paper presented to the annual meeting of the American Speech and Hearing Association, Las Vegas, Nevada, 1974 (unpublished)

Lenneberg, EH: *Biological Foundations of Language*. New York: Wiley, 1967

Lesser, R: *Linguistic Investigations of Aphasia*. London: Edward Arnold, 1978

Liepmann, H: Apraxie. *Ergbn der ges Med*, 1920, *1*, 516−543

Liepmann, H: Die linke hemisphaere und das handeln. *Muchener medizinische Wochenschrift*, 1905, *52*, 2322−2326, 2375−2378

Liepmann, H: Das Krankheitsbild der Apraxie (motorischen Asymbolie) auf Grund eines Falles von einseitiger Apraxie. *Monatsshrift fur Psychiatrie und Neurologie*, 1900, *8*, 15−40

Locke, JL: The inference of speech perception in the phonologically disordered child. Part I: A rationale, some criteria, the conventional tests. *J Speech Hear Disord*, 1980a, *45*, 431−444

Locke, JL: The inference of speech perception in the phonologically disordered child. Part II: Some clinically novel procedures, their use, some findings. *J Speech Hear Disord*, 1980b, *45*, 445−468

Lomas, J, & Kertesz, A: Patterns of spontaneous recovery in aphasic groups: A study of adult stroke patients. *Brain Lang*, 1978, *5*, 388−401

Longerich, MC, & Bordeaux, J: *Aphasia Therapeutics*. New York: Macmillan, 1954

Love, RJ, & Webb, WG: The efficacy of cueing techniques in Broca's aphasia. *J Speech Hear Disord*, 1977, *42*, 170−178

Lozano, RA, & Dreyer, DE: Some effects of delayed auditory feedback on dyspraxia of speech. *J Comm Disord*, 1978, *11*, 407−415

Luria, AR: *Traumatic Aphasia: Its Syndromes, Psychology and Treatment*. The Hague: Mouton, 1970

Luria, AR: *Restoration of Function After Brain Injury*. New York: Macmillan, 1963

Macaluso-Haynes, S: Developmental apraxia of speech: Symptoms and treatment, in Johns, DF (Ed.): *Clinical Management of Neurogenic Communicative Disorders*. Boston: Little, Brown and Co., 1978, pp. 243−250

MacKay, IRA: *Introducing Practical Phonetics*. Boston: Little, Brown, and Co., 1978

MacNeilage, PF: Motor control of serial ordering of speech. *Psychol Rev*, 1970, *77*, 182−196

Marcuse, H: Apraktische Symptome bei einem Fall von seniler Demenz. *Demenz Zentble Mervheilk Psychiat*, 1904, *27*, 737−751

Marks, M, Taylor, M, & Rusk, HA: Rehabilitation of the aphasic patient: A summary of three years' experience in a rehabilitation setting. *Arch Phys Med Rehabil*, 1957, *38*, 219−226

Marquardt, TP, Reinhardt, JB, & Peterson, HA: Markedness analysis of phonemic substitution errors in apraxia of speech. *J Comm Disord*, 1979, *12*, 481−494

Marshall, RC, & Phillips, DS: Prognoses for improved verbal communication in aphasic stroke patients. *Arch Phys Med Rehabil*, in press

Marshall, RC, Tompkins, CA, & Phillips, DS: Improvement in treated aphasia: Examination of selected prognostic factors. *Folia Phoniatrica*, 1982, *34*, 305−315

Martin, AD: Some objections to the term *apraxia of speech*. *J Speech Hear Disord*, 1974, *39*, 53–64

Martin, AD, & Rigrodsky, S: An investigation of phonological impairment in aphasia, Part 1. *Cortex*, 1974a, *10*, 317–328

Martin, AD, & Rigrodsky, S: An investigation of phonological impairment in aphasia, Part 2: Distinctive features analysis of phonemic commutation errors in aphasia. *Cortex*, 1974b, *10*, 329–346

Mateer, CK: Impairments of nonverbal oral movements after left hemisphere damage: A follow-up analysis of errors. *Brain Lang*, 1978, *6*, 334–341

Mateer, C, & Kimura, D: Impairment of nonverbal oral movements in aphasia. *Brain Lang*, 1977, *4*, 262–276

Mayo Clinic Procedures for Language Evaluation, (unpublished)

McDonald, ET: *A Deep Test of Articulation: Sentence Form.* Pittsburgh: Stanwix House, 1964

McHenry, LC: *Garrison's History of Neurology.* Springfield: Charles C Thomas, 1969

McNeil, MR, & Prescott, TE: *Revised Token Test.* Baltimore: Univ. Park Press, 1978

McReynolds, LV, & Bennett, S: Distinctive feature generalization in articulation training. *J Speech Hear Disord*, 1972, *37*, 462-470

McReynolds, LV, & Kearns, KP: *Single-subject Experimental Designs in Communicative Disorders.* Baltimore: Univ. Park Press, 1983

Messerli, P, Tiscot, A, & Rodriguez, J: Recovery from aphasia: Some factors of prognosis, in Lebrun, Y, & Hoops, R (Eds.): *Neurolinguistics 4: Recovery in Aphasics.* Amsterdam: Swets and Zeitlinger BV, 1976, pp. 124–135

Mever, A: *Historical Aspects of Cerebral Anatomy.* London: Oxford Univ. Press, 1971

Mlcoch, AG, & Noll, JD: Speech production models as related to the concept of apraxia of speech, in Lass, N (Ed.): *Speech and Language: Advances in Basic Research and Practice.* New York: Academic Press, 1980, 201–237

Mohr, JP: Revision of Broca aphasia and the syndrome of Broca's area infarction and its implications in aphasia theory, in Brookshire, RH (Ed.): *Clinical Aphasiology: Conference Proceedings.* Minneapolis: BRK Publishers, 1980, pp. 1–16

Mohr, JP: Rapid amelioration of motor aphasia. *Arch Neurol*, 1973, *28*, 77–82

Mohr, JP, Pessin, MS, Finkelstein, S, et al.: Broca aphasia: Pathologic and clinical aspects. *Neurol*, 1978, *28*, 311–324

Monrad-Krohn, GH: Altered melody of language ("dysprosody") as an element of aphasia. *Acta Psychiat, Scand.*, 1947, *46*, 204–212

Moore, WM: Assessment of oral, nonverbal gestures in normal and selected brain-injured sample populations. Doctoral dissertation, Univ. of Colorado, 1975 (unpublished)

Moore, WM, Rosenbek, JC, & LaPointe, LL: Assessment of oral apraxia in brain-injured adults, in Brookshire, RH (Ed.): *Clinical Aphasiology: Conference Proceedings.* Minneapolis: BRK Publishers, 1976, pp. 64–79

Moss, CS: *Recovery With Aphasia: The Aftermath of My Stroke.* Urbana: Univ. of Illinois Press, 1972

Nailling, KR, & Horner, J: Reorganizing neurogenic articulation disorders by modifying prosody. Paper presented to the American Speech and Hearing Association, Atlanta, Georgia, 1979 (unpublished)

Nathan, PW: Facial apraxia and apraxic dysarthria. *Brain*, 1947, *70*, 449–478

Nebes, RD: The nature of internal speech in a patient with aphemia. *Brain Lang*, 1975, *2*, 489–497

Nespoulous, JL, Lecours, AR, Deloche, G, et al.: On the non-oneness of phonemic deviations of aphasic patients with and without phonetic disintegration. Paper presented to the Academy of Aphasia, London, Ontario, 1981 (unpublished)

Netsell, R: Speech motor control: Theoretical issues with clinical impact. Paper presented to the Clinical Dysarthria Conference, Tucson, Arizona, 1982 (unpublished)

Netsell, R: Physiologic recordings in the evaluation and rehabilitation of dysarthria. Commun Dis: An Audio Journal for Continuing Education. New York: Grune & Stratton, Inc., 1978

Netsell, R: Physiological bases of dysarthria. Final report for Research Grant NS 09627. Bethesda, Institute of Neurological and Communicative Disorders and Stroke, 1976 (unpublished)

Netsell, R, & Daniel, B: Dysarthria in adults: Physiologic approach to rehabilitation. *Arch Phys Med Rehabil*, 1979, *60*, 502-508

Ohala, JJ: Production of tone, in Fromkin, V (Ed.): *Tone: A Linguistic Survey*. New York: Academic Press, 1978, pp. 5−39

Ohigashi, Y, Hamanaka, T, Ohashi, H, et al.: A propos de l'heterogeneite de l'apraxie bucco-facile. *Folia Psychiatr Neurol Jpn*, 1980, *34*, 35−43

Ostreicher, HJ, & Hafmeister, LB: The use of simultaneous gestural−verbal technique with aphasic and apraxic adults. *Aphasia, Apraxia, Agnosia*. 1980, *2*, 31−44

Penfield, W, & Roberts, L: *Speech and Brain Mechanisms*. Princeton: Princeton Univ. Press, 1959

Pick A: Studien uber Motorische Apraxie und ihre Mahestehende Erscheinunger. Leipzig: Deuticke, 1905

Poeck, K, & Kerschensteiner, M: Analysis of the sequential motor events in oral apraxia, in Zulch, KJ, Creutzfeldt, O, & Galbraith, GC (Eds.): *Cerebral Localization*. Berlin: Springer-Verlag, 1975, pp. 98−109

Poncet, M, Degos, C, Deloche, G, et al.: Phonetic and phomemic transformations in aphasia. *Int J Ment Health*, 1972, *1*, 45−54

Porch, BE: *Porch Index of Communicative Ability, Volume 2, Third Edition*. Palo Alto: Consulting Psychologists Press, 1981

Porch, BE: *The Porch Index of Communicative Ability*. Palo Alto: Consulting Psychologists Press, 1967

Porch, BE, & Callaghan, S: Making predictions about recovery: Is there HOAP?, in Brookshire, RH (Ed.): *Clinical Aphasiology: Conference Proceedings*. Minneapolis: BRK Publishers, 1981, pp. 187−200

Porch, BE, Collins, MJ, Wertz, RT, et al.: Statistical prediction of change in aphasia. *J Speech Hear Res*, 1980, *23*, 312−322

Porch, BE, Wertz, RT, & Collins, MJ: A statistical procedure for predicting recovery from aphasia, in Porch, BE (Ed.): *Clinical Aphasiology: Conference Proceedings*. Albuquerque: Veterans Administration, 1974, pp. 27−37

Porch, BE, Wertz, RT, & Collins, MJ: Recovery of communicative ability: Patterns and prediction. Paper presented to the Academy of Aphasia, Albuquerque, New Mexico, 1973 (unpublished)

Prins, R, Snow, C, & Wagenaar E: Recovery from aphasia: Spontaneous speech versus language comprehension. *Brain Lang*, 1978, *6*, 192−211

Raven, JC: *Coloured Progressive Matrices*. London: H.K. Lewis, 1962

Riese, W: *Selected Papers on the History of Aphasia*. Amsterdam: Swets and Zeitlinger BV, 1977

Riese, W: *History of Neurology*. New York: MD Publications, 1959

Riese, W: The early history of aphasia. *Bull Hist Med*, 1947, *23*, 322

Rizzolatti, G, Bertoloni, G, & Buchtel, HA: Interference of concomitant motor and verbal tasks on simple reaction: A hemispheric difference. *Neuropsychologia*, 1979, *17*, 323−330

Rose, C, Boby, V, & Capildeo, R: A retrospective survey of speech disorders following stroke

with particular reference to the value of speech therapy, in Lebrun,Y, & Hoops, R
(Eds.): *Neurolinguistics 4: Recovery in Aphasics*. Amsterdam: Swets and Zeitlinger
BV, 1976, pp. 189–197

Rosenbek, JC: Treating apraxia of speech, in Johns, DF (Ed.): *Clinical Management of
Neurogenic Communicative Disorders*. Boston: Little, Brown, and Co., 1978, pp.
191–241

Rosenbek, JC, Collins, MJ, & Wertz, RT: Intersystemic reorganization in the treatment of
apraxia of speech, in Brookshire, RH (Ed.): *Clinical Aphasiology: Conference Proceedings*. Minneapolis: BRK Publishers, 1976, pp. 255–260

Rosenbek, JC, & LaPointe, LL: Motor speech disorders and the aging process, in Beasley,
DS, & Davis, GA (Eds.): *Aging: Communication Processes and Disorders*. New York,
Grune & Stratton, 1981, pp. 159-174

Rosenbek, JC, & LaPointe, LL: The dysarthrias: Description, diagnosis and treatment, in
Johns, DF (Ed.): *Clinical Management of Neurogenic Communicative Disorders*.
Boston: Little, Brown, and Co., 1978, pp. 251–310

Rosenbek, JC, Lemme, ML, Ahern, MB, et al.: A treatment for apraxia of speech in adults. *J
Speech Hear Disord*, 1973a, *38*, 462–472

Rosenbek, JC, & Merson, RM: Measurement and prediction of severity in apraxia of speech.
Paper presented to the American Speech and Hearing Association, Chicago, Illinois,
1971 (unpublished)

Rosenbek, JC, & Wertz, RT: Veterans Administration Workshop on Motor Speech Disorders. Madison, Wisconsin, 1976 (unpublished)

Rosenbek, JC, Wertz, RT, & Darley, FL: Oral sensation and perception in apraxia of speech
and aphasia. *J Speech Hear Res*, 1973b, *16*, 22–36

Rottenberg, D, & Hochberg, F: *Neurological Classics in Modern Translation*. New York:
Hafner, 1977

Roy, EA: Apraxia: A new look at an old syndrome. *J Human Movement Studies*, 1978, *4*,
191–210

Rubow, RT, Rosenbek, JC, Collins, MJ, et al.: Vibrotactile stimulation for intersystemic
reorganization in the treatment of apraxia of speech. *Arch Phys Med Rehabil*, 1982, *63*,
150–153

Russell, DG: Spatial location cues and movement production, in Stelmach, GE (Ed.): *Motor
Control: Issues and Trends*. New York: Academic Press, 1976, pp. 67–85

Sagan, C: *Broca's Brain: Reflections on the Romance of Science*. New York: Random
House, 1979

Sands, ES, Freeman, FJ, & Harris, KS: Progressive changes in articulatory patterns in verbal
apraxia: A longitudinal case study. *Brain Lang*, 1978, *6*, 97–105

Sands, ES, Sarno, MT, & Shankweiler, D: Long-term assessment of language function in
aphasia due to stroke. *Arch Phys Med Rehabil*, 1969, *50*, 202–206, 222

Sarno, J, Sarno, MT, & Levita, E: Evaluating language improvement after completed stroke.
Arch Phys Med Rehabil, 1971, *52*, 73–78

Sarno, MT: *The Functional Communication Profile: Manual of Directions*. New York:
Institute of Rehabilitation Medicine, New York Univ. Medical Center, 1969

Sarno, MT, & Levita, E: Recovery in treated aphasia during the first year post-stroke. *Stroke*,
1979, *10*, 663–670

Sarno, MT, & Levita, E: Natural course of recovery in severe aphasia. *Arch Phys Med
Rehabil*, 1971, *52*, 175–179

Sarno, MT, Silverman, M, & Levita, E: Psychosocial factors and recovery in geriatric
patients with severe aphasia. *J Am Geriat Soc*, 1970, *18*, 405–409

Sasanuma, S: Speech characteristics of a patient with apraxia of speech. *Annual Bulletin,
Research Institute of Logapedics and Phoniatrics, Univ. of Tokyo*, 1971, *5*, 85–89

Schmidt, RA: The schema as a solution to some persistent problems in motor learning theory, in Stelmach, GE (Ed.): *Motor Control: Issues and Trends*. New York: Academic Press, 1976, pp. 41-65

Schnitzer, ML: Generative Phonology: Evidence from Aphasia. Doctoral dissertation, Univ. of Rochester, 1971 (unpublished)

Schuell, H: *Differential Diagnosis of Aphasia with the Minnesota Test, Second Edition, Revised.* Minneapolis: Univ. of Minnesota Press, 1973

Schuell, H: *Differential Diagnosis of Aphasia with the Minnesota Test.* Minneapolis: Univ. of Minnesota Press, 1965a.

Schuell, H: *The Minnesota Test for Differential Diagnosis of Aphasia.* Minneapolis: Univ. of Minnesota Press, 1965b

Schuell, H, Jenkins, JH, & Jiménez-Pabón, E: *Aphasia in Adults: Diagnosis, Prognosis, and Treatment.* New York: Harper & Row, 1964

Shane, HC, & Darley, FL: The effect of auditory rhythmic stimulation on articulatory accuracy in apraxia of speech. *Cortex,* 1978, *14,* 444-450

Shane, SA: *Generative Phonology.* Englewood Cliffs: Prentice-Hall, 1973

Shankweiler, D, & Harris, KS: An experimental approach to the problem of articulation in aphasia. *Cortex,* 1966, *2,* 277-297

Shankweiler, D, Harris, KS, & Taylor, ML: Electromyographic studies of articulation in aphasia. *Arch Phys Med Rehabil,* 1968, *49,* 1-8

Shewan, CM: Verbal dyspraxia and its treatment. *Human Communications,* 1980, *5,* 3-12

Shulak, CB: The integrity of internal speech in phonologically impaired brain-injured adults with minimal aphasia. Masters thesis, Univ. of California, Santa Barbara, 1979 (unpublished)

Silverman, FH: *Research Design in Speech Pathology and Audiology.* Englewood Cliffs: Prentice Hall, 1977

Simmons, NN: Finger counting as an intersystemic reorganizer in apraxia of speech, in Brookshire, RH (Ed.): *Clinical Aphasiology: Conference Proceedings.* Minneapolis: BRK Publishers, 1978, pp. 174-179

Singer, RN: *Motor Learning and Human Performance: An Application to Motor Skills and Movement Behaviors.* New York: Macmillan, 1980

Singh, S, & Polen, S: Use of a distinctive feature model in speech pathology. *Acta Symbolica,* 1972, *3,* 17-25

Skelly, M: *Ameri-Ind Gestural Code Based on Universal American Indian Hand Talk.* New York: Elsevier, 1979

Skelly, M, Schinsky, L, Smith RW, et al.: American Indian Sign (Amerind) as a facilitation of verbalization for the oral verbal apraxic. *J Speech Hear Disord,* 1974, *39,* 445-456

Smith, A: Diagnosis, intelligence, and rehabilitation of chronic aphasics: Final Report. Ann Arbor: Department of Physical Medicine and Rehabilitation, Univ. of Michigan, 1972

Sparks, R, Helm, NA, & Albert, M: Aphasia rehabilitation resulting from melodic intonation therapy. *Cortex,* 1974, *10,* 303-316

Sparks, RW, & Holland, AL: Method: Melodic intonation therapy for aphasia. *J Speech Hear Disord,* 1976, *41,* 287-297

Spreen, O, & Benton, AL: *Neurosensory Center Comprehensive Examination for Aphasia.* Victoria B.C.: Univ. of Victoria Neuropsychology Laboratory, 1969

Square, PA, Darley, FL, & Sommers, RI: An analysis of the productive errors made by pure apractic speakers with differing loci of lesions, in Brookshire, RH (Ed.): *Clinical Aphasiology: Conference Proceedings.* Minneapolis: BRK Publishers, 1982, pp. 245-250

Square, PA, Darley, FL, & Sommers, RI: Speech perception among patients demonstrating apraxia of speech, aphasia, and both disorders, in Brookshire, RH (Ed.): *Clinical Aphasiology: Conference Proceedings.* Minneapolis: BRK Publishers, 1981, pp. 83-88

Square, PA, & Weidner, WE: Oral sensory perception in adults demonstrating apraxia of speech. Paper presented to the American Speech and Hearing Association, Houston, Texas, 1976 (unpublished)

Stedman's Medical Dictionary (21st Ed.). Baltimore: Williams and Wilkins, 1966

Stelmach, GE (Ed.): *Motor Control: Issues and Trends.* New York: Academic Press, 1976

Stoicheff, M: Motivating instructions and language performance of dysphasic subjects. *J Speech Hear Res,* 1960, *3,* 75−85

Stookey, B: Jean-Baptiste Bouillaud and Earnest Auburtin. *J Am Med Assoc,* 1963, *184,* 1024−1029

Stryker, S: *Speech After Stroke.* Springfield: Charles C Thomas, 1975

Summers, JJ, & Sharp, CA: Bilateral effects of concurrent verbal and spatial rehearsal on complex motor sequencing. *Neuropsychologia,* 1979, *17,* 331−343

Taylor, J (Ed.): *Selected Writings of John Hughlings Jackson, Vol. 2.* London: Hodder and Stoughton, 1932

Templin, MC, & Darley, FL: *The Templin-Darley Tests of Articulation.* Iowa City: Bureau of Educational Research and Service, Extension Division, State Univ. of Iowa, 1960

Thomas, L: *The Lives of a Cell: Notes of a Biology Watcher.* New York: Bantam, 1974

Tompkins, CA, Golper, LA, Lambrecht, KJ, et al.: Persisting language deficit and the minor Broca syndrome (Abstract), in Brookshire, RH (Ed.): *Clinical Aphasiology: Conference Proceedings.* Minneapolis: BRK Publishers, 1981, pp. 322−326

Tonkovich, JD, & Marquardt, TP: The effects of stress and melodic intonation on apraxia of speech, in Brookshire, RH (Ed.): *Clinical Aphasiology: Conference Proceedings.* Minneapolis: BRK Publishers, 1977, pp. 97−102

Trost, JE: Patterns of articulatory deficits in patients with Broca's aphasia. Doctoral dissertation, Northwestern Univ., 1970 (unpublished)

Trost, JE, & Canter, GJ: Apraxia of speech in patients with Broca's aphasia: A study of phoneme production accuracy and error patterns. *Brain Lang,* 1974, *1,* 63−79

Ulatowska, H, & Baker, WD: On a notion of markedness in linguistic systems: Application to aphasia, in Brookshire, RH (Ed.): *Clinical Aphasiology: Conference Proceedings.* Minneapolis: BRK Publishers, 1975, pp. 153−164

Van Riper, C, & Irwin, J: *Voice and Articulation.* Englewood Cliffs: Prentice Hall, 1958

Vaughn, GR, & Clark, RM: *Speech Facilitation: Extraoral and Intraoral Stimulation Technique for Improvement of Articulation Skills.* Springfield: Charles C. Thomas, 1979

Vignolo, LA: Evolution of aphasia and language rehabilitation: A retrospective exploratory study. *Cortex,* 1964, *1,* 344−367

Warren, R: Rehearsal for naming in apraxia of speech, in Brookshire, RH (Ed.): *Clinical Aphasiology: Conference Proceedings.* Minneapolis: BRK Publishers, 1977, pp. 80−90

Warrington, EK: Constructional apraxia, in Vincken, P, & Bruyn, G (Eds.): *Handbook of Clinical Neurology.* Amsterdam: North Holland, 1969, pp. 67−83

Warrington, EK, James, M, & Kinsbourne, M: Drawing disability in relation to laterality of cerebral lesion. *Brain,* 1966, *89,* 53−82

Watamori, TS, Itoh, M, Fukusako, Y, & Sasanuma: Oral apraxia and aphasia. *Ann Bull RILP,* 1981, *15,* 129−146

Webb, WG, & Love, RJ: The efficacy of cueing techniques with apraxic-aphasics. Paper presented to the American Speech and Hearing Association, Las Vegas, Nevada, 1974 (unpublished)

Weinstein, S: Experimental analysis of an attempt to improve speech in cases of expressive aphasia. *Neurol,* 1969, *9,* 632−635

Weintraub, S, Mesulam, MM, & Kramer, L: Disturbances of prosody. *Arch Neurol,* 1981, *38,* 742−744

Weisenberg, TH, & McBride, KE: *Aphasia: A Clinical and Psychological Study.* New York: Commonwealth Fund, 1935

Wepman, JM: The relationship between self-correction and recovery from aphasia. *J Speech Hear Disord*, 1958, *23*, 302–305

Wepman, JM: *Recovery from Aphasia*. New York: Ronald Press, 1951

Wepman, JM, & Jones, LV: *Studies in Aphasia: An Approach to Testing*. Chicago: Education-Industry Service, 1961

Wertz, RT: Response to treatment in patients with apraxia of speech, in Rosenbek, JC, McNeil, MR, & Aronson, AE (Eds.): *Apraxia of Speech*, in press

Wertz, RT, Collins, MJ, Weiss, D, et al.: Veterans Administration cooperative study on aphasia: A comparison of individual and group treatment. *J Speech Hear Res*, 1981, *24*, 580–594

Wertz, RT, Deal, LA, & Deal, JL: Prognosis in aphasia: Investigation of the high-overall (HOAP) and the short-direct (HOAP slope) method to predict change in PICA performance, in Brookshire, RH (Ed.): *Clinical Aphasiology: Conference Proceedings*. Minneapolis: BRK Publishers, 1980, pp. 164–173

Wertz, RT, & Lemme, ML: Input and output measures with aphasic adults. Research and Training Center 10, Final Report, Social Rehabilitation Services, Washington, D.C., 1974 (unpublished)

Wertz, RT, & Porch, BE: Effects of masking noise on the verbal performance of adult aphasics. *Cortex*, 1970, *6*, 399–409

Wertz, RT, & Rosenbek, JC: Appraising apraxia of speech. *J Colo Speech Hear Assoc*, 1971, *5*, 18–36

Wertz, RT, Rosenbek, JC, & Collins, MJ: Identification of apraxia of speech from PICA verbal tests and selected oral–verbal apraxia tests, in Brookshire, RH (Ed.): *Clinical Aphasiology: Collected Proceedings 1972–1976*. Minneapolis: BRK Publishers, 1978, pp. 6–16

Wertz, RT, Rosenbek, JC, & Deal, JL: A review of 228 cases of apraxia of speech: Classification, etiology, and localization. Paper presented to the American Speech and Hearing Association, New York, New York, 1970 (unpublished)

White, EB: *The Trumpet of the Swan*. New York: Harper and Row, 1970

Wilson, P: Temporal relationships in therapy for apraxia, in Brookshire, RH (Ed.): *Clinical Aphasiology: Conference Proceedings*. Minneapolis: BRK Publishers, 1977, pp. 119–123

Wilson, SAK: A contribution to the study of apraxia. *Brain*, 1908, *31*, 164–216

Winitz, H: *Articulatory Acquisition and Behavior*. New York: Appleton-Century-Crofts, 1969

Wolk, L: A markedness analysis of initial consonant clusters in aphasic phonological impairment: A case study. *Die Suid-Afrikaanse Tyskvif vir Kommunikasieafwykings*, 1978, *25*, 81–100

Wood, KS: Measurement of progress in the correction of articulatory speech defects. *J Speech Hear Disord*, 1949, *14*, 171–174

Yarnell, P, Monroe, P, & Sobel, L: Aphasia outcome in stroke: A clinical neuroradiological correlation. *Stroke*, 1976, *7*, 514–522

Young, EH, & Hawk, SS: *Moto-Kinesthetic Speech Training*. Stanford: Stanford Univ. Press, 1955

Index